Pediatric Nail Disorders

Pediatric Diagnosis and Management
Series Editors: James F. Bale Jr. and Stephen D. Marks

NEW AND FORTHCOMING TITLES

James F. Bale, Jr., Joshua L. Bonkowsky, Francis M. Filloux, Gary L. Hedlund, Paul D. Larsen, and Denise C. Morita, *Pediatric Neurology, Second Edition*

Robert Baran, Smail Hadj-Rabia, and Robert Silverman, *Pediatric Nail Disorders*

Juan Ferrando and Ramon Grimalt, *Pediatric Hair Disorders: An Atlas and Text, Third Edition*

Chloe Macaulay, Polly Powell, and Caroline Fertleman, *Learning from Paediatric Patient Journeys: What Children and Their Families Can Tell Us*

Stephan Strobel, Lewis Spitz, and Stephen D. Marks, *Great Ormond Street Handbook of Paediatrics, Second Edition*

Pediatric Nail Disorders

Robert Baran, MD
Nail Diseases Center
Cannes, France

Smail Hadj-Rabia, MD, PhD
Department of Dermatology
Reference Center for Rare Diseases
Necker—Enfants Malades Hospital
Paris, France

Robert Silverman, MD
Department of Pediatrics
Georgetown University Medical Center
Washington, DC, USA

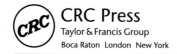

CRC Press
Taylor & Francis Group
Boca Raton London New York

CRC Press is an imprint of the
Taylor & Francis Group, an **informa** business

CRC Press
Taylor & Francis Group
6000 Broken Sound Parkway NW, Suite 300
Boca Raton, FL 33487-2742

Printed and bound in India by Replika Press Pvt. Ltd.

Printed on acid-free paper
Version Date: 20160825

International Standard Book Number-13: 978-1-4987-2045-8 (Paperback)

Visit the Taylor & Francis Web site at
http://www.taylorandfrancis.com

and the CRC Press Web site at
http://www.crcpress.com

Contents

Preface

Medicine has always raised clinical challenges, and this work is our latest attempt to deal with one of these.

A specific book on pediatric nail disorders has never been written before, and although the subject is quite narrow, the gap in the clinical practice that it concerns is large. Parents are understandably disturbed about any abnormality in the shape, color, size, or texture of their child's nails. Whether or not the appearance is significant, clinicians are generally ill prepared to address these concerns. Dermatologists, pediatricians, and family physicians may all be called on to treat these patients, but they may well feel uncertain about aspects that they may think belong to other specialists.

We hope all these groups of readers will benefit from the labors of the group of esteemed physicians from many fields who have focused their efforts to bring detailed and useful information on such a small appendage of the body. We also thank our publisher for having granted us confidence to complete our task.

Robert Baran
Smail Hadj-Rabia
Robert Silverman

Contributors

Paula Aguilera
Department of Dermatology
University of Barcelona
Barcelona, Spain

Marc Al Ahmar
Université Paris Descartes, Sorbonne Paris Centre
Service de Radiologie B Hôpital Cochin
Paris, France

Hiroko Arai
ARAI Dermatology Clinic
Tokyo, Japan

and

Department of Environmental
    Immuno-Dermatology
Yokohama City University Graduate School of
    Medicine
Yokohama, Japan

Robert Baran
Nail Diseases Center
Cannes, France

Didier Bessis
Department of Dermatology
University of Montpellier
Montpellier, France

Marie Caucanas
Clinique Saint-Jean Languedoc
Toulouse, France

Jean-Luc Drapé
Université Paris Descartes, Sorbonne Paris Centre
Service de Radiologie B Hôpital Cochin
Paris, France

Smail Hadj-Rabia
Department of Dermatology, Reference Center
    for Rare Diseases
Necker-Enfants Malades Hospital
Paris, France

Eckart Haneke
Department Dermatol, Inselspital
University of Bern
Bern, Switzerland

and

Dermatol Practice Dermaticum
Freiburg, Germany

and

Centro Dermatol, Inst CUF
Porto, Portugal

and

Kliniek voor Huidziekten, Acad Hosp
Ghent University
Gent, Belgium

Roderick Hay
Department of Dermatology
Kings College Hospital NHS Trust
London, United Kingdom

Jean-Philippe Lacour
Department of Dermatology
University of Nice Sophia-Antipolis
Nice, France

Gerard Lorette
Department of dermatology, Pediatric Unit
University François-Rabelais
Tours, France

Annabel Maruani
Department of Dermatology, Pediatric Unit
University François-Rabelais
Tours, France

Jose M. Mascaró Sr.
Department of Dermatology
University of Barcelona
Barcelona, Spain

Valérie Merzoug
Université Paris Descartes, Sorbonne Paris Centre
Service de Radiologie B Hôpital Cochin
Paris, France

and

Université Paris Sud
Service de radiologie pédiatrique, Hôpital
    Bicêtre
Le Kremlin-Bicêtre, France

Iria Neri
Dermatology—Department of Specialised
    Experimental and Diagnostic Medicine
University of Bologna
Bologna, Italy

Marcel Pasch
Department of Dermatology
Radboud University Medical Center
Nijmegen, The Netherlands

Bianca Maria Piraccini
Dermatology—Department of Specialised
    Experimental and Diagnostic Medicine
University of Bologna
Bologna, Italy

Bertrand Richert
Brugmann, Saint-Pierre and Queen Fabiola
    Children's University Hospitals
Université Libre de Bruxelles
Brussels, Belgium

Robert Silverman
Department of Pediatrics
Georgetown University Medical Center
Washington, DC

Michela Starace
Dermatology—Department of Specialised
    Experimental and Diagnostic Medicine
University of Bologna
Bologna, Italy

Luc Thomas
Service de Dermatologie Centre Hospitalier
    Lyon Sud
and
Université Claude Bernard Lyon 1
and
Centre de Recherche sur le Cancer de Lyon
Lyons, France

Stephane Vignes
Lymphology Unit
Referral Center for Rare Vascular Diseases
    (Primary lymphedema)
Cognacq-Jay Hospital
Paris, France

Ximena Wortsman
Department of Radiology and Department of
    Dermatology
Institute for Diagnostic Imaging and Research of
    the Skin and Soft Tissues Clinica Servet
University of Chile
Santiago, Chile

1

Embryology and Inherited Disorders

Smail Hadj-Rabia

Introduction

Despite the advances in diagnosis, management, and care of nail diseases, much remains unknown about the initial nail development and its morphogenesis. Nail changes are reported in many genodermatoses. They might be isolated or combined with other organs or tissue features. In many genetic disorders, the diagnosis is based on the anomalies of other organs. Rarely, changes in nails are characteristic, representing a major clue for the diagnosis. The description of the nail feature represents a striking difficulty. Different terms used to describe are sloppy, such as *onychodystrophy* or *onychodysplasia. Onycholysis* is rarely used. The number of nails involved is mentioned rarely.

Nail Embryology

Development

The development of nail apparatus begins during the eighth week of gestation and is completed by the fifth month (20 weeks) of intrauterine development. The rectangular surface of the future nail bed is delineated by a continuous shallow groove at the proximal, lateral, and distal grooves during 8–10 weeks of gestation. The nail bed on the dorsal digit is the first skin structure to keratinize at around 11 weeks. Keratinization begins distally and then continues over the nail bed toward the proximal nail fold. After 12 weeks, the presumptive nail matrix cells, which will later produce the differentiated nail plate, are found ventral to the proximal nail fold. After 14 weeks of gestation, the whole nail bed develops a granular layer. After 15 weeks, the nail plate emerges from the nail matrix and grows distally by the accumulation of flattened keratinocytes. The granular layer of the nail bed disappears gradually. Keratinocytes of the nail bed are integrated into the underside of the nail plate. After 16 weeks, the outline of the nail digit is established. The nail plate completely covers the nail bed during the fifth month. After 22 weeks, it grows over the distal ridge called the hyponychium.[1]

Involved Genes and Pathways

Epidermal appendages embryology is under the influence of many genes and pathways. It requires communication between cells (at least gap junction), between tissues (epidermis and dermis or ectoderm and mesoderm), and structures (no bone no nail) (Figure 1.1). Initiation of development, morphogenesis, and spatial orientation require many specific protein factors, which are mostly unknown. Structural components, such as keratins, are also important. Deregulation of these pathways is associated with many diseases. Two major pathways involved in the nail morphogenesis are as follows:

1. The Wnt pathway is involved in the appendage unit induction. Both Respondin 4 (RSPO4) and FDZ6 belong to this pathway. They cause nonsyndromic congenital nail disorders (NDNCs).

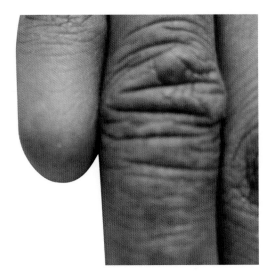

FIGURE 1.1 Importance of communication between tissues (epidermis and dermis or ectoderm and mesoderm) and structures. Note the total absence of last phalange and therefore, of the nail in the fifth digit.

Expression of *RSPO4* in digit mesenchyme during embryogenesis is thought to influence induction of the nail unit in the overlying epithelium.

2. The NFκB pathway is involved in the initiation of the ectodermal appendages morphogenesis. IKKγ (NEMO) belongs to this pathway. *IKKγ (NEMO)* mutation causes incontinentia pigmenti (IP).

Other pathways participate in the spatial organization and/or interlink with other organs. Anomalies of these pathways manifest through multivisceral anomalies. In the skin, p63 is required for the cross talk between the developing epidermis and dermis. Mutations in the gene encoding p63 are associated with various manifestations involving epidermal appendages, ear, nose, and throat (ENT), or gastrointestinal tract. Dorsoventral limb patterning is under the influence of *LMX1B*, involved in nail–patella syndrome (NPS).

Diseases

Intrauterine development is divided into two periods: embryogenesis before 20 weeks of gestation and fetal development afterward. Genetic diseases occur during the first period and belong to the large group of embryopathies. Nail anomalies associated with genetic disorders develop during this period. Excluding the pathognomonic aspect of the nail in NPS, nail examination might be helpful for the diagnosis. Genetic conditions may constitute differential diagnosis of frequent diseases such as mucoepithelial dysplasia (Figure 1.2a and b) and nail lichen planus (LP). The disorders are described as follows:

- Genetic disorders restricted to the nail apparatus
- Genetic diseases involving the nail and associated only with skin manifestations
- Genetic diseases involving the nail and other organs
- Genetic diseases in which nail might be involved

Genetic Diseases Restricted to the Nail Apparatus

They correspond to NDNC which is classified into 10 different forms of abnormal nail development (from anonychia to nail dysplasia). Leukonychia is also included.[2] We have choosen to include both Iso-Kikuchi syndrome and isolated congenital nail clubbing (ICNC) in this group (Table 1.1). Although bone anomalies are reported, nails involvement is the major feature.

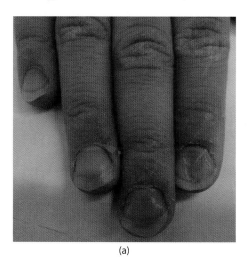
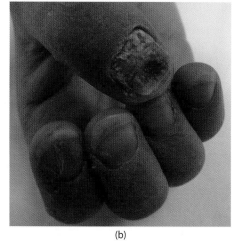

(a)   (b)

FIGURE 1.2   (a) and (b) Mucoepithelial dysplasia. Mucoepithelial dysplasia is a rare autosomal dominant disorder characterized by ocular and cutaneous involvement. Skin lesions mimic napkin psoriasis and are associated to alopecia. Nail involvement is similar to lichen planus.

TABLE 1.1

Nonsyndromic Congenital Nail Disorders

Type MIM Number	Clinical Manifestations	Mode of Inheritance, Gene, Mapping	Other Manifestations
NDNC-1, MIM161050	Trachyonychia	AD	Nails are variably involved. Thinning, thickening, pitting, opalescence, absence of thumb nails, longitudinal ridges, discoloration is possible. Koilonychia reported sometimes.
NDNC-2	Koilonychia	AD	
NDNC-3, MIM 151600	Leukonychia	AR and AD, *PLCD1*, 3p21.3	True, apparent, or pseudoleukonychia belong to this group.
NDNC-4, MIM 206800	Anonychia, hyponychia congenita	AR, *RSPO4*	Possible remnants or rudimentary nail plates.
NDNC-5, MIM 164800	Distal onycholysis	AD	Increased transverse curvature and absent lunulae are possible.
NDNC-6, MIM 107000	Partial absence of nails	AD	Thumbs and great toe are severely affected; anonychia is reported.
NDNC-7, MIM 605779	Longitudinal streaks	AD, 17p13	Thinning of nail plate, poorly developed, or absent lunulae, vulnerability of the free nail margins.
NDNC-8, MIM 607523	Isolated toenail dystrophy	AD, (3p21.3, *COL7A1*)[a]	Two compound heterozygous families.
NDNC-9, MIM 614149	Anonychia of toenails and onycholysis of fingernails	AR, 17q25	Normal fingers and toes at birth. When 7–8 years old, onychodystrophy started on finger and toenails.
NDNC-10, MIM 614157	Nail dysplasia	AR, 8q22.3, *FZD6*	Started at birth, slow rate of nail growth. When 10 years old, claw-like structure is reported.
ICNC, MIM 119900	Isolated congenital nail clubbing	AR, 4q32-q34, *HPGD*	Bilateral, symmetric, congenital, all nails affected
Iso-Kikuchi (congenital onychodysplasia of the index finger)	Anonychia, micronychia, polyonychia of the index finger. Rolled nail	AD	Y-shaped bifurcation of the distal phalanx.

Abbreviations: NDNC, nonsyndromic congenital nail disorder; AD, autosomal dominant; AR, autosomal recessive; ICNC, isolated congenital nail clubbing.

Genetic Diseases Involving the Nail and Associated with Skin Manifestations Only

Various forms of epidermolysis bullosa (EB) (Figure 1.3)[3] and their associated nail changes, which might aid diagnosis, are listed in Table 1.2 (Figures 1.4 through 1.6).[4–6] In EB, nail trauma might explain some clinical aspects.

Genetic Diseases Involving the Nail and Other Organs

Most of the genodermatoses belong to this group. A special mention is made of NPS, which presents itself with pathognomonic nail manifestations.

Nail–Patella Syndrome (MIM161200, LMX1B Gene)

NPS is a rare autosomal dominant disease characterized by nail, skeletal, and renal manifestations. The nail changes are most pronounced on the ulnar side of the thumbs and decrease toward the fifth finger. The toenails are rarely affected. Fingernails are affected in 98% of the patients. The nails, especially on the thumbs, might be absent or may be short, narrow, spoon shaped, soft, and/or fragile. Triangular- or V-shaped lunula (Figure 1.7) alone or in combination with missing dorsal creases of distal finger joint are the particular characteristics of NPS. The patella is aplastic or luxated in 90% of patients. The radius head is small that can cause limitation in elbow motion or subluxation. Bilateral posterior iliac horns are pathognomonic. Renal involvement is seen in 42% of the cases with various degrees of dysfunction. Proteinuria, the most prominent symptom, occurs in adults. Heterochromia of the iris with hyperpigmentation of the papillary margin is a helpful key feature for diagnosis.[7]

Ectodermal Dysplasias

Ectodermal dysplasia (ED) is clinically and genetically a heterogeneous condition, characterized by abnormal development of two or more of the following ectodermal derived structures: hair, teeth, nails, and sweat glands (Table 1.3).[8] Anomalies in other organs and systems may also be observed. Anhidrotic or hypohidrotic ectodermal dysplasia (EDA/HED), the most common phenotype of ED, is characterized by a triad of signs comprising sparse hair (hypotrichosis), abnormal or missing teeth (anodontia, oligodontia or hypodontia), and inability to sweat (anhidrosis or hypohidrosis), or intolerance to heat. When

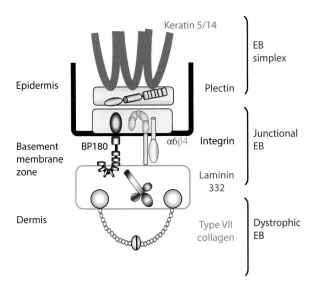

FIGURE 1.3 Three major categories of epidermolysis bullosa (EB). Recent advances in research on EB have led to the identification of mutations in 18 different genes, which encode basement membrane proteins and account for the clinical heterogeneity in EB. (From Sawamura D et al., *J Dermatol*, 37, 214–219, 2010. With permission.)

TABLE 1.2

Nails in Patients with Inherited Epidermolysis Bullosa

Major Types		Subtype	Inheritance, Gene, Mapping, MIM number	Nails	Comments
EB simplex	Suprabasal	Acral peeling skin syndrome type 2	AR, *TGM5*, 15q15 609796	None	
		EBS superficialis	AD 607600	Dystrophic nails (frequency 70%)	
		Acantholytic EBS	AR, *DSP*, 6p24 607600 AR, *JUP*, 17q21	Nail loss (frequency 100%)	
		EBS-plakophilin deficiency (Skin fragility-ED syndrome)	AR, *PKP1*, 1q32 604536	Thickened dystrophic nails (frequency 100%)	
	Basal	EBS localized	AD, *KRT5*, *KRT14*, 12q13, 17q12-q21 131800	Blistering may cause onycholysis and onychomadesis, with normal regrowth or thickened dystrophic nails (uncommon, 12%?). Mostly normal	Previously called Weber-Cockayne.
		EBS generalized severe	AD, *KRT5*, *KRT14*, 12q13, 17q12-q21 131760	Onychomadesis, pachyonychia, onychogryphosis, pincer nails or absent nails (frequency > 75%). Loss with regeneration. End result dystrophic or normal	
		EBS genralized intermediate	AD, *KRT5*, *KRT14*, 12q13, 17q12-q21 131900	Onychomadesis, with normal regrowth, pachyonychia, thickened great toenail (frequency = 14%)	Includes patients previously with EBS Koebner
		EBS with mottled pigmentation	AD, *KRT5*, 13q13 131960	Peculiar curving, Dystrophic nails, small toenail (frequency uncommon)	Pigmentation of the neck and the abdomen
		EBS migratory circinate	AD, *KRT5*, 12q13 609352	none	
		EBS AR	AR, *KRT14*, 17q12-q21 601001	Hyperkeratotic nails, horizontal ridging, anonychia	
		EBS with muscular dystrophy	AR, *PLEC1*, 8q24 226670	Onychomadesis, pachyonychia, onychogryphosis, pincer nails, anonychia (frequency = 50%)	

(Continued)

TABLE 1.2 (*Continued*)

Nails in Patients with Inherited Epidermolysis Bullosa

Major Types		Subtype	Inheritance, Gene, Mapping, MIM number	Nails	Comments
EB simplex	Basal	EBS with pyloric atresia	AR, *PLEC1, ITGA6, ITGβ4,* 8q24, 2q31.1, 17q11-qter 612138	None	
		EBS-Ogna	AD, *PLEC1,* 8q24 131950	Onychogryphosis of big toe in adulthood	
		EBS-BP230 deficiency	AR, *DST,* 6p12-p11 615425	Nail dystrophy of all toenails (particularly the toenail)	One case reported
		EBS-exophilin 5 deficiency	AR, *EXPH5,* 11q22 615028	None	
Junctional EB	Generalized	severe or intermediate	AR, *LAMA3, LAMB3, LAMC2* 18q11.2, 1q32, 1q25-q31 226700	Sometimes heaped up. Easily shed,	
		Generalized intermediate	AR, *COL17A1,* 10q24.3 226650	Anonychia, dystrophic nails (frequency > 75%)	
		With pyloric atresia	AR, *ITGA6, ITGβ4,* 2q31.1, 17q11-qter 226650	Nail thinning and atrophy or absent nails	
		Late onset JEB	AR, *COL17A1,* 10q24.3 226650	Onycholysis, nail loss, Beau Line's	
		Respiratory and renal involvement	AR, *ITGA3,* 17q21 614748	Toenail dystrophy evident from five months	
	Localized	Localized	AR, *LAMA3, LAMB3, LAMC2, COL17A1, ITGA6, ITGβ4,*	see above generalized junctional EB	
		Inversa	AR, *LAMA3, LAMB3, LAMC2,* 18q11.2, 1q32, 1q25-q31 —	Dystrophic or absent nails (frequency > 50%)	
		Laryngo-onycho cutaneous syndrome	AR, *LAMA3,* 18q11.2 245660	Nail thickening, nail erosions with granulation tissue, anonychia (frequency 100%)	
Dystrophic EB		DDEB generalized	AD, *COL7A1,* 3p21.3 131750	Nail thickening, onychogryphosis, anonychia, pseudosyndactyly (frequency > 75%)	

(*Continued*)

TABLE 1.2 (*Continued*)

Nails in Patients with Inherited Epidermolysis Bullosa

Major Types	Subtype	Inheritance, Gene, Mapping, MIM number	Nails	Comments
	Acral DDEB or RDEB	AD/AR, *COL7A1*, 3p21.3 131750; 226600	Nail thickening, anonychia (frequency > 75%)	
	Pretibial DDEB or RDEB	AD/AR, *COL7A1*, 3p21.3 131850; 226600	Nail thickening (frequency > 75%), short	
	Pruriginosa DDEB or RDEB	AD/AR, *COL7A1*, 3p21.3 604129	Nail thickening, anonychia (frequency > 75%)	
	DDEB nails only	AD, *COL7A1*, 3p21.3 131750	Pachyonychia, thickened dystrophic nails, anonychia (frequency 100%)	
	DEB, bullous dermolysis of the newborn	AD/AR, *COL7A1*, 3p21.3 131705	Nail thickening, anonychia, pseudosyndactyly (frequency 25–50%)	
	RDEB generalized severe	AR, *COL7A1*, 3p21.3 226600	Anonychia, pseudosyndactyly (frequency > 75%)	
	RDEB generalized intermediate	AR, *COL7A1*, 3p21.3 226600	Dystrophic or absent nails (frequency > 75%)	
	RDEB inversa	AR, *COL7A1*, 3p21.3 226600	Nail thickening (frequency > 75%)	
	RDEB localized	AR, *COL7A1*, 3p21.3 226600	Nail dystrophy or thickening	
	RDEB centripetalis	AR, *COL7A1*, 3p21.3 226600	Dystrophic or absent nails (frequency > 75%)	
Kindler syndrome		AR, *KIND-1*, 20p13 173650	Nail dystrophy, parrot beak nail deformity, absent nails	

Abbreviations: AD, autosomal dominant; AR, autosomal recessive

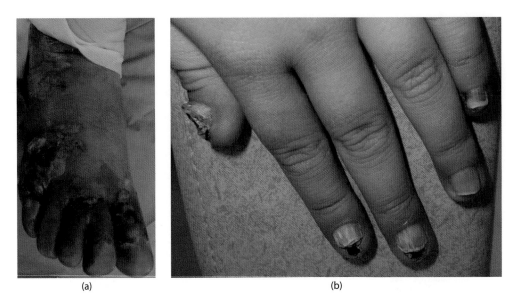

(a)   (b)

FIGURE 1.4 EB simplex with heterozygous mutation in (a) *KTR5* and (b) *KRT14* genes encoding keratin 5 and keratin 14, respectively. (a) Corresponds to Figure 1.5b (partial absence of laminin 332; (b) corresponds to Figure 1.5c (LOC syndrome).

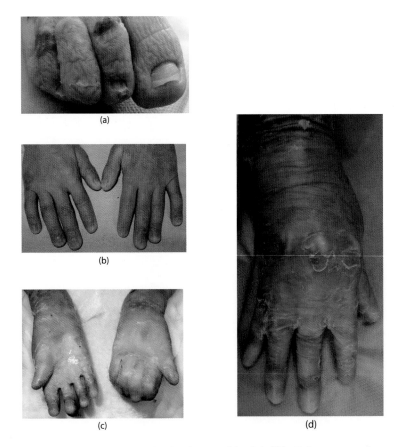

FIGURE 1.5 Junctional EB. Total (a) or partial (b) absence of laminin-332. (c) Laryngo-onycho-cutaneous (LOC) syndrome. (d) Total absence of collagen XVII. (a) Corresponds to Figure 1.4a KRT5 mutation; (b) corresponds to Figure 1.4b keratin 14 mutation; (c) corresponds to Figure 1.6a; (d) corresponds to Figure 1.6b.

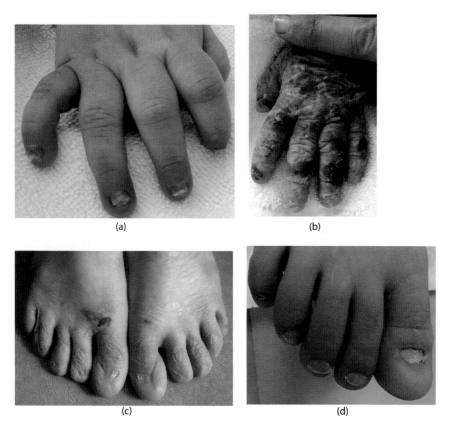

(a)

(b)

(c)

(d)

FIGURE 1.6 Dystrophic EB (DEB). (a)–(c) Different forms of autosomal recessive DEB and (d) autosomal dominant DEB. (a) Corresponds to Figure 1.5a total absence of laminin 332; (b) corresponds to Figure 1.5d (total absence of collagen XVII).

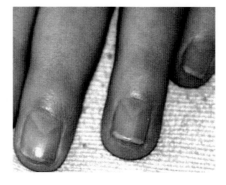

FIGURE 1.7 Nail–patella syndrome. Triangular lunula might be the only manifestation.

EDA1 (encoding ectodysplasin A), *EDAR* (ectodysplasin receptor), and *EDARADD* (EDAR associated death domain) genes are involved, nails are frequently found to be normal. Growing might be accelerated. Depressed nasal bridge (saddleback nose), large and conspicuous nostrils, high cheekbones, and a narrow lower face are observed characteristics. On the other hand, hypoplastic, brittle nail (Figure 1.8a and b), and koilonychia which are associated with mild palmoplantar keratoderma (PPK) are associated with *WNT10A* mutations. This last group represents 20% of the HED patients.

Other ectodermal syndromes where cleft lip and palate dominate the picture are Rapp–Hodgkin syndrome, ankyloblepharon-ectodermal defects-cleft (AEC) syndrome, and ectrodactyly-ectodermal

TABLE 1.3

Ectodermal Dysplasias

Condition	Inheritance, Gene, Mapping MIM No	Nails	Hair	Skin with palmoplantar hyperkeratosis	Teeth	Ear	Eye	Other findings
Cardio-facio-cutaneous syndrome	AD, *KRAS*, *BRAF*, *MAP2K1*, *MAP2K2*, 12p12.1, 7q34, 15q21, 19p13.3 115150	Thin, koilonychia, dysplastic	Sparse, thin scalp, eyelashes, eyebrows	Ichthyosiform or follicular hyperkeratosis	Normal or dysplastic	Angulated, prominent helices	Palpebral fissures	Congenital heart defects, cranial vault, depressed bridge of nose
Dyskeratosis congenita, Zinsser–Engman–Cole syndrome	XR, *DKC1*, Xq28 30500	Short, atrophic after late childhood, most prominent on fingers where they often are lost	Normal or scarring alopecia	Mainly palmar hyperkeratosis; hyperhidrosis of palms and soles; reticulated hyperpigmentation of neck, face, and chest	Sometimes malformed	Deafness	Blepharitis with loss of cilia, leucoplakia on conjunctivae, lacrimal duct obstruction	Acrocyanosis, aplastic anaemia, pancytopenia, oral lesions and leukoplakia, immunological abnormalities, testicular atrophy, avascular necrosis of femur
Ectrodactyly–clefting (EEC1) syndrome	AD, 7q11.2–q21.3 129900	Deformed, thin, brittle, striated; pitted and terminated irregular (Figure 11.8)	Wiry, hypopigmented	Fair, hypopigmented, scaly skin with comedo-naevus	Dysplasia, partial anodentia, caries		Blue sclera, photophobia, absence of lacrimal puncta, tearing, blepharitis, Meibomian glands deficient, corneal scarring, blindness	Cleft lip + palate, short stature, ectrodactyly + syndactyly, claw-shaped hands, genital and urinary tract abnormalities, growth hormone deficiency

(Continued)

TABLE 1.3 (Continued)

Ectodermal Dysplasias

Condition	Inheritance, Gene, Mapping MIM No	Nails	Hair	Skin with palmoplantar hyperkeratosis	Teeth	Ear	Eye	Other findings
Focal dermal hypoplasia, Goltz–Gorlin syndrome	XD, *PORCN*, Xp11.23 305600	Thin, spoon-shaped, can be absent in 50%, no lunula	Sparse in focal areas of scalp and pubis	Focal thin skin with herniation of fat, linear hypo- and hyperpigmentation, papillomas	Hypodontia, oligodontia, enamel hypoplasia, delayed eruption	Protruding simple ears, low set ears. Narrow auditory canals, hearing loss mixed	Multiple severe anomalies	Small stature; asymmetric face; cranial, spinal, and bone anomalies; cleft lip and palate; papillomas of mucous membranes; urinary abnormality
Hidrotic ED, Clouston syndrome	AD, *GJB6*, 13q12	Thick on toes or dystrophic. Grow slowly. Change more marked with age. Onycholysis, pits ridges. Often small and conical. Paronychia. Hyperkeratotic nailbed looks like thickened nails	In 50% sparse, short and thin. Eyebrows and eyelashes often absent	Normal sweat. Hyperpigmentation especially over joints. Clubbing of fingers	Normal but occasionally hypodontia and natal teeth		Occasionally strabism, conjunctivitis, blepharitis, and cataracts	Short stature. Nakamura and Ishikawa reported a particular form without mutation in the known genes[11]
Incontinentia pigmenti, Bloch–Sulzberger syndrome	XD *308300, *NEMO*, (*IKBKG*) Xq28	Dystrophic. In 7% koilonychia. At 15 years subungual tender tumors which clear spontaneously	Alopecia of the vertex	Classical four stages rash	Abnormal shape and oligodontia are reported	-	Retinal detachment, strabismus, microphtalmia	Anomalies of nervous system, teeth. Mainly lethal in males. Rare reports of postzygotic *NEMO* mutations in affected males. *NEMO* is involved in ED with immunodeficiency *(Continued)*

TABLE 1.3 (Continued)

Ectodermal Dysplasias

Condition	Inheritance, Gene, Mapping MIM No	Nails	Hair	Skin with palmoplantar hyperkeratosis	Teeth	Ear	Eye	Other findings
Pachyonychia congenita type 1 of Jadassohn–Lewandowsky	AD, *KRT16*, *KRT6A*, 17q12-q21, 12q13 167200	Yellow or brown at age 3–5 months, followed by thickening of nail bed. Paronychia common. Onycholysis	Normal	Palmoplantar hyperhidrosis often with blisters. Follicular hyperkeratosis with hyperpigmentation. Leukokeratosis of tongue	Natal teeth (caries or normal)	Deafness	Cataract and corneal dyskeratosis	Short statute. Mental retardation. Hoarseness
Pachyonychia congenita type 2 of Jackson and Lawler	AD, *KRT17*, *KRT6B*, 17q12-q21, 12q13 167210	Thick subungual hyperkeratosis at early age	Dry, kinky, sometimes alopecia	Palmoplantar hyperhidrosis. Follicular keratosis	Teeth present at birth	—	—	Epidermal cysts, sebocystomatoses
Pachyonychia congenita with amyloidosis and hyperpigmentation	AD —	Thick and discolored in infancy but improving in adulthood	Normal	Diffuse rippled and macular. Hyperpigmentation of neck, axilla, trunk, thighs, and popliteal fossa. Fading when adult. Amyloid deposits in papillary dermis of hyperpigmented areas	Normal	Normal	Normal	—
Pachyonychia congenita with leuconychia	AR 260130 225000	Proximal leuconychia with obliteration of lunula after age 12. Mild onycholysis of toes with slight elevation of nail plate	—	Blister on plantar surface. Punctate keratoderma. Hyperkeratotic papules on dorsa of toes and fingers. Angular cheilitis	Normal	Normal	Normal	—

(Continued)

TABLE 1.3 (*Continued*)

Ectodermal Dysplasias

Condition	Inheritance, Gene, Mapping MIM No	Nails	Hair	Skin with palmoplantar hyperkeratosis	Teeth	Ear	Eye	Other findings
Schopf–Schutz–Passage syndrome. PPK with cystic eyelids, hypodontia and hypotrichosis	AR, *WNT10A*, 2q35 *224750	Fragile with longitudinal and oblique furrows, thin, narrow nails, onycholysis	Sparse on vertex	—	Hypodontia	—	Cyst on upper and lower eyelids (hydrocystoma), senile cataract	Squamous cell carcinoma on a finger in one patient, basal cell carcinoma
AEC syndrome Limb mammary and Hay–Wells syndromes are included	AD, *TP63*, 3q27 106260	Absent or dystrophic	Partial or complete loss	Dry. Partial anhidrosis, often thick palms and soles; hidrocystoma	Widely spaced	Auricular deformities	Ankyloblepharon, lacrimal duct atresia	Cleft lip and palate. Syndactyly, supernumerary nipples. Adhesions between jaws can occur
ADULT syndrome. Acro-Dermato-Ungual-Lacrimal-Tooth syndrome	AD, *TP63*, 3q27 103285	Concave dysplastic	Blond, thin scalp, sparse axillary, premature hair loss (>30 years)	Atrophic, thin, dry, and photosensitive. Freckling	Hypodontia, oligodontia, small teeth, premature loss	—	Conjunctivitis, lacrimal duct obstruction	Breast hypoplasia, absent or hypoplastic and widely spaced nipples, mammary gland hypoplasia
Rapp–Hodgkin syndrome	AD, *TP63*, 3q27 *129400	Small, disfigured with distal soft tissue. Subungual keratosis	On scalp sparse, short, slow growing, wiry or pili torti. Sparse eyelashes, eyebrows, and body hair	Mild palmoplantar keratosis. One or more café-au-lait spots. Keratoderma or normal	Slow development. Hypodontia conical shaped. Caries	—	Aplasia of lacrimal punctae	Absence of lingual frenulum. Short stature + cleft lip and palate. Hypospadias. Syndactyly

(*Continued*)

TABLE 1.3 (*Continued*)

Ectodermal Dysplasias

Condition	Inheritance, Gene, Mapping MIM No	Nails	Hair	Skin with palmoplantar hyperkeratosis	Teeth	Ear	Eye	Other findings
Hypohidrotic ED anhidrotic ED. Christ Siemens–Touraine syndrome	XR, *EDA1*, Xq12-q13 305100	Often normal, may be dystrophic	Thin, sparse on scalp and body	Thin, dry shiny. No or decreased sweating. Dermoglyphic changes	Delayed eruption. Hypodontia. Peg-shaped, conical	—	—	Saddle-shaped nose. Small nostrils. Oral dryness causes hoarseness.
Hypohidrotic ED anhidrotic ED	AD, AR *EDAR*, *EDARADD*, AR, *WNT10A*, 2q11-q13, 1q42-43, 2q35	Small, concave koilonychia, sometimes rapid growing	Thin and sparse	Mild hypohydrosis, intolerance to heat	Adontia, hypodontia or normal teeth	—	Ocular dryness, mild photophobia	As above Heterozygous carrier of *WNT10A* mutation might be symptomatic

Inheritances are indicated as follows: AD, autosomal dominant; AR, autosomal recessive; XD, X-linked dominant; XR, X-linked recessive; ?, still unclear. Pachyonychia congenita is still named according to the old classification. Further studies will clarified their classification (see the section *Pachyonychia Congenita*).

dysplasia-cleft (EEC) syndrome. Genitourinary anomalies can also occur with these syndromes, which are related to *TP63* gene mutations (Figure 1.9a and b). Focal dermal hypoplasia is characterized by the association of atrophy and linear pigmentation of the skin, herniation of fat through the dermal defects, and multiple papillomas of the mucous membranes or skin. In addition, digital, oral, ocular anomalies and mental retardation are also described. Striated bones are probably a nearly constant feature (Figure 1.10).

Incontinentia Pigmenti

Incontinentia pigmenti (MIM308300) is a rare X-linked dominant genodermatosis that is usually lethal in male fetuses and primarily affects females. IP belongs to the ED group. Mutations in NF-κB essential modulator (*NEMO* or *IKKγ*) gene induces a loss of function of NF-κB signaling pathway and causes IP. The cutaneous lesions, classically observed since birth, remarkably occur in four successive stages. Erythema, vesicles, and pustules (stage 1), followed by verrucous and keratotic lesions (stage 2), linear hyperpigmentation (stage 3), and pale, hairless, scarring patches (stage 4). All stages do not necessarily occur and may overlap. The lesions follow Blaschko lines. Neurological manifestations like early seizures and ophthalmological manifestations like retinal detachment explain the severity of the disease. Early hypoplastic nail during infancy and subungual tumor is reported (Figure 1.11).[9]

Pachyonychia Congenita

Pachyonychia congenita (PC) is a group of disorders characterized by increase in nail thickness and hyperkeratosis involving the palms, soles, knees, and elbows. PC is an ED disorder and mostly is inherited as a dominant trait. Initially divided into PC1 and PC2, a new classification proposes five subtypes,

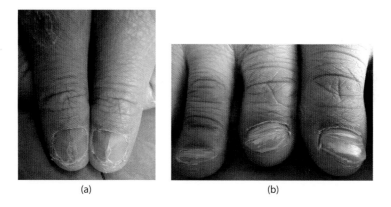

(a)   (b)

FIGURE 1.8 Ectodermal dysplasia. Patient with a *WNT10A* heterozygous (a) or a bi-allelic (b) mutation.

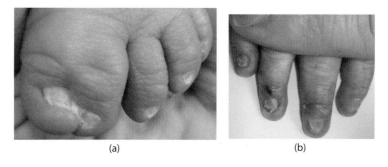

(a)   (b)

FIGURE 1.9 p63-related ectodermal dysplasia. (a) Note the syndactyly and synostosis. (b) Changes might be limited to nails.

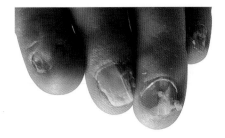

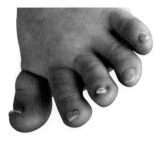

FIGURE 1.10   Focal dermal hypoplasia.   **FIGURE 1.11**   Incontinentia pigmenti.

each corresponding to the involved keratin, i.e., PC-K6a, PC-K6b, PC-K6c, PC-K16, and PC-K17. Toenail dystrophy is one of the characteristics. Clinical appearance frequently shows the V-shaped thickening involving hallux and the fifth toenail (role of trauma). At birth, about half of the neonates had changes occurring in the toenail. During the first year, the dystrophy of finger and toenails occurs in most of the affected infants. The PPK, often painful, is seen in two-thirds of the patients by the time they are 5 years old. The combination of age of onset, presence of PPK, concomitant involvement of toe and finger nails, and mucous membrane manifestations might help to classify PC. Nail dystrophy at birth, especially involving all the nails predict PC-K6a or PC-K17. The occurrence of natal teeth indicates PC-K17, while hoarseness and leukokeratosis during the first year indicate PC-K6a. PC-K16 is characterized by the development of PPK during childhood with late-onset of other characteristic features. Localized nail involvement is common in PC-K6c.[10]

Genetic Diseases in Which the Nail Might Be Involved

In this group of disorders, nail might be involved (Table 1.4). Nail examination might help in the diagnosis (for example, tuberous sclerosis, Figure 1.12). Lesh–Nyhan syndrome, neurofibromatosis, keratinization disorders, and familial pytiriasis rubra pilaris (PRP) belong to this group.

TABLE 1.4

Hereditary Disorders with Secondary Nail Changes

Disease	Inheritance MIM	Nails	Comments
Darier–White disease	AD, *ATP2A2*, 12q23-q24 *124200	Brown, red or white.	Usually as longitudinal white and red streaks. Subungeal, V-shaped keratoses
Lesh–Nyhan syndrome	XL, *HPRT*, Xq26-q27 *308950	Destroyed.	Self-mutilation
Neurofibromatosis type 1 (Recklinghausen)	AD, *NF1*, 17q11.2 *162200	One or more hypertrophic fingers or toes with dislocation of nails. Subungual glomus tumors are reported.	Multiple neurofibromas, cutaneous pigmentation, central nervous involvement
Pityriasis rubra pilaris	AD, *CARD14* *173200	One or more hypertrophic fingers brachyonychia.	
Tuberous sclerosis, epiloia, (Bourneville–Pringle)	AD, *TSC1, TSC2*, 9q34, 16p13 *191100	Koenen's tumors. Peri and subungual fibroma dislocating nails. Red comets. Longitudinal leukonychia.	Epilepsy, mental retardation. Angiofibroma of face and oral mucosa, intracranial calcification

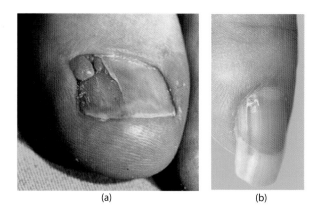

(a)　　　　　　　　　(b)

FIGURE 1.12　(a) and (b) Tuberous sclerosis of Bourneville: Koenen tumor is more frequent on toenails compared to fingernails.

REFERENCES

1. de Berker DAR and Baran R. Science of the nail apparatus. In Baran R, Dawber RPR, de Berker DAR et al. (eds.), *Baran and Dawber's Diseases of the Nails and Their Management*, Fourth Edition. Oxford, United Kingdom: Wiley Blackwell; 2012. pp. 3–5.
2. Khan S, Basit S, Habib R et al. Genetics of human isolated hereditary nail disorders. *Br J Dermatol.* 2015; 173: 922–929.
3. Sawamura D, Nakano H, and Matsuzaki Y. Overview of epidermolysis bullosa. *J Dermatol.* 2010; 37: 214–219.
4. Tosti A, de Farias DC, and Murrell DF. Nail involvement in epidermolysis bullosa. *Dermatol Clin.* 2010; 28: 153.
5. McGrath JA. Recently identified forms of epidermolysis bullosa. *Ann Dermatol.* 2015; 27: 658–666.
6. Fine JD, Bruckner-Tuderman L, Eady RA et al. Inherited epidermolysis bullosa: Updated recommendations on diagnosis and classification. *J Am Acad Dermatol.* 2014; 70: 1103–1126.
7. Hadj-Rabia S, Juhlin L, and Baran R. Hereditary and congenital nail disorders. In Baran R, Dawber RPR, de Berker DAR et al. (eds.), *Baran and Dawber's Diseases of the Nails and Their Management*, Fourth Edition. Oxford, United Kingdom: Wiley Blackwell; 2012. pp. 487–489.
8. Visinoni AF, Lisboa-Costa T, Pagnan NA, and Chautard-Freire-Maia EA. Ectodermal dysplasias: Clinical and molecular review. *Am J Med Genet A.* 2009; 149A: 1980–2002.
9. Hadj-Rabia S, Froidevaux D, Bodak N et al. Clinical study of 40 cases of incontinentia pigmenti. *Arch Dermatol.* 2003; 139: 1163–1170.
10. Shah S, Boen M, Kenner-Bell B et al. Pachyonychia congenita in pediatric patients: Natural history, features, and impact. *JAMA Dermatol.* 2014; 150: 146–153.
11. Nakamura M and Ishikawa O. A patient with alopecia, nail dystrophy, palmoplantar hyperkeratosis, keratitis, hearing difficulty and micrognathia without *GJB2* or *GJB6* mutations: a new type of hidrotic ectodermal dysplasia? *Br J Dermatol.* 2007; 156(4): 777–779.

2

Nail Anatomy

Robert Baran

The nail plate is the permanent product of the nail matrix. Its normal appearance and growth depend on the integrity of the perionychium and the bony phalanx (Figure 2.1).[1] The *nail* is a semihard horny plate, relatively smooth, covering the dorsal aspect of the tip of the digit curved in both the longitudinal and transverse axes. In the ventral aspect of the nail, longitudinal ridges are present that correspond to the complementary ridges of the nail bed. The nail is inserted proximally in an invagination that is practically parallel to the upper surface of the skin and laterally to the lateral nail grooves. This pocket-like invagination has a roof, the proximal nail fold and a floor, the matrix from which the nail is derived. Newborn nails mostly reach the end of fingertips but seldom reach the end of toes. The shapes of the nails vary from one child to another. The fingernails and toenails do not necessarily resemble each other.[2]

The *matrix* extends approximately 6 mm under the proximal nail fold, and its distal portion is only visible as the white semicircular lunula. Interestingly, the shape of the lunula determines the nail plate. The general shape of the matrix is a crescent, concave in its posteroinferior portion. The lateral horns of this crescent are more developed in the great toe and located at the coronal plane of the bone. The ventral aspect of the proximal nail fold encompasses both, a lower portion which continues the matrix, and an upper portion (roughly three-quarters of its length) called the *eponychium*. The germinal matrix forms the bulk of the nail plate. In the great toes, the extensor tendon lies between the matrix and the phalanx and extends dorsally to the distal aspect of the distal phalanx.[3] Consequently the nail matrix of the great toe is not attached to the periosteum of the dorsal aspect of the base of the distal phalanx. The proximal element produces the superficial third of the nail plate, whereas the distal element provides two-thirds of its inferior. The matrix is the sole subungual location of the functioning melanocytes. The longitudinal axis of the matrix becomes the vertical axis of the nail plate. The ventral surface of the proximal nail fold adheres closely to the nail for a short distance and forms a gradually desquamating tissue, the cuticle, made up of the stratum corneum of both the dorsal and the ventral sides of the proximal nail fold. The cuticle seals and protects the nail cul-de-sac against irritants, solvents, and other agents that might disturb matrix function and hence, nail growth. The average rate of growth of fingernails is 0.1 per day (Figure 2.2). Toenails grow at one-half to one-third of the rate of fingernails.

The rate of nail growth peaks between the ages of 10 and 14 and begins an inexorable decrease with age after the second decade, Rate of growth of the nail plate is usually undertaken as a simple measure of longitudinal elongation, using the lunula as a reference structure.[4,5]

The nail plate is bordered by the paronychium made of the proximal nail fold, which is continuous with the similarly structured lateral nail fold on each side.

The *nail bed* that has parallel longitudinal ridges extends from the lunula to the hyponychium. However, in contrast to the matrix, the nail bed has a firm attachment to the nail plate and avulsion of the overlying nail denudes the nail bed. Colorless but translucent, this highly vascular connective tissue containing glomus organs transmits a pink color through the nail. The distal margin of the nail bed which has a contrasting hue in comparison with the rest of the nail bed is called the *onychocorneal band*. Normally this is a transverse band of 1–1.5 mm of a deeper pink (Caucasian) or brown (Afro-Caribbean) followed by a relatively avascular pale band. It represents a band of increased structural

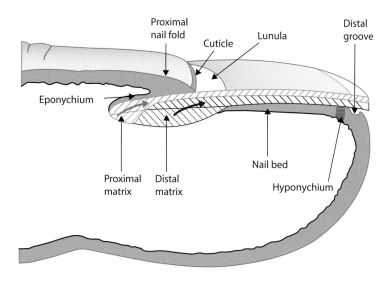

FIGURE 2.1 Longitudinal section of the distal digit showing the different components of the nail apparatus.

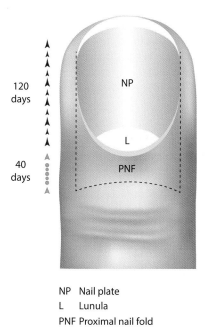

NP   Nail plate
L   Lunula
PNF Proximal nail fold

FIGURE 2.2 Linear nail growth.

adherence between nail and nail bed and acts as a first barrier to the penetration of materials beneath the nail plate. Its color or presence may vary with disease, or with compression, which influences the vascular supply.[6] Nail bed dermis is sparse, with little fat, firm collagenous adherence to the underlying periosteum, and no sebaceous or follicular appendages. Sweat ducts can be seen at the distal nail bed, using dermoscopy.

Distally, adjacent to the nail bed, lies the *hyponychium*, an extension of the volar epidermis under the nail plate, which marks the point at which the nail separates from the underlying tissue. The distal nail groove, which is convex anteriorly, separates the hyponychium from the fingertip. The hyponychium and the onychodermal band may be the focus or the origin of subungual keratosis in some diseases. The hyponychium and overhanging free nail provide a crevice. This is a reservoir for scabies, antigens, and microbes.[1]

The *circulation* of the nail apparatus is supplied by two digital arteries that course along the digits and give off branches to the distal and proximal arcades. The proximal matrix is also supplied by a branch of the digital artery coming off at the midportion of the middle phalanx and proceeding directly to the matrix, providing a collateral circulation. The normal nail fold capillary network in children resembles that observed in adults with some differences, such as a lower number of loops per millimeter, a higher subpapillary venous plexus visibility score, and a higher frequency of atypical loops. This information is important for the diagnostic evaluation of children in the context of autoimmune rheumatic diseases.[6]

The *sensory nerves* to the distal phalanx of the three middle fingers are derived from fine, oblique, dorsal branches of the volar collateral nerves. Longitudinal branches of the dorsal collateral nerves supply the terminal phalanx of the fifth digit and also the thumb. The distal digit has sensory and autonomic nerves. Autonomic nerves are not myelinated and end in fine arborizations. Sensory nerves end in either free nerve endings or special and organ receptors. The nail bed, richly innervated, contains Vater–Pacini corpuscles, Meissner corpuscles, and Merkel–Ranvier endings. They are numerous in the transition between nail bed and tip of the digit.[7]

The nail should be seen as a *musculoskeletal appendage*. Enthesis is defined as the site of insertion of a tendon, ligament, or joint capsule to bone. Among its multiple functions, the nail provides counter pressure to the pulp that is essential for the touch sensation involving the fingers and for the prevention of hypertrophy of the distal soft tissue leading to anterior ingrown nails. Physical characteristics of the nail are explained by its composition (Table 2.1) and the element content of the nails has been reported to be altered in certain disease states (Table 2.2).

TABLE 2.1

Nail Composition

Lamellar sheets of tightly adherent dead corneocytes
Protein (78%)
Water (18%)
Lipid (<5%)
Zn, Cu, Fe, Mg present in small quantities
DNA in fingernails can now be amplified for genetic analysis and has become a standard forensic identification technique

Source: Silverman, RA and Baran, R, Nail and appendageal abnormalities. In Schachner LA, Hansen RC (eds.), *Pediatric Dermatology*, Fourth Edition, Vol. 1, Chapter 12, Mosby-Elsevier, Philadelphia, 2011.

TABLE 2.2

Trace Elements in Nail Clippings from Patients with Systemic Diseases

Disease	Element	Level
Cystic fibrosis	Na, K	Increased
Wilson's disease	Cu	Increased
Iron-deficiency anemia	Fe	Decreased
Acrodermatitis enteropathica	Zn	Decreased

Source: Silverman, RA and Baran, R, Nail and appendageal abnormalities. In Schachner LA, Hansen RC (eds.), *Pediatric Dermatology*, Fourth Edition, Vol. 1, Chapter 12, Mosby-Elsevier, Philadelphia, 2011.

REFERENCES

1. De Berker D. Nail anatomy. *Clin Dermatol.* 2013; 31: 509–515.
2. Seaborg B, Bodurtha J. Nail size in normal infants establishing standards for healthy term infants. *Clin Pediatr.* 1989; 28: 142–145.
3. Paloma-Lõpez P, Becerro de Bengoa Vallejo R, Lõpez Lõpez D et al. Anatomic relationship of the proximal nail matrix to the extensor hallucis longus tendon insertion. *J Eur Acad Dermatol Venereol.* 2015; 29(10): 1967–1971.
4. Fleckman P. Anatomy and physiology of the nail. *Dermatol Clinics.* 1985; 3: 373–381.
5. De Berker D, Forslind B. The structure and properties of nails and periungual tissues. In Forslind B, Linberg M, Norlén L (eds.), *Skin, Hair, and Nails, Structure and Function.* New York, NY: Marcel Dekker; 2004. pp. 409–464.
6. Terreri MTRA, Andrade LEC, Puccinelli ML et al. Nail fold capillaroscopy: Normal findings in children and adolescents. *Semin Arthritis Rheum.* 1999; 29: 36–42.
7. Morgan AM, Baran R, Haneke E. Anatomy of the nail unit in relation to the distal digit. In Krull EA, Zook EG, Baran R, Haneke E (eds.), *Nail Surgery: A Text and Atlas.* Philadelphia, PA: Lippincott; 2000. pp.1–28.

3

Nail Contour Variations

Robert Baran

Congenital and hereditary nail dystrophies are classified according to the defects occurring in the nail matrix, the nail field, or the nail bed.[1]

The nail field is the area where the nail matrix and the nail bed develop. A defect in the matrix is the most common cause of abnormal nails. The matrix can have an abnormal position, size, or quality. Proliferation of the nail bed will produce a thickened nail which, as in pachyonychia congenita, is not evident until early childhood (Table 3.1).

Physical Signs

Ainhum (Amniotic Syndrome)

Ainhum presents as a painful constricting band, which, most often, encircles the fifth toe with eventual spontaneous amputations (Figure 3.1). It may be unilateral, but 75% of cases are bilateral. It affects the black population of the subtropical regions of America, Africa, and Asia. The condition often leads to an abnormality in the foot vessels producing an abnormal blood supply, alone or in combination with chronic trauma and infection. Similar changes occur in pseudoainhum caused by constriction of external forces, such as hair or threads encountered in children, or mentally deranged adults.[2–4]

Anonychia

Anonychia implies the absence of all or part of one or several nails (Figures 3.2 through 3.4). Total absence of all nails from birth is rare. Often, there are rudimentary nails on some digits; therefore, there is frequently only a quantitative difference between anonychia and hyponychia, and they often occur together in a patient.

Rudimentary nails of 1–2 mm long with a thin plate and even thinner free margin can be observed. This type of nail never grows.

Isolated anonychia without other symptoms can be inherited as an autosomal dominant or recessive trait or acquired (Table 3.2). If an X-ray is undertaken, absence of bone or underlying bone abnormality is generally found in congenital cases.[5–8]

Congenital anonychia corresponds to total absence of one or several nails. It is usually permanent. In the isolated type, it may be associated with the total or partial absence of the distal bony phalanx. Normally, the interaction of mesoderm and ectoderm simultaneously infers the epidermal thickening producing the nail and the mesenchymal condensation producing the distal phalanx. The size of the nail surface depends on the shape of the terminal phalanx. Thus, this combination is governed by subtle proteinic mechanisms. For the time being, two genes are incriminated in the autosomal recessive form: *RSP04*, coding a receptor on chromosome 20, and *FZD6* coding its ligand. Both belong to the Wnt signaling pathway. Of note, other protein partners of this pathway are associated with syndromic anonychias: *LMX1B* (nail–patella syndrome [NPS]) and *WNT10A* (various types of hypohidrotic ectodermal dysplasias [HEDs]).

TABLE 3.1

Conditions Producing Nail Contour Variations

Ainhum	Hoof nail deformity
Anonychia	Koilonychia
Brachyonychia	Macronychia and micronychia
Circumferential fingernail	Pachyonychia
Clubbing—shell nail	Polydactyly
Curved nail of the fourth toe	Racquet nail
Dolichonychia	Rudimentary supernumerary digit
Double little toenail	Transverse overcurvature
Ectopic nail	Trapezoid nails

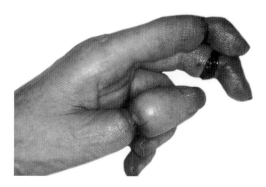

FIGURE 3.1   Ainhum. (Courtesy of Morand JJ.)

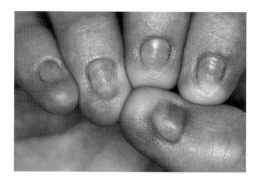

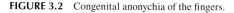

FIGURE 3.2   Congenital anonychia of the fingers.

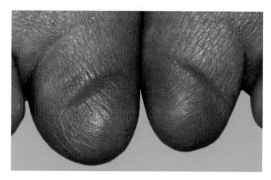

FIGURE 3.3   Congenital anonychia of the big toenails.

A prosthetic treatment has been suggested.

In Coffin–Siris syndrome, there is an absence of the fifth fingernail. In Iso-Kikuchi syndrome (IKS), anonychia may involve the index finger.

In patients with brachydactyly, syndactyly, zygodactyly (union of digits by soft tissues without bony fusion of the phalanges), the nails are sometimes malformed or absent. When the distal phalanges are involved, the nails are longitudinally convex and/or broad. Skeletal changes are also found in syndromes with ectodermal dysplasia and with chromosomal anomalies. Ectopic nails should be differentiated from rudimentary polydactyly, from congenital onychodysplasia of the index fingers (COIF) syndrome, and from the nail matrix doubling syndrome of Vigh and Pinter.

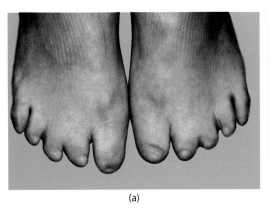
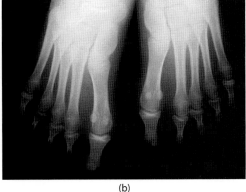

(a)   (b)

FIGURE 3.4   (a) Anonychia of the 10 toenails. (b) Same patient showing absence of the distal phalanx.

TABLE 3.2

Anonychia

Coffin–Siris syndrome	Craniofacial malformation syndromes
Cooks syndrome (MIM 106995)	Mammary digital nail syndrome
Deafness, onychodystrophy, osteodystrophy, and mental retardation (DOOR syndrome)	Tood syndrome
	Ectrodactyly–ectodermal dysplasia–cleft (EED) syndrome
Iso-Kikuchi syndrome	Ankyloblepharon-ectodermal dysplasia-cleft lip/palate (AEC) syndrome
Nail–patella syndrome	Hypohidrotic ectodermal dysplasia
Acquired Anonychia	
Postinflammatory nail loss	Stevens–Johnson syndrome
	Severe paronychia
	Epidermolysis bullosa
Pterygium formation	Lichen planus
	Scleroderma
Traumatic	Onychotillomania
	Lesch–Nyhan syndrome

Brachyonychia

Racquet nail has been reported in association with multiple malignant Spiegler tumors. Disorders associated with brachyonychia include cartilage–hair hypoplasia, acroosteolysis (Table 3.3), Larsen syndrome, pyknodysostosis, and acrodysostosis. Acroosteolysis may also be acquired in bitten nail or associated with bone resorption in scleroderma, hyperparathyroidism, psoriatic arthropathy, and frostbite[9] associated with shortening of the nail (Figure 3.5), and sometimes periungual swelling. In these conditions, acroosteolysis is present radiologically with longitudinal acroosteolysis and leads to a "pencilling" like deformity in contrast to idiopathic acroosteolysis. Of note, two children have developed latent epiphysial destruction in the middle and distal phalanges after frostbite, with one case developing brachyonychia.[10] In phalangeal microgeotic syndrome, which is usually present with frostbite-like symptoms, swelling and redness of the phalanges occurs after exposure to cold, such as during winter in Japan and Europe, when the ambient temperature often drops below freezing point. The radiological findings in this syndrome are compatible with acroosteolysis.[11] Due to the width of the nail plate, the lateral fold may be very narrow. The appearance of a racquet thumb nail can be improved in narrowing the nail and creating lateral nail folds: an excision of both sides of the thumbnail and lateral segments of the matrix is performed, followed by creation of lateral nail folds after back-stitching is performed on the lateral soft aspects of the distal phalanx that have been dissected from the bone.

TABLE 3.3

Cause of Acroosteolysis

Primary	Mucopolysaccharidosis
Farber disease	Multicentric reticulohistiocytosis
Hajdu–Cheney syndrome	Neoplasma
Hereditary sensory autonomic neuropathy type II	Neuropathic disease (especially, diabetes, leprosy, tabes
Phalangeal acroosteolysis (Joseph and Shinz disease)	dorsalis, syringomyelia, meningomyelocele)
Mandibuloacral dysplasia	Nutritional deficiencies
Massive osteolysis (Gorham's disease)	Pachydermoperiostosis
Multicentric osteolysis	Pachyonychia congenita type I
Winchester syndrome	Phalangeal microgeodic syndrome
	Physical injury (burn, frostbite, fulguration, mechanical stress)
Secondary	Porphyria
Acrodermatitis continua of hallopeau	Progeria
Acromegaly	Psoriatic arthritis
Adjuvant	Pycnodysostosis
Bureau–Barrière disease	Raynaud's disease
Carpal tunnel syndrome	Reactive arthritis
Collagen disease (Mad cow disease [MCD], polymyositis,	Renal osteodystrophy
dermatomyositis, scleroderma, rheumatoid arthritis [RA])	Rothmund's syndrome
Ehlers–Danlos syndrome	Sarcoidosis
Epidermolysis bullosa	Self-mutilation after spinal cord injury
Gout	Sezary syndrome
Haim–Munk syndrome	Spine tumors
Hereditary sensory automatic neuropathy types I and IV	Syphilis
Hyperparathyroidism	Vascular disease (ainhum, atherosclerosis,
Ichthyosiform erythroderma	Buerger's disease)
Infections	Van Bogaert–Hozay syndrome
Juvenile hyaline fibromatosis	Vinyl chloride disease
Metastases	Werner syndrome

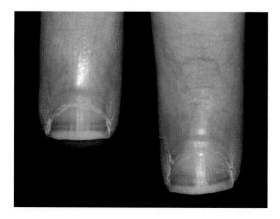

FIGURE 3.5 Brachyonychia following frostbite in a child. (Courtesy of El-Komy M.)

A hallmark of the Rubinstein–Taybi syndrome (RTS), an autosomal dominant genodermatosis, is the presence of broad thumbs and great toes. These patients also have growth and mental retardation, and multiple facial abnormalities. This syndrome is associated with mutations in the *CREBBP* and *EP300* genes.

Circumferential Fingernail

Circumferential fingernail is an extremely rare congenital malformation associated with other bony and soft tissue abnormalities of the affected limb. The tubular nail plate resembles a punch biopsy[12] (Figure 3.6).

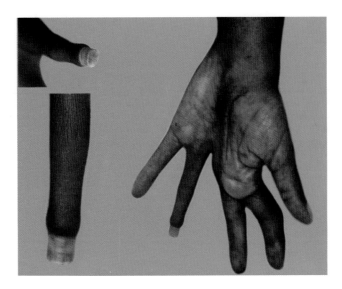

FIGURE 3.6   Circumferential fingernail. (Courtesy of Griffith WA.)

There is another type of circumferential fingernail with well-formed nails on both the dorsal and palmar surfaces of the small fingers.[13]

Clubbing

Clubbing is defined as increased transverse and longitudinal nail curvature with hypertrophy of the soft tissue components of the digits pulp, hyperplasia of the fibrovascular tissue at the base of the nail, allowing the plate to be "rocked" and sometimes local cyanosis (Figure 3.7a and b).

In normal individuals, the opposition of the dorsum of two fingers from opposite hands delineates a diamond-shaped "window" formed at the base of the nail beds. Early clubbing obliterates this window and creates a prominent distal angle between the ends of the nails. Almost 80% of cases are due to intrathoracic disorders. Chronic mucocutaneous candidosis may be present with pseudoclubbing.

In addition to clubbing, *hypertrophic pulmonary osteoarthropathy* is associated in adolescence with acromegalic limb changes, pseudoinflammatory symmetric large joint arthropathy, bilateral proliferative periostitis, peripheral cyanosis and paresthesia, local pain, and swelling. The latter may be relieved by treating the underlying disease. Pachydermoperiostosis is a rare type of idiopathic hypertrophic osteoarthropathy. It may be associated with characteristic facial features such as prominent skinfold on the forehead and cheeks.[14]

Shell nail syndrome occurs in some cases of bronchiectasis and looks like clubbing.[15] It differs from the latter because it is associated with atrophy of the nail bed and the underlying bone.

In a 5-year-old girl with bronchiectasis, avulsion of the nail plate revealed atrophy of the nail bed instead of hypertrophy observed in true clubbing.

Curved Nail of the Fourth Toe

Curved nail of the fourth toe is often bilateral (Figure 3.8a). There are cases without other anomalies of the extremities, but sometimes hypoplasia of the bone and soft tissues are present.[1,16] The primary defect is congenital shortening of the distal phalanx, and the curved nail plate is a secondary phenomenon. Young children may feel slight pain when they wear shoes.[17] Another curved nail anomaly is Kirner's deformity, but this is usually absent before 12 years of age.

Congenital curved nail of the fourth toe[18] is inherited in an autosomal recessive manner.

Differential diagnosis includes osteoid osteoma, which is painful (Figure 3.8b).

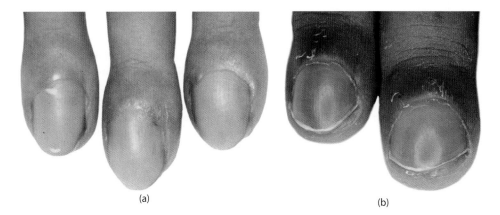

FIGURE 3.7   (a) Clubbing involving the fingernails of a child. (b) Clubbing with cyanosis in congenital heart disease.

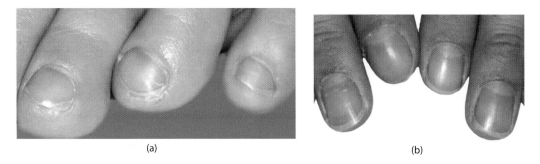

FIGURE 3.8   (a) Curved nail of the fifth toe. (b) Convex nail in osteoid osteoma affecting the right index finger.

Dolichonychia

Normally the quotient between the length and the width of the nail is 1 ± 0.1. In dolichonychia it is greater: the nails appear long and narrow. This condition is observed in Ehlers–Danlos syndrome, Marfan syndrome, HED, in association with eunuchoidism or hypopituitarism.

Double Little Toenail (Inherited Accessory Nail of the Fifth Toe)

A rudimentary accessory or double nail of the little toe is not rare (Figure 3.9).[19,20] Most cases are accidentally detected and only few patients come because they have discomfort or pain. Symptoms do not necessarily depend on the width of the nail but rather on the severity of accompanying foot anomalies.

Some patients have a positive family history, but most patients cannot give any information concerning heredity. This condition is not a special racial or ethnic feature despite some authors' opinion on the former subject.[21] It appears to be autosomal dominant, occurring in families, both in males and females.

Clinically, the nail of the little toe is abnormally wide and is either split or shows a longitudinal depression corresponding to a slight protuberance of the cuticle. The condition may be bilateral. Histopathology shows a complete, though short nail. The treatment of choice is the segmental excision of the entire accessory nail unit with mobilization of the lateral skin and primary suture or phenolization of the accessory matrix. The differential diagnosis comprises of traumatic double nail, ectopic nail, and nail spicule after incomplete extirpation of the lateral matrix horn.

Ectopic Nail (Onychoheterotopia, Polyonychia Congenita Sine Polydactylia)

Onychoheterotopia is a rare condition in which the nail tissue grows outside the classic nail apparatus on the dorsal fingers or toes. It presents as either small outgrowths of a deviant nail or a complete double fingernail malformation.[22] It may be associated with multiple malformations such as Pierre Robin syndrome. It is most often seen on the fifth digit of the hand (Figure 3.10) but the palm or sole may be involved. A case with multiple congenital ectopic nails of the toes has been reported.[23] Ectopic nail occurs both congenitally or as a result of trauma (acute or repeated minor injuries).

Physical examination shows a keratotic horn with a variable orientation, vertical or flat. Vertical growth is more often caused by incomplete, or lack of a proper nail fold or the nail bed.[22]

Ectopic nail has been described as claw-like finger and toes, circumferential nail, curved nail, double nail with onychodystrophy, congenital palmar nail syndrome, and clam nail.[24]

The differential diagnosis includes a foreign body, teratoma, hamartoma, split, nail deformity, and cutaneous horn,[22] IKS, the nail matrix doubling syndrome of Vigh and Pinter. Ectopic nail should be differentiated from rudimentary polydactylia. The former is the ectopic presence of nail tissue growing at the same speed as that of normal nails, while the latter is a digit with or without vestigial nail tissue.

The best treatment is the surgical resection of the ectopic nail to remove it completely.

Hoof Nail Deformity

This nail deformity was a family trait as patient's relatives had a similar alteration. There was no consanguineous marriage. Over four generations, six members of the family appeared to have had the same nail abnormality of varying severity affecting the same digits. Specifically, a father and two of his three daughters were afflicted with malformed second toenails. The nails bilaterally appear to arise from a subunit of the distal phalanx when viewed from the plantar surface. The subunit is well delineated within the distal tip and has a circumferential trough-like groove that imparts a "hoof-like appearance" to the toe.[25] When viewed from the dorsal aspect, the nail is thickened, hypercurved longitudinally, extensively ridged, and opaque with no apparent lunula. Lateral nail folds are missing. The nail plate appears shortened (brachyonychia). X-ray reveals absence of bony abnormalities of the distal phalanges.

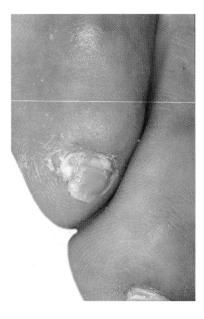

FIGURE 3.9   Double little toenail.

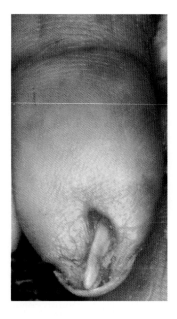

FIGURE 3.10   Ectopic nail.

Koilonychia

Koilonychia describes a transverse and longitudinal concave nail dystrophy where the nail plate is depressed centrally and everted laterally (spoon nail) (Figure 3.11a).[1] As the nail loses its curvature, the nail may first appear flat and broad resulting in platonychia or a "petaloid nail." In dermatology practice, koilonychias is often a sign of an inflammatory dermatosis or onychomycosis. Otherwise, koilonychias may be seen with iron deficiency in Plummer–Vinson syndrome, as a normal variant in children, or as a familial syndrome.

The etiologies of koilonychias are diverse (Table 3.4) but can be divided into hereditary (Figure 3.11b), acquired, and idiopathic causes. There is a congenital type shaped like the catch of a safety pin (Figure 3.11c).

Transient acquired koilonychia is relatively common. It is normally observed in up to 5% of 2-year-olds. A presentation of isolated koilonychia of the toenails in children is usually idiopathic, although, this remains a diagnosis of exclusion (Figure 3.11d).

The fingernails of the first three digits are preferentially affected, except in early childhood and congenital etiologies.

To help confirm the diagnosis of mild koilonychia, the clinician may place a drop of water on the nail plate.

If koilonychia develops later in the first year of life, anemia and nutritional deficiencies should be considered. Trauma is a common cause of koilonychias in children, often due to tightly fitting shoes or thumb/finger sucking. Nail growth normalizes with behavior modification.

Familial koilonychia, while rare, has been appreciated in several pedigrees and is inherited in an autosomal dominant fashion with a high degree of penetrance and no-predilection for sex. Keratosis pilaris, total leukonychia, and syndermatotic cataract have been associated with it, but in most cases there is no named underlying disorder. Rarely, koilonychias may also be seen as a part of genodermatoses. In acquired forms, most cases are reversible.

Macronychia and Micronychia

The nails are larger (macronychia) or smaller (micronychia) (Figure 3.12) than normal and affect one or more digits with wide or narrow nail bed and matrices. They occur as an isolated defect or in association with megadactyly.

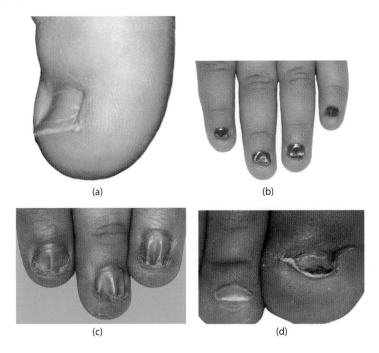

(a)

(b)

(c)

(d)

FIGURE 3.11 (a) Big toe koilonychia of a child. (b) Congenital koilonychia in a young child. (c) Congenital koilonychia shaped like the catch of a safety pin. (d) Transient acquired koilonychia in a young child.

TABLE 3.4

Classification of Koilonychias in Children and Adults

I Hereditary and Congenital Forms

Genodermatoses and congenital conditions
Chondroectodermal dysplasia (Ellis–van
  Creveld syndrome)
Congenital koilonychia associated with dome-shaped
  epiphyses and vertebral platyspondylia
Ectodermal dysplasia with anhidrosis
Familial-autosomal dominant
Familial koilonychia with keratosis pilaris
Familial koilonychia with syndermatotic cataract
Familial severe twenty-nail dystrophy
Prenatal exposure to polychlorinated
  biphenyl (PCB)
Fissured nails, in adenoma sebaceum
Focal dermal hyperplasia (Goltz syndrome)
Gottron's syndrome (acrogeria)
Hereditary osteo-onychodysplasia (nail–patella
  syndrome)
Idiopathic age-associated, particularly in big toes in
  early childhood
Incontinentia pigmenti
Isolated congenital dysplasia with longitudinal
  angular ridging
Kindler's syndrome
LEOPARD syndrome
Leukonychia and sebaceous cysts
Monilethrix
Neonatal ichthyosis-sclerosing cholangitis (NISCh)
Nezelof's syndrome (immunological defect)
Oliver–McFarlane syndrome
  (congenital trichomegaly)
Palmoplantar keratoderma (Meleda type)
Trichorhinophalangeal syndrome
Trichothiodystrophy
Witkop's tooth and nail syndrome
Nonfamilial twenty nail dystrophy

II Acquired Forms

Dermatologic
Cronkhite–Canada syndrome, Darier's syndrome,
  acanthosis nigricans
Lichen planus, psoriasis, trachyonychia, alopecia areata,
  Porphyria cutanea tarda
Scleroderma, Raynaud's disease, systemic lupus
  erythematosus

Cardiovascular and hematological
Banti's syndrome/portal hypertensive biliopathy (PHB)
Coronary disease
Hemochromatosis
Iron deficiency anemia
Polycythemia vera
Primary amyloid
Pyruvate kinase deficiency
Sickle cell disease

Infectious disease
Fungal diseases (onychomycosis)
Scabies
Syphilis
Endocrine
Acromegaly
Diabetes
Hyperthyroidism, thyrotoxicosis
Hypothyroidism

Traumatic and occupational
Acids, alkalis, thioglycolate (hairdressers) (chemical hair
  removal products)
Nail-biting, thumb/finger sucking, poorly fitting shoes
Petrol, solvents
Rickshaw boys, mushroom growers
Thermal burns

High altitude

Avitaminosis/nutritional
Nutrients
Niacin, zinc, copper
Protein deficiency/low albumin
Sulfur-containing amino acids: methionine, cysteine
Vitamin B12
Vitamin C
Populations
Kidney transplantation, end-stage renal disease
Poor nutrition, cachexia

Liver cell adenoma

Erythropoietin-producing tumors

Carpal tunnel syndrome

III Idiopathic

Source: Walker JL et al., *J Eur Acad Dermatol Venereol*, in press.

Most commonly macrodactyly manifests in the middle and index finger, usually corresponding to the territory supplied by the branches of the median nerves, designated as "nerve territory-oriented macrodactyly." This is frequently noted as a part of the syndrome (Table 3.5).

Duplication of the distal phalanx is usually accompanied by a wide digit with a bivalve nail, fissured or confluent (Figure 3.13a and b).

Macrodactyly (Figure 3.14) most commonly manifests in the middle and index finger, usually corresponding to the territory supplied by the sensory branches of the median nerves, which was designated as "nerve territory-orientated macrodactyly."

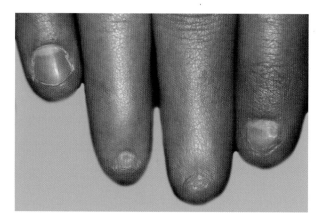

FIGURE 3.12   Micronychia involving several digits.

TABLE 3.5

Macrodactyly as Part of Syndromes

1. Congenital lymphoedema
2. Congenital partial gigantism
3. Klippel–Trenaunay–Weber syndrome
4. Macrodactyly fibrolipomatosis
5. Mafucci syndrome
6. Ollier disease
7. Tuberous sclerosis
8. von Recklinghausen disease

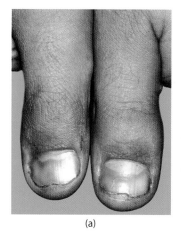   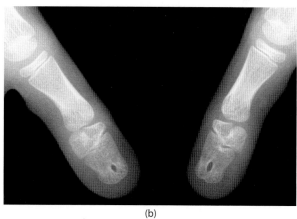

(a)   (b)

FIGURE 3.13   (a and b) Macronychia resulting from duplication of the distal phalanx associated with confluent nail.

Apparent micronychia may be due to overlapping of the nail surface by thickened lateral nail fold. This is sometimes seen in Turner syndrome, in which the whole paronychium may be swollen as in recalcitrant chronic paronychia. Micronychia is often observed in Zimmermann–Laband syndrome.

Congenital enlargement of a digit or digits is frequently noted as a part of the following syndromes.

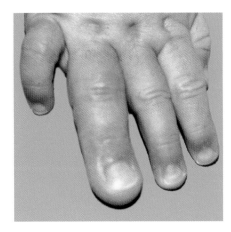

FIGURE 3.14   Macrodactyly in Proteus syndrome.

Nail Hypoplasia—Onychatrophy

Nail hypoplasia may be sporadic, inherited, or associated with malformation, such as in Coffin–Siris (micronychia of the fifth finger) or toxin exposure (dilantin, polychlorinated biphenyls).

Onychogryposis

See Chapter 4.

Pachyonychia (Onychauxis)

Pachyonychia is characterized by thickening of the nail. When the thickening is regular and confined due to the involvement of the matrix, it is called onychauxis. This sign has been reported in association with the eunuchoid state.

Hyperplastic subungual tissues, especially of the hyponychium, can alter the nail plate and nail consistency may be hard, as in pachyonychia congenital, or soft, as in psoriasis, pityriasis rubra pilaris (PRP), chronic eczema, and onychomycosis. In pachyonychia congenita (Jadassohn–Lewandowsky syndrome), the nails are yellow-brown in color and extremely hard (Figure 3.15a and b). There is increased transverse overcurvature with a free-edge shape like a horseshoe or a barrel. All the nails may be affected but the toenails are less severely involved. Recurrent paronychia results in repeated shedding of the nails. The nail plate is normal or moderately thickened.

Polydactyly

Supernumerary digits may be observed on the hands or feet (Figure 3.16a and b).

Racquet Nail

In racquet nail, the width of both the nail bed and the nail plate is greater than their length. The racquet thumb is usually inherited as an autosomal dominant trait due to premature obliteration of the epiphyseal line at the age of 13–14 years in girls and slightly later in boys.

Rudimentary Supernumerary Digits

The so-called rudimentary supernumerary digit is usually present at birth, often bilaterally symmetrical and almost located at the base of the metacarpophalangeal joint. Surgical excision is easy and solves the problem.

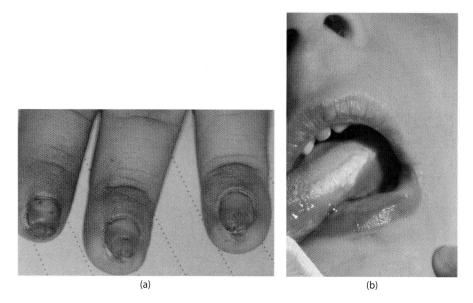

FIGURE 3.15 (a and b) Pachyonychia congenita in a young child—tongue of the patient, some years later.

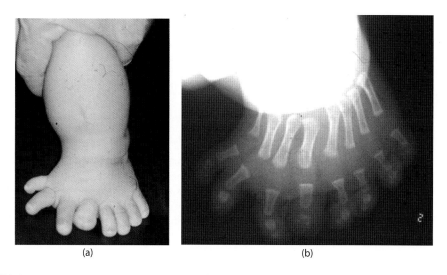

FIGURE 3.16 (a and b) Polydactyly. (Courtesy of Jouvè JL.)

Transverse Overcurvature of the Nail

Excessive transverse overcurvature may give the effect of an ingrowing toenail, often causing discomfort. In hydrotic ectodermal dysplasia, the nails are conical with distal ingrowing and increased convexity.

Three main types of overcurvature of the nail can be observed as follows:

1. Arched, pincer, trumpet, or omega nail (see Chapter 16). In this variety, the transverse overcurvature increases along the longitudinal axis of the nail plate and reaches its greatest proportion at the distal portion. At this point, the lateral borders tighten around the soft tissues, pinched without necessarily breaking through the epidermis.

They may even join together forming a tunnel or may roll around themselves taking the form of a cone of nail bed tissue, which can be extremely painful.

After a while, the soft tissue may disappear and this may be accompanied by resorption of the underlying bone. The origin of this dystrophy probably resides in the developmental anomaly and may be an inherited disorder,[26] but underlying pathology should be looked for, such as ill-fitting shoes, subungual exostosis, tinea unguium,[27] and β-blockers.[28]

2. The tile-shaped nail is present with an increase in the transverse curvature but the lateral edges of the nail plate remains parallel.

3. The plicated overcurvature is present with a surface almost flat, while one or both lateral edges are sharply angled forming vertical parallel side. Sometimes the angle may reach almost 180° if the lateral margin turns close to the ventral aspect of the plate.

Trapezoid Nails (Fan Nails)

The fan nail is a congenital nail deformation where the nail plate, too wide for its bed, appears to widen distally as its proximal part remains hidden by the proximal portion of the lateral nail folds.[29] The condition is always symmetrical and affects both great toenails. Unlike racquet thumbs, no bony alteration is associated.

REFERENCES

1. Telfer NR. Congenital and hereditary nail disorders. *Seminar Dermatology*, 1991; 10: 2–6.
2. Dent DM, Fatar S, and Rose AG. Ainhum and angiodysplasia. *Lancet*, 1981; 11: 396–397.
3. Kamalan A and Thambiah AS. Ainhum trichoporosis and Z-plasy. *Dermatologica*, 1981; 162: 372.
4. Maggitt SJ, Harper J, Lacour M, and Taylor AEM. Raised limb bands in infancy. *Br J Dermatol*, 2002; 147: 359–363.
5. Mesrati H, Amouri M, Loukils H et al. Isolated congenital anonychia about seven cases. Nail meeting programme, Marrakesh 2nd ISND, 2013; p 147.
6. Baran R and Juhlin L. Bone dependent nail formation. *Br J Dermatol*, 1986; 114: 371–375.
7. Priolo M, Rosaia L, Seri M et al. Total anonychia congenita in a woman with normal intelligence. *Dermatology*, 2000; 200: 84–85.
8. Al Hawsawi K, Al Aboud K, Alfadley A, and Al Aboud D. Anonychia congenital totalis: A case report and review of the literature. *Int J Dermatol*, 2002; 41(7): 397–399.
9. El-Komy MHM and Baran R. Acroosteolysis presenting with brachyonychia following exposure to cold. *J Eur Acad Dermatol Venereol*, 2015; 29(11): 2252–2254. doi: 001:10.1111/jdv.12826.
10. Nakazato T and Ogino T. Epiphyseal destruction of children's hands after frostbite: A report of two cases. *J Hand Surg Am*, 1986; 11: 289–292.
11. Van Ackere T, Eykens A, Wouters C, and Toelen J. The phalangeal microgeodic syndrome in childhood: Awareness leads to diagnosis. *Eur J Pediatr*, 2013; 172: 763–767.
12. Alves GE, Roon E, John J et al. Circumferential fingernail. *Br J Dermatol*, 1999; 140: 960–962.
13. Kalisman M, Goldberg R, and Ship AG. Dorsal skin and fingernails on the volar aspect of the hand: An unusual anatomic deformity. *Plast Reconstr Surg*, 1982; 69: 694–696.
14. Bhaskaranand K, Shetty RR, and Bhat AK. Pachydermoperiostosis: Three case reports. *J Orthop Surg*, 2001; 9: 61–65.
15. Cornelius CE and Shelley WB. Pincer nail syndrome. *Arch Surg*, 1968; 96: 321–322.
16. Higashi N and Kume AT. Congenital curved nail of the 4th toe. *J Pediatr Dermatol*, 1999; 18: 99–101.
17. Iwasawa M, Hirose T, and Matsuo K. Congenital curved nail of the 4th toe. *Plast Reconstr Surg*, 1991; 87: 569–574.
18. Kang JH, Kim M, Chobk et al. A congenital curved nail of the 4th toe. *J Dermatol*, 2015; 72(Suppl 1): AB 110.

19. Haneke E. Double nail of the little toe. *Skin Appendage Disorders*, 2015; 1:163–7.

20. Chi CC and Wang SH. Inherited accessory nail of the fifth toe cured by surgical matricectomy. *Dermatol Surg*, 2004; 30: 1177–1179.

21. Hundeiker M. Hereditare Nageldysplasie der 5. *Zehe Hautarzt*, 1969; 20: 281–282.

22. Riaz F, Rashid RM, and Khachemoune A. Onychoheterotopia: Pathogenesis, presentation, and management of ectopic nail. *J Am Acad Dermatol*, 2011; 64: 161–166.

23. Yadav S, Khullar G, and Dogra S. Congenital onychoheterotopia involving multiple toenails. *J Am Pod Med Assoc*, 2013; 5: 445–447.

24. Kopera D, Soyer HP, and Kerl H. Ectopic calcaneal nail. *J Am Acad Dermatol*, 1996; 35(3): 484–485.

25. Jung GW and Salopek TG. Hoof-nail deformity: A previous unknown hereditary nail malformation. *Br J Dermatol*, 2013; 169: 946–947.

26. Chapman RS. Overcurvature of the nails—An inherited disorder. *Br J Dermatol*, 1973; 89: 317–318.

27. Higashi N. Pincer nail due to tinea unguim. *Hifu*, 1990; 32: 40–44.

28. Greiner D, Schofer H, and Milbradts R. Reversible transverse overcurvature of the nails (pincer nails) after treatment with a beta-blocker. *J Am Acad Dermatol*, 1998; 39: 486–487.

29. Richert B, Choffray A, and De La Brassinne M. Cosmetic surgery for congenital nail deformities. *J Cosm Dermatol*, 2008; 7: 304–308.

4

Nail Surface, Direction, Thickness, and Consistency Variations

Robert Baran and Stephane Vignes

Nail Surface Variations

Transverse Grooves (Beau's Lines)

There are various causes of grooves, ridges, and pits, including local trauma to the nail matrix, and acute febrile systemic disease. Poor nutrition to the matrix leads to a defective band of nail formation resulting in a *transverse groove* on the thin nail plate (Beau's line) (Figure 4.1). Recurrent disease will produce recurrent transverse grooves separated by the normal nail. The depression may extend all the way to the nail plate, leading to temporary latent onychomadesis (Figure 4.2), followed by loss of nail. By measuring the position of the transverse grooves, it is possible to date the previous illness. Transverse grooves sometimes found in psoriasis may be present in isolation or multiple. These should be differentiated from *washboard* nails (Figure 4.3), in which there is also a longitudinal depression usually affecting one or both thumb nails and resulting from a habit-tic pushing back of the cuticle.

Longitudinal Ridges

Longitudinal ridges are small rectilinear projections extending from the proximal nail fold to the free edge of the nail (Figure 4.4a and b). They may be interrupted at regular intervals, giving rise to a beaded appearance. A *longitudinal groove* may run all or some part of the length of the nail. *Median canaliform dystrophy of Heller* (Figure 4.5a and b) is the most distinctive nail surface anomaly. It may be split in the midline, with a fir tree–like appearance of ridges angled backward. Thumbs that are most commonly

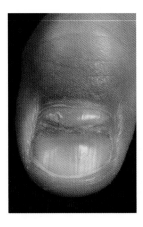

FIGURE 4.1 Beau's line.

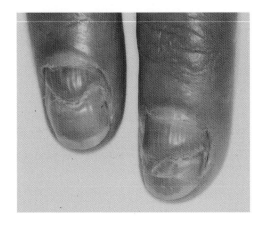

FIGURE 4.2 Latent onychomadesis.

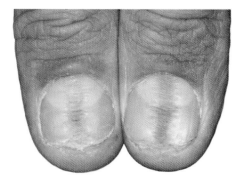

FIGURE 4.3 Transverse grooves resulting from habit-tic pushing back of the cuticle.

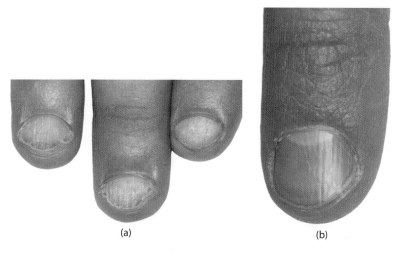

(a) (b)

FIGURE 4.4 (a) Excess longitudinal ridges in twenty-nail dystrophy. (b) Longitudinal ridges replacing progressively oblique lines.

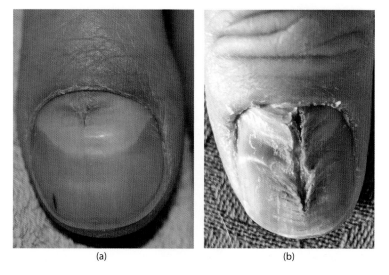

(a) (b)

FIGURE 4.5 (a) Median canaliform dystrophy at the beginning stage. (b) Median canaliform dystrophy at the late stage.

involved usually show an enlarged lunula resulting probably from pressure repeatedly exerted on the base of the nail; some familial cases have been reported.[1] Interestingly, median nail dystrophy may follow isotretinoin and may be associated with ritonavir and alitretinoin therapy.[2]

A single, wide groove or *canal* (Figure 4.6a and b) develops from a permanent or intermittent pressure on the matrix due to a tumor-like myxoid cyst involving the proximal nail fold. *Ridging* becomes pronounced in old age; rheumatoid arthritis, peripheral vascular disease (PVD), and Darier's disease are common in pediatric lichen planus (LP).

Nail Pits

Nail pits are superficial punctate depressions in the dorsum of the nail (Figure 4.7). Sometimes they may be shallow, irregular, rarely deep, suggesting the involvement of the distal portion of the matrix in addition to the proximal portion. The clusters of cells with retained nuclei which develop in the superficial layers of the nail are sloughed off as it grows out, leaving pits on its top.

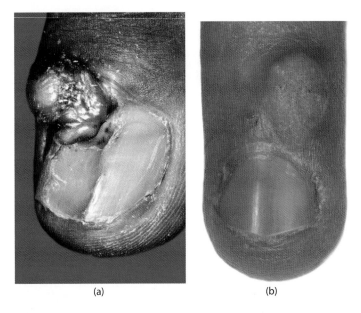

(a)   (b)

FIGURE 4.6   (a) Wide groove due to pressure from fibrokeratoma, emerging under the proximal nail fold in epiloia. (b) Wide canal due to pressure from wart involving the proximal nail fold.

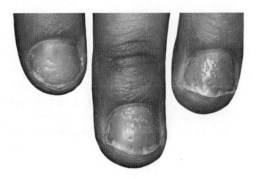

FIGURE 4.7   Pitting caused by psoriasis.

Pitting is not specific to any one disease, but the most common associated condition is psoriasis. However, it may also be found in alopecia areata, eczema, LP, vitiligo, lichen nitidus, reactive arthritis, and chronic renal failure, and even in onychomycosis.

Pits are arranged haphazardly, often seen in psoriasis, or in regular patterns as longitudinal or transverse lines in alopecia areata.

Trachyonychia

Trachyonychia is characterized by a roughness in the nail surface (Figure 4.8a). The nail plate becomes brittle and splits at the free edge. Trachyonychia can involve a single fingernail resulting from external chemical action; other forms are idiopathic, familial, congenital, and acquired. Clinically we have classified it into two main types as follows:

The first type is characterized by opaque, sandpapered nails due to excessive longitudinal ridging and roughness with consequent loss of luster[3] (Figure 4.8b). The second type is characterized by shiny, opalescent nails. This fine stippled appearance reflects light and is clearly demonstrated on photographs.

Twenty-nail dystrophy of childhood is a misnamed syndrome,[4] considered to be a self-limited abnormality that slowly resolves with age. It may be observed in adults and usually disappears spontaneously after a few months or years , which explains the success of the drugs prescribed at the "right" time preceding the disappearance of this condition.

When biopsy was performed, histology demonstrated changes in representing the underlying associated dermatosis, such as LP and psoriasis. Multiple causes may involve the nails, such as alopecia areata, twenty-nail dystrophy, atopic dermatitis, vitiligo, ichthyosis vulgaris, incontinentia pigmenti (IP), primary biliary cirrhosis (PBC), and immunoglobulin A deficiency (IgAD).

In alopecia areata and vitiligo spongiotic, changes are identical to those found in eczema/atopic dermatitis. It is to be noted, alopecia areata and LP have been reported in the same 11-year-old child affected by trachyonychia.[5] Unilateral trachyonychia has been observed in a patient with reflex sympathetic dystrophy.[6]

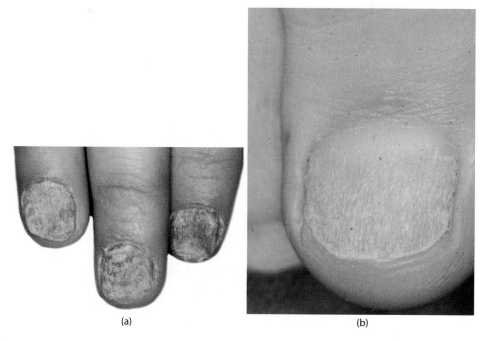

(a) (b)

FIGURE 4.8 (a) Trachyonychia with severe roughness in twenty-nail dystrophy. (b) Longitudinal sandpapered trachyonychia.

A majority of cases of pediatric trachyonychia are isolated and improve with time, regardless of treatment.[7]

Oblique Lines/Chevron Nail/Herringbone Nail

In early childhood, the ridges may be oblique and converge distally toward the center (Figure 4.9).

Sometimes, in teenagers, in one longitudinal half of the nail, oblique lines may be present while the other half is covered with longitudinal ridges.

The oblique lines disappear with adulthood in contrast to that of gorilla, where they remain lifelong.[8]

The significance of chevron nail[9] or herringbone nail[10] is still debatable.[11]

Transverse Lamellar Changes at the Free Edge (Splitting) Onychoschizia

This condition can be observed in newborns (Figure 4.10a). In the first few years it is common for nails to be fragile with transverse lamellar changes at the free edge (Figure 4.10b).

In a survey of 160 schoolchildren, the most common features seen in 5- to 7-year-old children were herringbone nails, nail-biting fingers, lamellar nail dystrophy, koilonychias, malalignment, and nail thickening in the toes.[12]

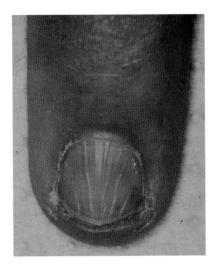

FIGURE 4.9   Oblique lines.

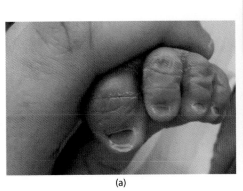

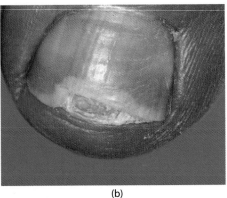

(a)   (b)

FIGURE 4.10   (a) Onychoschizia of the free edge in a 6-day newborn. (Courtesy of Chinazzo M.) (b) Splitting of distal end into layers in an adolescent.

Triangular Worn-Down Nail Syndrome

Worn-down nail syndrome has first been described as the *bidet nail syndrome*, in women affected by a unilateral nail disorder characterized by a triangular defect of the fingernails with its base at the free edge of the nail.[12] All these women displayed an obsessive behavior toward excessive genital hygiene, which resulted in injuries in the three middle fingernails caused by the constant friction against the porcelain of the bidet while cleaning their genital area. This worn-down condition may be observed in children as a habit-tic (Figure 4.11a). However, it may involve both hands, as in the following case: an 8-year-old girl with triangular thinning of the distal shiny nail plate of all the fingers with the base distally located and accompanied by a pink erythema of the distal nail bed.[13] In each nail, thinning progressed proximally to anteriorly, resulting in a fragile irregular free edge of the nail. Dermoscopy of the nail showed erythema of the nail bed with dilated capillaries and pinpoint hemorrhages of the thinned areas. The patient's history revealed that, while at school, she had the habit of scratching the desk with her nails and fingertips.

Worn-down nail syndrome may be included in the group of disorders observed in childhood, such as onychotillomania, onychophagia, and trichotillomania. Behavior modification of the child is necessary for successful treatment.

Runner's big toenail shows similar triangular thinning (Figure 4.11b and c).

Elkonyxis

The nail appears punched out at the lunula and subsequently the disorder moves distally with the growth of the nail. It has been observed in syphilis, psoriasis, reactive arthritis, reflex sympathetic dystrophy, histiocytosis X, post-trauma, and graft-versus-host disease. It has been diagnosed with etretinate, isotretinoin, alitretinoin, and penicillamine.

Nail Direction Variations

Claw-Like Nail

One or both little toenails are often rounded like a claw. This condition usually predominates in women wearing high heels and narrow shoes. Congenital claw-like finger and toenails have been reported.[14] Claw-like nails may be curved dorsally showing a concave upper surface.[1]

Hook Nail

This reflects bowing of the nail bed due to lack of support from the short bony phalanx. Hook nail usually occurs due to a traumatic cause.

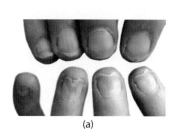
(a)

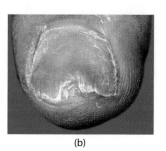
(b)

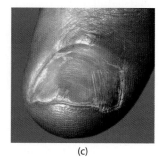
(c)

FIGURE 4.11 (a) Worn-down nail syndrome involving one hand. (b) and (c) Worn-down nail syndrome involving runner's big toes.

Iso-Kikuchi Syndrome

In Iso-Kikuchi syndrome (IKS) or congenital onychodysplasia of the index fingers (COIF), the five criteria characterizing are: (1) congenital occurrence, (2) unilaterally or bilaterally affected index fingers, (3) variability in nail appearance, (4) Y-shaped bifurcation of the distal phalanx visible on lateral X-ray pictures, and (5) possible role of hereditary factors.

The micronychia is usually sited medially (Figure 4.12a) instead of a centrally placed small nail, except for a less common type, termed *rolled micronychia*, where the nail is centrally located. Nail malalignment or anonychia can also be observed. In addition, asymmetrical lunula leads to hemi-onychogryphosis[15] (Figure 4.12b).

A new type has been described presenting a congenital bifid nail deformity with two separate nail matrices and symmetric nail plates, each with corresponding lateral nail folds, separated by a fibrous

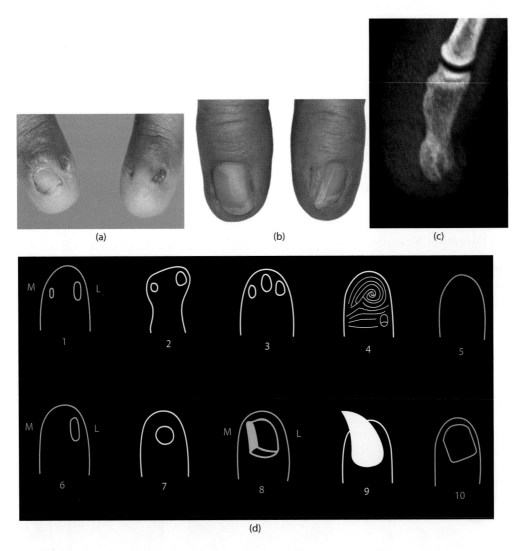

(a)   (b)   (c)

(d)

FIGURE 4.12 (a) Iso-Kikuchi syndrome with micronychia. (b) Iso-Kikuchi syndrome: left deviation leading to onychogryphosis, and right deviation leading to malalignment of a narrow nail. (c) Y-shaped bifurcation of the distal phalanx. (d) Scheme of Iso-Kikuchi syndrome with differential diagnosis. 1: Polyonychia in IKS (M: medial; L: lateral); 2: Polyonychia in syndactyly; 3: Polyonychia in congenital skin disease; 4: Ectopic nail (Ohya's type); 5: Anonychia in IKS; 6: Micronychia in IKS; 7: Usual micronychia; 8: "Rolled" micronychia in IKS; 9: Hemionychogryposis in IKS; 10: Malalignment in IKS.

band. There was a deformity in the distal tuft of the index phalanx with a *Y-shaped configuration* on the lateral view[16] (Figure 4.12c).

The differential diagnosis is shown in Figure 4.12d.

Malalignment of the Nail Plate

Inherited, congenital malalignment of the great toenail which is often misdiagnosed is not an uncommon condition (see Chapter 15). It consists of a lateral deviation of the long axis of nail growth relative to the distal phalanx (see Chapter 17). When the second toenail is misdirected, the deviation is usually medial. Malalignment of the nail plate may occur after experiencing a trauma in the matrix area or following a lateral longitudinal nail biopsy wider than 3 mm in adolescence. The nail may become slightly deviated toward the operated side.

Triangular Nail of Hallux in Newborn

It is probably a mild variant of congenital malalignment, where the apparent hypertrophy of the nail folds seems to be secondary due to the lack of pressure of the nail plate on the subungual tissue[17] (Figure 4.13).

Onychogryphosis (Onychogryposis)

In this disorder, the nail is severely distorted, thickened, opaque, brownish, spiraled, and not attached to the nail bed. The nail of the great toe is particularly vulnerable; it is often shaped like a ram's horn or an oyster. Nail keratin is produced by the nail matrix at uneven rates, with the faster-growing side determining the direction of the deformity. In rare cases, it may be produced by acute trauma, and is rarely inherited as an autosomal dominant trait. Hemi-onychogryphosis with lateral deviation of the nail plate results from congenital malalignment of the big toenail in IKS.

A congenital type of onychogryphosis was described on the left fifth finger as a thickened nail plate with gross hyperkeratosis, increased curvature, growing in an upward direction with a "leaning tower" appearance.[18]

Onychogryphosis may be hereditary or acquired. Involvement of fingernails is uncommon.

Parrot Beak Nails

Parrot beak nails refers to a peculiar, symmetrical overcurvature of the free edge of some fingernails, simulating the beak of a parrot.

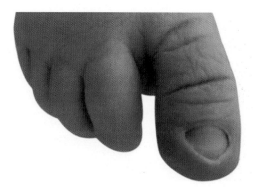

FIGURE 4.13   Triangular nail of the hallux in a newborn. (Courtesy of Chinazzo M.)

Soaking the nails in tepid water for about 30 minutes causes the overcurvature to disappear temporarily. If the patient trims the affected nails close to the line of separation from the nail bed, no abnormality would be noted clinically. Parrot beak nails can occur as a primary nail dermatosis or secondary to finger pulp atrophy.[19]

A new syndrome related to chronic crack cocaine includes the triad of perniosis, finger pulp atrophy of the distal digits, and parrot-beaked clawing of the nails.[20]

Vertical Little Toenail

This is a rare disorder that consists of a misdirected implantation of the matrix of the fifth toe. The nail is virtually growing vertically.[21] In addition to the aesthetic inconvenience, it generates a real discomfort; especially when pulling on stockings or socks, the nail being pushed backward. Female patients mostly complain of running their stockings. The treatment for the vertical little toenail is total nail ablation.

Up-slanting Nails (Upturned Nails, Ski Jump Nails)

The variation in nail contour (small: brachyonychy and concave) and in nail direction (returned small nails) may be observed in children or adolescent with lower-limb lymphedema. Lymphedema in adults is classically divided into two forms, primary and secondary, essentially after cancer treatment. The classification of isolated primary forms (Figure 4.14) includes the sporadic (the most frequent) and familial forms. When lymphedema is present at birth, it is called Milroy disease (due to *VEGFR-3* gene mutation) and when it appears later (during childhood or adolescence), it is called Meige disease. Pediatric lymphedema may be a part of syndromic form, with or without gene implication (Turner, Noonan, Hennekam syndromes and Waldmann disease)[22] (Table 4.1). Classically, lymphedema involves one limb or two limbs under the knee (foot, ankle, and calf). Lymphedema affects commonly the nail anatomy[23] with small hyperplastic concave nails and increased insertion angle. This increased angle of insertion can also be observed in secondary lymphedema.[24] It is interesting to note that there is no clear explanation as to why up-slanting toenail affects one or more toes (more frequently the second and the third one). In adolescents, primary lymphedema of the lower limbs is associated with the up-slanting toenails and soft upturned small nails in children. In Mosaic Turner syndrome, although an intermediate mean fingernail angle is noted, no clear correlation between mean fingernail angle and severity of other manifestations has been shown.

Small dysplastic upturned toenails, deep creases, and swollen sausage-like toes may be observed.[25] Moreover, other abnormalities are frequently associated with up-slanting toenail in patients with lower-limb lymphedema: cuticle disappearance, cutaneous dryness, hyperkeratosis of the proximal nail fold, papillomatosis on the lateral side of the toe, and eventually lymph vesicles with high risk of lymph oozing.[26] An up-slanting toenail represents a major problem with difficulty in cutting the nail and a risk of wrenching it off while pulling on stockings (the cornerstone of lymphedema management).

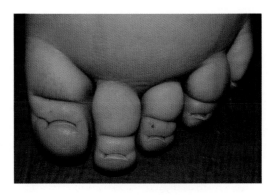

FIGURE 4.14   Up-slanting nail in an isolated form of primary lymphedema.

TABLE 4.1

Syndromic Diseases Including Lymphedema

Disease or Syndrome	MIM Number	Mode of Inheritance/Gene(s)
Aagenes syndrome (lymphedema and neonatal cholestasis)	214900	AR, uk
Emberger syndrome (myelodysplasia and lymphedema)	614038	AD, *GATA2*
Hennekam syndrome	235510	AD, *CCBE1*
Hypotrichosis–lymphedema–telangiectasia syndrome	607823	AR, *SOX18*
Lymphedema–distichiasis syndrome	153400	AD, *FOXC2*
Microcephaly +/− chorioretinopathy +/− lymphedema	152950	AD, *KIF11*
Osteopetrosis–lymphedema–anhidrotic ectodermal dysplasia–immunodeficiency (OL-EDA-ID syndrome)	300301	XLR, *NEMO (IKBKG)*
Noonan syndrome type 1	MIM#163950	AD, *PTPN11, PTP2C, SHP2, NS1, JMML, METCDS* AD ?, uk
Waldemann disease	MIM#152800	AD ?, uk
Yellow nail syndrome	MIM#153300	
Turner syndrome	–	Complete or Mosaïc 45, X0

Abbreviations: AD, autosomal dominant; AR, autosomal recessive; uk, unknown gene; XLR, X-linked recessive; ?, unknown or uncertain mode of inheritance; MIM, Mendelian in man.

Nail Consistency Variations

Changes in nail consistency may be due to impairment of one or more factors on which the health of the nail depends and includes elements like variations in the water content or the keratin constituent. Changes in the intercellular structures, cell membranes, and intracellular changes in the arrangement of keratin fibrils have been revealed by electron microscopy. Normal nails contain approximately 18% water. After prolonged immersion in water, this percentage increases and the nail becomes soft; this makes toenail trimming much easier. A low lipid content may decrease the nail's ability to retain water. If the water content is considerably reduced, the nail becomes brittle. Splitting, which results from this brittle quality, probably is partly due to repeated uptake and drying out of water.

The nail shows a layered structure when examined histologically. The different orientation of keratin fibrils within the layers appears to lend characteristics of both toughness and flexibility.

Hardness of Nail

Hard nails are a major characteristic of the pachyonychia congenita syndrome and the yellow nail syndrome. A study of hardness of fingernails in well-nourished and malnourished populations revealed that the hardest nails were those of Filipino infants and children suffering from protein–energy deficiency.[27] The softest nails were those of children in Guatemala recovering from protein–energy deficiency. In children up to 12 years of age, hardness did not appear to be influenced by the age, sex, and racial origins of individuals, or the environmental conditions to which nail specimens were exposed.

> Thickening of the toenails should not be over interpreted in children under the age of 10 years. In the early stages of walking, toenails thickening can represent a reactive change equivalent to the development of a hammertoe. The immature muscles of the foot can direct the toe so that the pulp is plantar-flexed, making the free edge of the nail tap against the ground. The nail reacts with hypertrophy and, sometimes, subungual hyperkeratosis. For this reason, it is important to examine young children as they move about the consulting room unhindered, so that the natural positions of the toes are apparent.[12]

Soft Nail

In neonates, nails are soft, which explains koilonychias particularly obvious on the toenails. In young children, koilonychias may occur due to contact with water and/or chemicals. For very soft nails, the term hapalonychia is used: such nails may be thinner than usual and bend easily and break or split at the free edge. Soft nail disease is an unusual, congenital nail dystrophy with anatomical and junctional defect of the nail matrix.[28]

Nail Thickness (Pachyonychia, Onychauxis)

Hypertrophy of the nail may be acquired, as a result of dermatologic or systemic conditions, including trauma, or occur as a developmental abnormality. When the thickening is regular and confined to the nail plate, it is due to the involvement of matrix and is sometimes called onychauxis, a sign reported in association with the eunuchoid state. Hyperplastic subungual tissues, especially of the hyponychium can alter the nail plate, and nail consistency may be hard as in pachyonychia congenita or soft as in psoriasis, pityriasis rubra pilaris, chronic eczema, and onychomycosis.

Brittle Nails

We consider that usually the *brittle nail syndrome* encompasses six main types which are as follows[29]:

1. Onychorrhexis is made of shallow parallel furrows running in the superficial layer of the nail. It may result in an isolated split at the free edge, which sometimes extends proximally. This is observed in LP, for example.
2. A single longitudinal split of the entire nail plate is sometimes observed. It may also be produced by focal matrix LP.
3. Multiple crenellated splitting, which resembles the battlements of a castle. Triangular pieces may easily be torn from the free margin.
4. Lamellar splitting of the free edge of the nail into fine layers (Figure 4.10a and b). It may occur in isolation, or associated with the other types. Proximal lamellar splitting may occasionally be observed in LP and during etretinate or acitretin therapy.
5. Transverse splitting and breaking of the lateral edge is usually close to the distal margin.
6. The changes in brittle, friable nails are often confined to the surface of the nail plate; this occurs in superficial white onychomycosis and in nail enamel friability as keratin granulation.

For very soft nails, the term *hapalonychia* is sometimes used.

Hard nails are seen in pachyonychia congenita and yellow nail syndrome. They must be soaked in warm water for prolonged periods before they can be trimmed.

REFERENCES

1. Sweeney SA, Cohen PR, Schulze KE et al. Familial median canaliform nail dystrophy. *Cutis.* 2005; 75: 161–165.
2. Schmutz JL and Tréchot P. Median nail dystrophy and ritonavir. *Ann Dermatol Vénéréol.* 2014; 141: 485–486.
3. Baran R and Dawber R. Twenty-nail dystrophy of childhood: A misnamed syndrome. *Cutis.* 1987; 39: 481.
4. Baran R and Dupré A. Vertical striated sandpaper nails. *Arch Dermatol.*1977; 113(11): 1613.
5. Fenton D and Samman PD. Twenty nail dystrophy of childhood associated with alopecia areata and lichen planus. *Br J Dermatol.* 1988; 119(Suppl 33): 63.

6. Kumar MG, Ciliberto H, and Bayliss SJ. Long-term follow-up of pediatric trachyonychia. *Pediatr Dermatol.* 2015; 32: 198–200.

7. Pucevich B, Spencer L, and English JC. Unilateral trachyonychia in a patient with reflex sympathetic dystrophy. *J Am Acad Dermatol.* 2008; 58: 320–322.

8. Pinkus F. Die normale anatomie der Haut. In Jadassohn J (ed.), *Handbuch der Haut und Geschlechtskrankheiten.* Berlin, Germany: Springer; 1927. p. 278.

9. Schuster S. The significance of chevron nails. *Br J Dermatol.* 1996; 135: 151–152.

10. Parry EJ, Morley WN, and Dawber RPR. Herringbone nails: An uncommon variant of nail growth in childhood? *Br J Dermatol.* 1995; 132(6): 1021–1022.

11. Applin CG and de Berker DAR. Chevron nails are a common finding in childhood: A nail survey. *Br J Dermatol.* 2002; 147(Suppl 62): 6.

12. Baran R and Moulin G. The bidet nails: A French variant of the worn-down nail syndrome. *Br J Dermatol.* 1999; 140: 377.

13. Patrizi A, Tabanelli M, Neri I et al. Worn-down nail syndrome in a child. *J Am Acad Dermatol.* 2008; 59: S45–S46.

14. Egawa T. Congenital claw-like fingers and toes. Case report of two siblings. *Plast Reconstr Surg.* 1977; 59: 569–574.

15. Baran R and Stroud JD. Congenital onychodysplasia of the index finger (Iso-Kikuchi syndrome). *Arch Dermatol.* 1984; 120: 243–244.

16. Crowe D and Disano K. Congenital onychodysplasia of the index finger presenting as a congenital bifid nail. *Dermatol Online J.* 2014; 20: 11.

17. Milano A, Cutrone M, Laforgia N et al. Incomplete development of the nail of the hallux in the newborn. *Dermatol Online J.* 2010; 16(6): 6.

18. Nath AK and Udayashankar C. Congenital onychogryphosis: Leaning tower nail. *Dermatol Online J.* 2011; 17: 11.

19. Kandal E. Parrot beak nails. *Lebanese Medical J.* 1971; 24: 433.

20. Payne-James JJ, Munro MH, and Rowland-Payne CM. Pseudosclero dermatous triad of perniosis pulp atrophy and "parrot beaked" clawing of the nails: A newly recognised syndrome of chronic crack cocaine use. *J Forensic Leg Med.* 2007; 14: 65–71.

21. Richert B, Choffray A, and De La Brassinne M. Cosmetic surgery for congenital nail deformities. *J Cosm Dermatol.* 2008; 7: 304–308.

22. Brouillard P, Boon L, and Vikkula M. Genetics of lymphatic anomalies. *J Clin Invest.* 2014; 124: 898–904.

23. Lowenstein EJ, Kim KH, and Glick SA. Turner syndrome in dermatology. *JAAD.* 2004; 50: 767–776.

24. Le Fourn E, Duhard E, Tauveron V et al. Changes in the nail unit in patients with secondary lymphoedema identified using clinical, dermoscopic and ultrasound examination. *Br J Dermatol.* 2011; 164: 765–770.

25. Carver C, Brice G, Mansour S et al. Three children with Milroy disease and de novo mutations in VEGFR3. *Clin Genet.* 2007; 71(2): 187–189.

26. Vidal F, Arrault M, and Vignes S. Pediatric primary lymphoedema: A cohort of 155 children and newborns. *Br J Dermatol.* 2016, doi:10.1111/bjd.14556.

27. Robson JRK. Hardness of fingernails in well-nourished and malnourished populations. *Br J Nutr.* 1974; 32: 389–394.

28. Prandi G and Ciccialanza M. An unusual congenital nail dystrophy ("soft nail disease"). *Clin Exp Dermatol.* 1977; 2: 265–269.

29. Baran R and Schoon D. Nail fragility syndrome and its treatment. *J Cosm Dermatol.* 2004; 3: 131–137.

5

Nail and Periungual Color Variations

Robert Baran

Chromonychia

The term *chromonychia* may indicate a trifold abnormality in the color of the substance and/or the surface of the nail plate and/or the periungual tissues.

Examination of abnormal nails should be done with the fingers completely relaxed and not pressed against any surface. To differentiate between discoloration of the nail plate and the vascular nail bed, the fingertip should be blanched to determine if the pigmented abnormality is grossly altered. If the pigment originates from the blood vessels (e.g., in methemoglobinemia), it will usually disappear. If the pigmentation is not altered in the blanching test, it may be obliterated by a penlight pressed against the pulp, meaning that the pigment is deposited in the nail bed; the exact position of the discoloration can then be identified more easily. All digits are usually involved when pigmentation is due to systemic absorption of a chemical through the skin. When the cause is endogenous, the discoloration often corresponds to the shape of the *lunula* (Figure 5.1). By contrast, when the discoloration follows the shape of the *proximal nail fold* (*PNF*) (Figure 5.1), it corresponds to the stigmata of an external contactant. In that case, finger pressure producing blanching does not alter the pigmentation, nor does a penlight placed against the finger pulp. The discoloration can sometimes be removed by scraping or cleaning the nail plate with a solvent like acetone. To determine if the color is within the nail, a piece of it should be excised and examined while it is immersed in water. In deeper or subungual impregnation of the nail keratin, microscopic studies (potassium hydroxide [KOH], periodic acid–Schiff [PAS] stain) may be indicated.

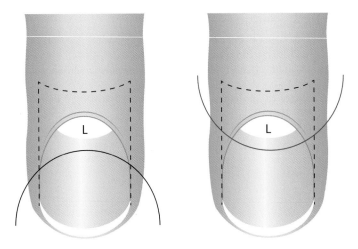

FIGURE 5.1 Scheme explaining the shape of pigmentation.

Leukonychia

True Leukonychia

This is a white discoloration of the nail attributable to matrix dysfunction and presents six patterns described as follows[1]:

1. Total leukonychia (usually inherited) (Figure 5.2a).
2. Subtotal leukonychia, in which the distal portion of the nail appears normally pink.
3. Transverse leukonychia, in which there is a 1- to 2-mm-wide transverse arcuate band, reflecting a systemic disorder when several nails are involved, and this is the most common form; it may occur in isolation or with any other form, involving several digits (Figure 5.2b).

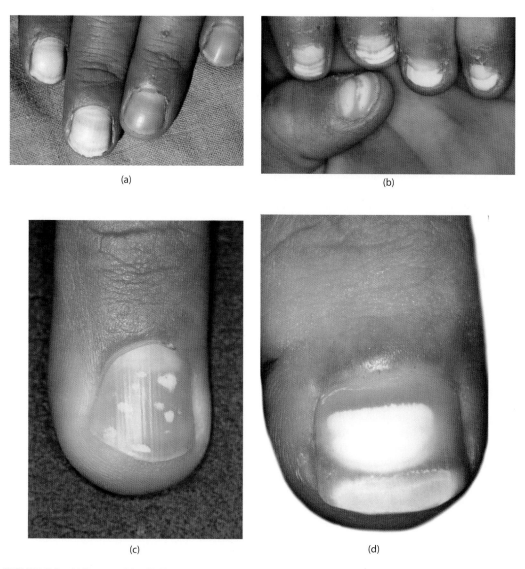

(a)

(b)

(c)

(d)

FIGURE 5.2 (a) Leuconychia. (b) Transverse leuconychia. (c) Punctate leuconychia. (d) Leuconychia resulting from freezing a wart on the proximal nail fold.

4. Punctate leukonychia, in which white spots result, usually from minor trauma: pushing back the cuticles (Figure 5.2c) or after treating warts on the PNF with cryotherapy (Figure 5.2d). Interestingly, both transverse striate leukonychia and punctate leukonychia are among the most commonly nail conditions noted in childhood. Because punctate leukonychia can be associated with alopecia areata or thyroid disease, they can also be an indirect manifestation of autoimmunity. These benign, single, or multiple white spots frequently result from minor injury to the nail cuticle or matrix. Parents should be reassured that these markings are temporary and need no definitive therapy.

5. Longitudinal leukonychia is associated with Darier's disease, Hailey–Hailey disease, tuberous sclerosis complex, or in adulthood with onychopapilloma and even Bowen's disease.

6. Double longitudinal pachyleukonychia[2] is an epidermal hamartoma involving the nail apparatus as a sole characteristic that appeared between the age of 9 and 30 years. This dysplasia is isolated (see Chapter 4).

7. Autonomic leuconychia.[3] This true leukonychia is associated with cold and sweaty hands and pallor of the fingers unrelated to ambient or body dysfunction.

Pseudoleukonychia

This term is used when the nail plate alteration has an external origin, such as in onychomycosis or in keratin granulations observed after nail enamel applications in adolescent girls.

Apparent Leukonychia

The white appearance of the nail is due to changes in the underlying tissue. The nail bed pallor is due to edema or lack of blood. Apparent leukonychia presents five patterns which are as follows:

1. *Terry's nail*, in which the white discoloration stops suddenly 1–2 mm from the distal edge, leaving a pink-brown area 0.5–3.0 mm wide. This condition, which involves all nail uniformly, is associated with cirrhosis of the liver and chronic congestive heart failure.

2. *Half-and-half nail*, which usually shows a sharp demarcation line between the two parts. The proximal area is dull white and the distal area (20%–60% of the total length) is brownish. It is reported in uremic patients, and it is unusual in children.

3. *Muehrcke's paired, narrow white bands*, which parallel the lunula across the nail bed and are commonly associated with hypoalbuminemia as well as chemotherapy.

4. *Anemia, especially hypochromic, exhibits nail bed pallor.*

5. *Raynaud's phenomenon* occurs with one or several white digits.

Splinter Hemorrhages

These longitudinal hemorrhages in the distal nail bed conform to the pattern of subungual vessels. Recently, emphasis has been given on their association with the antiphospholipid syndrome. Proximal splinter hemorrhages have been reported in bacterial endocarditis, trichinosis, and onychomatricoma. They may be seen in psoriasis and result from external trauma.

Green Nails

Green nails are rarely found in isolation (Figure 5.3a). They may be associated with onycholysis. They may also be a part of the triad characterizing the green nail syndrome: (1) green discoloration of the nail plate, (2) paronychia, and (3) *Pseudomonas* infection, often associated with fruity odor.

Pseudomonas species can invade any part of the nail apparatus. Sometimes *Pseudomonas* may be isolated in culture but what often happens is that the culture does not yield any bacteria.[4] Nevertheless,

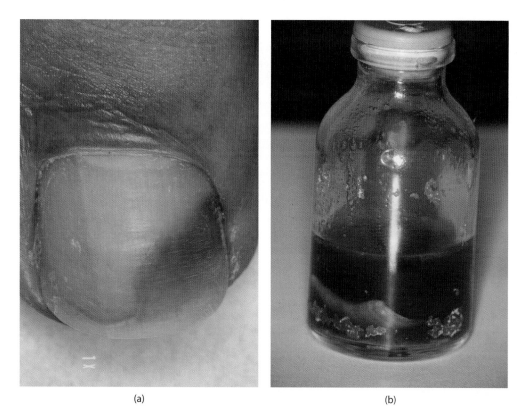

(a)   (b)

FIGURE 5.3   (a) *Pseudomonas* infection. (b) Green nail yielding its pigment in water.

the pigmentation that follows this colonization varies both with the species involved and the composition of the pigments produced. The colors vary from a light green to dark green/black.

The differential diagnosis includes the following:

1. Dark green pigmentation of *Proteus mirabilis*. This Gram-negative bacillus generates hydrogen sulfide. This compound reacts with traces of metals in the nail plate, such as zinc, nickel, cobalt, iron, manganese, tin, copper, and lead metal sulfides to blacken the nail plate.

2. Light greenish discoloration sometimes observed in psoriasis is due to serum glycoproteins. *Pseudomonas* infection can be diagnosed by soaking the fragments of nail in water or chloroform, and if these turn green, it reflects the discoloration is due to yielding of its pigment (Figure 5.3b). The need of oral antibiotics such as ciprofloxacin is rare. Topical treatment includes removal of the onycholytic portion of the nail, avoidance of wetness (finger sucking). Brushing of the nail bed twice daily with 2% sodium hypochlorite solution, or 2% acetic acid, or simply soaking the affected nails in 0.1% octenidine dihydrochloride solution for 6 weeks helps. In fact, the easiest treatment consists of vinegar soaks (10 parts water and 1 part white vinegar) for 5–10 minutes, twice daily.

"Bronze" Baby Syndrome

This syndrome is a rare complication of phototherapy for neonatal hyperbilirubinemia. Light in the blue portion of the visible spectrum corresponding to the maximum absorption of bilirubin (420–460 nm) is used in photooxidation of bilirubin transcutaneously.[5]

In the bronze baby syndrome, a gray-brown color develops in the skin and remains until the hyperbilirubinemia fades. The color of the skin and the nail beds, observed by transparency, resolve within 4–8 weeks after discontinuation of phototherapy.

Black Nails

Black nail is seen through the nail by transparency. Purpura fulminans is a rare syndrome that may occur as a very serious complication of varicella infection (Figure 5.4a and b). Intravascular thrombosis and hemorrhagic infarction of the skin lead to disseminated intravascular coagulation followed by necrosis of the tissue.

Blue Nails

Azure nails are classically described in silver toxicity.

Dark blue discoloration of the lunula is most commonly seen with drug therapy like zidovudine (human immunodeficiency virus [HIV] infection) and chemotherapy like cyclophosphamide (Figure 5.5), vincristine, doxorubicin, and hydroxyurea.

Systemic conditions manifesting blue nails include acrolabial telangiectasis, methemoglobinemia, ochronosis, and Wilson's disease.[6] Considering the latter possibility restricted to the proximal thumb nails of a 12-year-old boy, oral D-penicillamine (20 mg/kg/d) was administered. Outward shift of the discolored nail portion, owing to bad nail growth lead to its disappearance after 4 months of therapy.

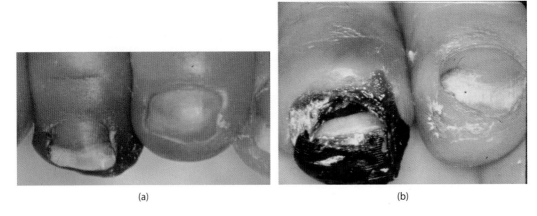

(a)   (b)

FIGURE 5.4   (a and b) Necrosis of the subungual and periungual tissue following purpura fulminans.

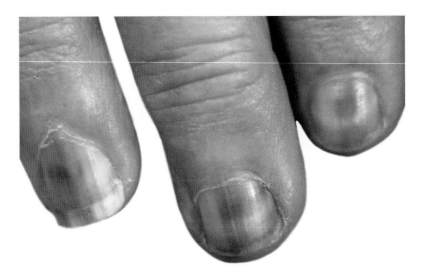

FIGURE 5.5   Dark bluish and white pigmentation due to cyclophosphamide.

Pseudo blue lunula has been observed in a 12-hour-old infant otherwise normal. The blue color of his lunula resolved spontaneously within 2 weeks.[7]

Acrodynia (Pink Disease)

"Acrodynia or pink disease is principally a disorder of infancy and early childhood in which many systemic and cutaneous symptoms are attributed to chronic exposure to mercury. In the earlier stage of the disease, the tips of the fingers, toes, and nose acquire a pink color, and later the hands and feet become a dusky pink. Pink disease, which was common earlier but is largely extinct now due to the discontinued use of mercury in tooth powders and anthelmintics."[8] Superficial desquamation of the palms and soles occur commonly during the course of acrodynia. Pain and pruritus of the extremities can lead to excoriation and lichenification as children constantly rub and scratch their skin. In some patients, this leads to self-mutilation.

Yellow Nail Syndrome

The yellow nail syndrome (YNS) is usually observed in adulthood,[1] but the incidence of this rare disease has increased in pediatric cases[9] (see section "Nail Direction Variations" in Chapter 4).

YNS is a triad made of specific nail changes, yellow, yellowish (Figure 5.6a), or yellow-green, absent lunula, increased transverse curvature with a "hump," slight longitudinal curvature, distal onycholysis, but above all, the nail plates are very hard and grow extremely slowly (0.1–0.25 mm/week instead 0.5–2 mm/week in normal nails). Consequently, the cuticle disappears and favors the appearance of chronic paronychia. Transverse ridging and distal onycholysis can be seen; nail loss is possible.

Lymphedema (Figure 5.6b) is the second sign and respiratory tract involvement the third main sign with bronchial hyperresponsiveness, bronchiectasis, and pleural effusion.

About 30 pediatric cases have been reported: roughly 20 above 10 years of age and among them, 7 are congenital.[10,11] It is noteworthy that exceptional cases of fetal hydrops have been labeled nonimmune

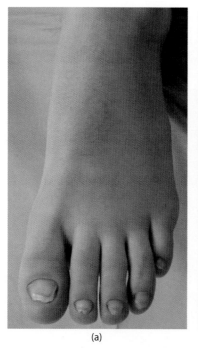 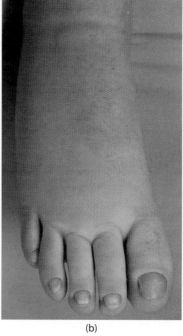

(a)   (b)

FIGURE 5.6 (a) Yellowish nails in yellow nail syndrome (YNS). (b) Yellow nails and lymphedema in YNS. (Courtesy Martin L.)

YNS in newborns who have survived and whose mother was affected by a complete YNS triad at the time of their birth. Subsequent reports have expanded the list of associations with yellow nails to include thyroid disease, nephrotic syndrome, immunoglobulin A (IgA) deficiency, mental retardation, Milroy's disease, and congenital lymphedema of Heige. Interestingly, primary lymphedema of the lower limbs occur simultaneously with the up-slanting (upturned) toenails and deep creases. In Turner syndrome (TS), lymphedema affects nail anatomy with small hypoplastic concave fingernails and increased insertion angle common in TS. It disappears at around 3 years of age.

Acquired Immunodeficiency Syndrome

Adult patients with AIDS might present a pseudo "YNS" with varying degrees of pigmentation, but the discoloration is limited to the distal one-half to one-third of the nail plate. However, the cases reported have not met the diagnostic criteria for YNS.[12]

HIV may produce longitudinal melanonychia as well as non-melanoma-Hutchinson's sign (Figure 5.7).

Mammalian Target of Rapamycin Inhibitors

They diffuse yellow nail discoloration. Given the role of mammalian target of rapamycin (mTOR) signaling downstream of epidermal growth factor receptor (EGFR), this similar effect is perhaps unsurprising.[13]

Hereditary Hemorrhagic Telangiectasia or Osler–Weber–Rendu Syndrome

This syndrome, inherited as an autosomal dominant, is characterized by familial occurrence of numerous telangiectasias on the skin and mucous membranes and repeated episodes of hemorrhage. This condition is rarest among blacks and commonest among persons of Jewish lineage. The telangiectasias may be pinpoint, spider-like, or papular, and bright-red, purple, or violaceous in color. An affected individual often looks pale because of frequent loss of blood with consequent anemia. The telangiectasias generally appear during the second decade of life and increases in number and size subsequently. *Spider* lesions are most often seen in older patients. In about 60% of the patients, the lesions are on the cheeks, nose, and ears, and in 30% on the lesions are on the fingers, toes, and in nail beds. Histologically, the lesions consist of dilated capillaries that are thought to be inherently weak rather than thin."[14]

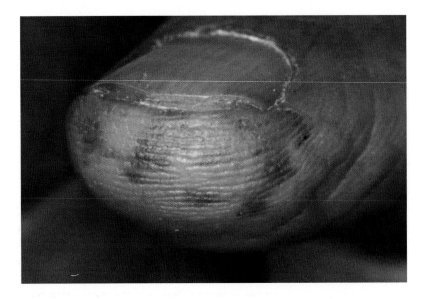

FIGURE 5.7   Non-melanoma-Hutchinson's pigmentation in HIV patient. (Courtesy Lacour JP.)

Acral Pigmentation

This includes nine different conditions.

Acromelanosis

Acromelanosis is an independent disease entity, characterized by increased skin pigmentation, usually located on the acral areas of the fingers and toes. It is mostly seen in newborns or during the first year of life. Periungual hyperpigmentation in newborns is a physiologic melanic pigmentation observed during the early months of life (Figure 5.8).

One hundred and fifty-three subjects constituted a homogeneous group of Caucasian neonates and infants from native Northern European, Italian, and Turkish families. Under 6 months of age, they were observed and presented a benign digital pigmentation.[15] The fingers were examined using Wood's light, which accentuates the light brown or ochre pigmentation situated between the proximal edge of the nails and the dorsal distal interphalangeal zone. The hyperpigmentation was mild in 31, moderate in 20, and intense in three. The prevalence of this hyperpigmentation is maximum between the ages of 2 and 6 months, and it declines before the age of 1 year. The same type of pigmentation was often observed in the toes.

A single publication mentions the existence of transient pigmentation of the perionychium and the dorsal aspect of the distal joint segment in 23% of premature black neonates.[16]

Another group of term newborns under 6 months of age were seen in the outpatient clinic for pediatric dermatology.[17] Of these 50, 40 were fair-skinned and 10 were dark-skinned. All of the dark-skinned patients showed periungual pigmentation of the distal phalanx in the finger and toes (Figure 5.9). Among the 40 fair-skinned patients, only 7 showed periungual pigmentation restricted to the fingers, starting to fade away after 2 years of age, which is longer than previously reported. Interestingly, the group of premature newborns did not show any hyperpigmentation. The intensity of the hyperpigmentation of the distal phalanges may vary among patients, but is not present in the toes.[15]

Acral pigmentation may be a predominant feature in uncommon disorders.[18]

Acromelanosis Progressiva

Acromelanosis progressiva is viewed as the epidermal counterpart of pigmentary disorders composed of dermal melanocytes, "epidermal melanocytosis."[19] Since birth, blue-black, irregular, dot-like macules were noted on the periungual areas of all fingers of the right hand.

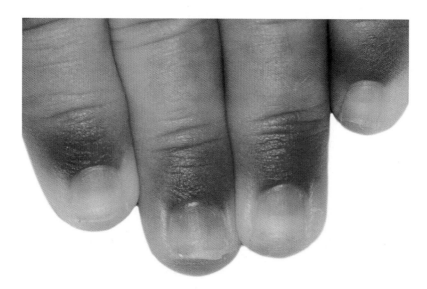

FIGURE 5.8 Physiological melanic pigmentation of the periungual area in a newborn.

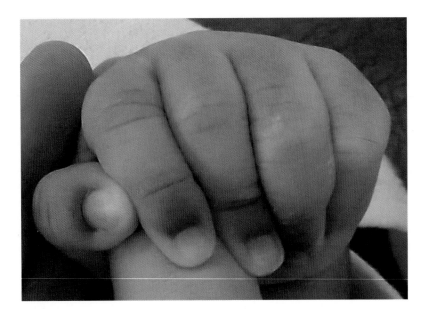

FIGURE 5.9   Periungual pigmentation of a dark-skinned patient (of African descent). (Courtesy Chinazzo M.)

Acropigmentation

Acropigmentation (Spitzenpigment) is a pigmentary condition of infancy restricted to the fingers and toes. It is characterized by brown undefined discoloration that usually diminishes gradually in intensity in the fifth year of life.[20]

Reticulate Acropigmentation

Reticulate Acropigmentation of Kitamura is a disorder usually seen during the first decade of life, in the extensor surfaces of the hands and feet.[21] The lesions present were freckle-like, reticulate, atrophic macules.

Acropigmentation of Dohi

Acropigmentation of Dohi[22] starts appearing in early childhood on the face and dorsal side of the hands and feet as freckle-like hyperpigmented spots occasionally associated with hypopigmented macules.

Universal Acquired Melanosis

Universal acquired melanosis[23] is a progressive dark brown pigmentation of the face and extremities with accentuation in the periungual area observed in a 15-day-old Caucasian Mexican boy. By the age of 3 years, the child had become universally black, including the ocular and mucous membranes.

Ethnic Nail Plate Pigmentation

Never described, this extremely rare condition, observed in Burkina Faso, is present at birth and does not tend to regress (Figure 5.10). The few biopsies that have been performed were reassuring.

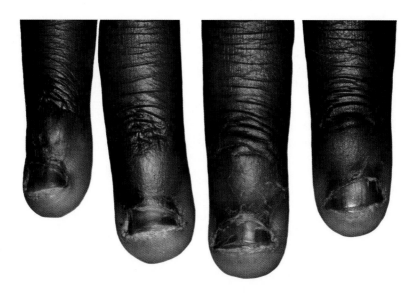

FIGURE 5.10 Ethnic nail pigmentation in a young child. (Courtesy Taieb A.)

TABLE 5.1

Clinical Manifestations of Nail Changes among the Patients and Controls

Types of Nail Changes	Number of Patients (%)
Longitudinal ridging	40 (43.9)
Leukonychia	18 (19.8)
Absent lunula	15 (16.5)
Pitting	9 (9.9)
Transverse ridging	6 (6.6)
Distal onycholysis	4 (4.4)
Chronic paronychia	2 (2.2)
Onychomycosis	2 (2.2)
Flag sign	5
Thinning	4
Terry's nail	3
Longitudinal band	2
Hyperpigmentation around the lunula	1

Source: Anbar T et al., *J Cosm Dermatol*, 12, 67–72, 2013. With permission.

Nail Changes in Vitiligo

In patients whose age ranged from 3 to 65 years, Egyptian authors[24] have found interesting nail changes in vitiligo (Table 5.1). They were observed in 62 out of 91 patients in comparison with 46 out of 91 control subjects. Nail trichrome vitiligo is a transitional pigmentary state with three stages of color: brown, tan, and white in the same patient.[25]

REFERENCES

1. Rubin AI and Baran R. Leukonychia. In Baran F, Dawber RPR (eds.), *Diseases of the Nail and Their Management,* Chapter 2. Oxford, UK: Wiley-Blackwell; 2012. pp. 8–91.
2. Moulin G, Baran R, and Perrin C. Epidermal hamartoma presenting as longitudinal pachyleuconychia: A new genodermatosis. *J Am Acad Dermatol.* 1996; 35: 675–677.
3. Newell L and De Berker DAR. Autonomic leuconychia. *Br J Dermatol.* 2013; 169(Suppl 1): 32.

4. LeFeber W and Golitz LE. Green foot. *Pediatr Dermatol.* 1984; 2: 38.

5. Kopelman AE, Brown RS, and Odell GB. The "Bronze" baby syndrome: A complication of phototherapy. *Pediatrics.* 1972; 81: 466–472.

6. Cohen PR. The lunula. *J Am Acad Dermatol.* 1996; 34: 943–953.

7. Siddiqui Y and Rashid RM. Pseudo-blue lunula and beyond: A normal variant. *Skinmed.* 2010; 8: 363–364.

8. Dinehart SM, Dillard R, Raimer SS et al. Cutaneous manifestations of Acrodynia (Pink disease). *Arch Dermatol.*1988; 124: 107–109.

9. Dessart P, Deries X, Guérin-Moreau M et al. Yellow nail syndrome: Two pediatric reports. *Ann Dermatol Venereol.* 2014; 141: 611–619.

10. Connell F, Brice G, Jeffery S et al. A new classification system for primary lymphatic dysplasias based on phenotype. *Clin Genet.* 2010; 77: 438–452.

11. Kitsou-Tzeli S, Vrettou C, Leze E et al. Milroy's primary congenital lymphedema in a male infant and review of the literature. *In vivo.* 2010; 24: 309–314.

12. Chernosky ME and Finley VK. Yellow nail syndrome in patients with acquired immunodeficiency disease. *J Am Acad Dermatol.* 1985; 13: 731–736.

13. Peuvrel L, Quéreux G, Brocard A et al. Oncyhopathy induced by temserolimus, a mammalian target of rapamycin inhibitors. *Dermatology.* 2012; 204: 8.

14. Gorlin RJ and Sedano HO. Hereditary hemorrhagic telangiectasia: The Rendu-Osler-Weber syndrome. *J Dermatol Surg Oncol.* 1978; 4: 864–865.

15. Crespel E, Plantin P, Schoenlaub P et al. Hyperpigmentation of the distal phalanx in healthy Caucasian neonates. *Eur J Dermatol.* 2001; 11: 120–121.

16. Feldman M, Abudi Z, and Yurman S. The incidence of birthmarks in Israeli neonates. *Int J Dermatol.* 1995; 34: 704–706.

17. Iorizzo M, Oranje AP, and Tosti A. Periungual hyperpigmentation in newborns. *Pediatr Dermatol.* 2008; 25: 25–27.

18. Gonzalez JR and Vasquez Botet M. Acromelanosis: A case report. *J Am Acad Dermatol.* 1980; 2: 128–131.

19. Furuya T and Mishima Y. Progressive pigmentary disorder in Japanese child. *Arch Dermatol.* 1962; 86: 412–418.

20. Thomas E. Ueber das spitzenpigment des kleinkindes. *München Med Wchnschr.* 1923; 70: 1102.

21. Woodley DT, Caro I, and Wheeler CE. Reticulate acropigmentation of Kitamura. *Arch Dermatol.* 1979; 115: 760–761.

22. Komaya G. Symmetrische pigmentanomalie der extremitaten. *Arch Dermatol Symph.* 1924; 147: 775–778.

23. Ruiz-Maldonado R, Tamayo L, and Fernandes-Diez J. Universal acquired melanosis. *Arch Dermatol.* 1978; 114: 775–778.

24. Anbar T, Hay RA, Abdel-Rannan A et al. Clinical study of nail changes in vitiligo. *J Cosm Dermatol.* 2013; 12: 67–72.

25. Di Chiacchio NG, Ferreira FR, de Alvarengo ML, and Baran R. Nail trichrome vitiligo: Case report and literature review. *Br J Dermatol.* 2013; 168: 668–669.

6

Nail and Periungual Tissue Abnormalities

Robert Baran and Didier Bessis

The ventral aspect of the proximal nail fold (PNF) adheres tightly to the dorsum of the nail plate, and its free border producing the cuticle seals the proximal nail invagination. The PNF can become acutely or chronically inflamed.

Acute Paronychia

Acute paronychia may follow a break in the skin. Acute paronychia is a common complaint usually due to staphylococcal infection, but herpes virus, Orf virus, and some fungi can also cause acute paronychia in children and adolescents. As it is important to distinguish nonbacterial from bacterial paronychia, cytologic examination of Tzanck smear may be useful diagnostically. It may result from local injuries, e.g., a thorn prick in a lateral nail groove, a splinter, torn hangnails (Figure 6.1a and b), or nail-biting, the latter two being the most common predisposing factors. It also occurs frequently as an episode during the course of chronic paronychia, when other organisms may be involved including *streptococci*, *Pseudomonas aeruginosa*, coliform organisms, and *Proteus vulgaris*.

The infection starts in the paronychium around the sides of the nail, with local redness, swelling, and pain (Figure 6.1c). If superficial, it may point close to the nail (Figure 6.1d), and can easily be drained by incision with a pointed (No. 11) scalpel without anesthesia. Sometimes a bullous pyoderma brings to light a narrow sinus. This may be part of a *collar-stud* abscess that may communicate with a deeper, necrotic zone. This must be laid open and excised. If the infection spreads to the nail bed, it may uplift the nail plate. If the infection does not show clear signs of response to penicillinase-resistant antibiotics within 2 days, partial avulsion of the base of the nail plate (Figure 6.1e) should be performed and soaking the finger twice a day in antiseptic solution would lead to rapid healing.

Complications of acute paronychia are rare but may include osteitis and amputation. Acquired periungual fibrokeratoma after staphylococcal paronychia has been reported.

As trauma and terminal phalanx fractures can mimic acute paronychia, radiography is advised when the latter occurs after trauma.

Subungual Abscess

Pockets of pus forming directly beneath the nail plate without coexisting paronychia are uncommon infections. There is a yellow discoloration of the nail. Onycholysis can affect the distal one-third of the nail. The severe throbbing pain is similar to that associated with a subungual hematoma and is caused by pressure.

The treatment is simple; a heated paper clip applied to the nail allows the release of the pus and bacterial culture. Partial avulsion of the abnormal nail area permits to treat the nail bed with chlorhexidine, mupirocin, or fusidic acid.

Orf Paronychia

Orf virus has been reported in subjects who have had a history of animal contact.

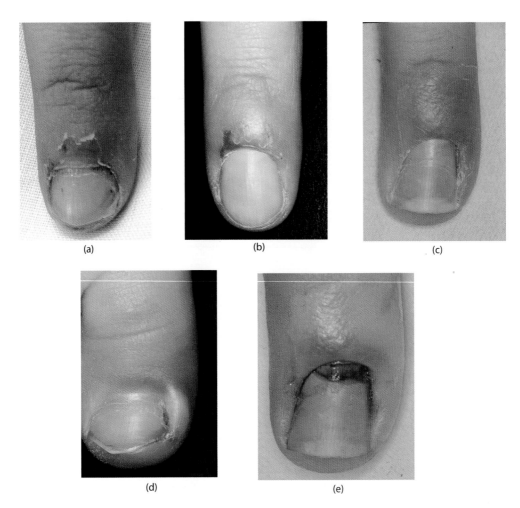

FIGURE 6.1   (a) Hangnail. (b) Torn hangnail. (c) Acute paronychia in an adolescent. (d) Acute paronychia with superficial lesions. (e) Avulsed proximal portion of the nail plate shown in (c). ([a] Courtesy of Zaraa I.)

Scabies

Epidemiologic history, distribution and types of lesions, and pruritus form the basis of the clinical diagnosis of scabies (Figure 6.2a). Head and neck are usually spared in healthy adults, however, in infants, elderly and immunocompromised, all skin surfaces are susceptible. The pathognomonic lesion is a linear burrow, 1–10 mm in length, highlighted by dermoscopy and best seen in the interdigital webs and wrists. Indurated, crusted nodules can be seen on intertriginous areas in children. In crusted scabies, hyperkeratotic plaques develop diffusely on the palmar and plantar regions with thickening and dystrophy of finger (Figure 6.2b and c) and toenails. Nails are important as the principal tools for scratching and may also act as a reservoir for mites and their eggs.[1]

Oral ivermectine is necessarily associated with topical treatment: permethrin twice a day following application of 40% ureal for chemical nail avulsion (partial or total). The local treatment should be repeated until complete cure of the nail unit.

Chronic Paronychia

This is a separate disorder prevalent in individuals whose hands are subjected to moist local environments in infancy, thumb-sucking being the most frequent predisposing factor, and may occur due to

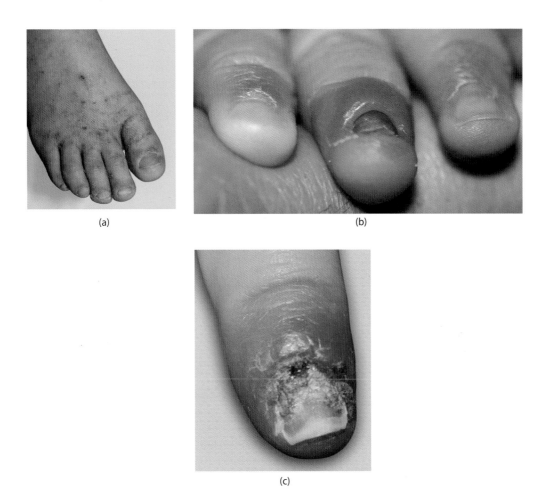

(a) (b)

(c)

FIGURE 6.2 (a) Classical lesion in scabies. (b) Paronychia in scabies. (c) Paronychia with infection leading to onychomadesis in scabies. (Courtesy of Boralevi F.)

contact dermatitis in adolescent. It manifests as a red, semicircular indurated cushion around the base of the nail, which is detached from the distal portion of the PNF (proximal nail fold) and has lost its cuticle. This is followed by secondary retraction of the posterior nail bed. From time to time, the persistent low-grade inflammation may flare into subacute painful exacerbations. Thick pustular material can often be expressed from the pocket under the fold. This causes disturbances of the nail plate that may produce discolored, often brownish, cross-ridged lateral edges, reflecting *Candida* invasion. Occasionally, greenish discoloration occurs when *P. aeruginosa* is present. The incidence of chronic paronychia is higher in diabetics, hypoparathyroidism, acrodermatitis enteropathica (AE), celiac disease, and chronic mucocutaneous candidiasis. Excessive sweating and atopic eczema favor *Candida* survival (Table 6.1).

Treatment is a combination of avoidance of precipitants, hand care, and medication. Perhaps, the most important part of the treatment, but the one most difficult to achieve, is to keep the hands dry.

General hand care with emollients and protection from trauma and irritants is helpful. If these precautions are not followed, the condition is unlikely to settle whatever medical treatment is given.

Topical therapy requires a combination of steroid and antimicrobial agents. A potent steroid may be used for short periods when there is adequate antimicrobial cover. Injected triamcinolone (2.5 mg/mL) is very useful in adolescents. Topical imidazoles are usually sufficient to treat *Candida* and may provide modest activity against some bacteria. More potent topical antibacterials may be needed occasionally. Twice a day application of Dakin solution (sodium hypochlorite) is very effective against *Pseudomonas* infection.

TABLE 6.1

Causes of Pathologic Reactions in Paronychium of Infants and Adolescents

Bacterial

   Classic organisms

   Erysipeloid

   Leprosy

   Milker's nodules

   Mycobacterium marinum infection

   Prosector's tuberculosis verrucosa cutis

   Pseudomonas

   Staphylococci

   Syphilis

   Tularemia

   Unusual organisms

   Actinobacillus actinomycetemcomitans

   Bartonella henselae

   Corynebacterium spp. (in 10% of the patients affected by pitted keratolysis)

   Eikenella corrodens

   Klebsiella pneumonia

   Serratia marcescens

   Torulopsis maris

Fungal

   Aspergillus niger

   Blastoschizomyces capitatus

   Candida spp.

   Fusarium spp.

   Microsporum gypseum

   Neoscytalydium spp.

   Scopulariopsis brevicaulis

   Trichosporum beigeilli

   Curvularia lunata

Parasitic

   Tungiasis

   Leishmaniasis

Viral

   Herpetic whitlow

   Milker's nodules

   Orf

   Warts

Occupational

   Animal origin (bristle, sea urchin, oyster shell)

   Harpists

   Pianists

   Violinist (nail dystrophy)

Drugs

   Acitretin

   Docetaxel

   Doxorubicin

   Cephalexin

Dermatological Diseases

   Artificial nails

   Atopic nails

   Contact dermatitis

   Darier disease

   Dyskeratosis congenita

   Erythema multiforme

   Finger sucking

   Frostbite

   Granulomas

   Hidrotic ectodermal dysplasia

   Ingrowing toenails

   Leukemia cutis

   Pachyonychia congenita

   Parakeratosis pustulosa

   Pemphigoid, pemphigus

   Pernio

   Psoriasis

   Repeated microtrauma

   Retronychia

   Rubinstein–Taybi syndrome

   Stevens–Johnson syndrome

   Toxic epidermal necrolysis

Systemic Disease

   Acrodermatitis enteropathica

   Acrodermatosis paraneoplastica

   Chronic mucocutaneous candidiasis

   Cushing syndrome

   Diabetis mellitus

   Digital ischemia

   Epidemic encephalitis

   Glucagonoma syndrome

   Graft-versus-host disease

   Hypoparthyroidism

   Immunosuppression

   Hyper IgE syndrome

   Langerhans histiocytosis

   Multiple mucosa neuroma syndrome

   Myeloma-associated systemic amyloidosis

   Neurofibromatosis, type 1

   Neuropathies (sensory or autonomic)

   Primary systemic amyloidosis

   Raynaud syndrome

   Sarcoidosis

   Schwannoma

   Systematized multiple fibrilar neuroma

   Systemic lupus erythematosus

(Continued)

TABLE 6.1 (*Continued*)

Causes of Pathologic Reactions in Paronychium of Infants and Adolescents

Cyclophosphamide/vincristine	Systemic sclerosis
Cyclosporine	Tricho-oculo–dermo-vertebral syndrome
Etretinate	Thromboangiitis obliterans
5-Fluorouracil	Wiskott–Aldrich syndrome
Indinavir	Yellow nail syndrome
Isotretinoin	Zinc deficiency
Lamivudine	**Tumors (primary or secondary of the nail unit)**
Methotrexate	Bizarre parosteal osteochondromatous proliferation of tubular bones
Sulphonamides	Bowen disease
Zidovidine	Enchondroma
	Glioma
	Keratoacanthoma
	Melanoma
	Metastases
	Myxoid pseudocyst
	Neurofibroma
	Osteoid osteoma
	Squamous cell carcinoma

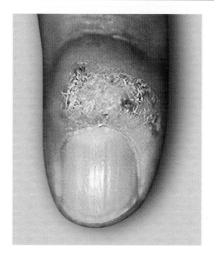

FIGURE 6.3 *Mycobacterium marinum.* (Courtesy of Arenas R.)

Drug-induced Paronychia

Some drugs like isotretinoin can involve multiple digits.

Mycobacterium Infections

For *Mycobacterium marinum*, the nail fold may be an entry point and the initial lesions appear as a developing paronychia followed by granulomatous infiltration or ulceration (Figure 6.3). *M. marinum* is best diagnosed by molecular methods, although it can be isolated in culture in almost half of the cases.

Treatment with clotrimazole or rifampicin, usually with a second drug such as clarithromycin, is effective.

Tungiasis

Clinical features of tungiasis consist initially of a pruritus, tender or painful, small, erythematous papules with a central black dot produced by the posterior part of the flea's abdominal segments. The fully developed lesion is a white pea-sized nodule with a central black or brown pit, or plug located in the subungual (Figure 6.4) and periungual areas of the toes.

Treatment varies from physically removing the flea with a sterile needle to application of 4% formaldehyde solution, paraffin, or turpentine. Systemic niridazole has been recommended if there are multiple sites of infections.

Pyogenic Granuloma, Pseudo Pyogenic Granuloma, and Excess of Granulation Tissue

Perionychial pyogenic granuloma (PPG) is a benign vascular tumor involving the nail area tissue which is prone to rapidly developing bleeding nodules and sometimes pain at the site of minor trauma during

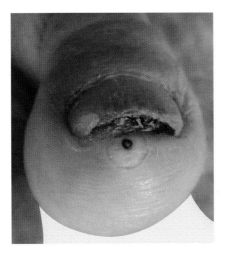

FIGURE 6.4   Tungiasis. (Courtesy of Bonatto D.)

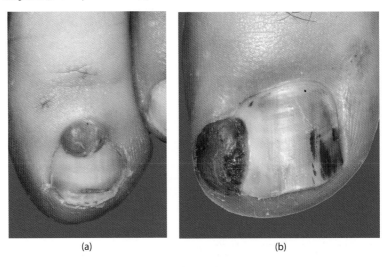

(a)   (b)

FIGURE 6.5   (a) Pyogenic granuloma. (b) Pseudopyogenic granuloma.

TABLE 6.2

Causes of Perionychial Pyogenic Granuloma and Pseudo Pyogenic Granuloma

---

Drug-induced Granulation Tissue

Retinoids (systemic isotretinoin, systemic etretinate, systemic acitretin, topical retinoic acid, and topical tazarotene); antiretrovirals[9] (indinavir and lamivudine); antineoplastic drugs (epidermal growth factor receptor inhibitors[10]: capecitabine, ciclosporin, docetaxel, doxorubicin, and mitoxantrone).

Mechanical Trauma

Periungual tissues are subject to trauma. They may be self-inflicted erosions of the nail folds in associations with neurosis. The ulnar side of the nail is most vulnerable, and there may be small, triangular tags of epiderma, *hangnails*, which are painful and vulnerable to secondary infection. A moisturizer cream applied after hand wash is helpful. As torn hangnails may become infected, they should be removed with sharp-pointed scissors and the affected skin area should be treated with mupirocine.

There are multiple causes of pathologic reactions in paronychium (Table 6.1).

Ingrown nails mainly (distal–lateral type, retronychia, and pincer nails), friction, onychophagia/onychotillomania, manicure, acute mechanical trauma, foreign body penetration.

Peripheral Nerve Injury

Bone fracture of the same limb (cast immobilization), reflex sympathetic dystrophy, prolonged staying in an intensive care unit, Guillain–Barré syndrome.

PPG due to inflammatory systemic disease is only observed in adulthood.

Inflammatory Systemic Diseases

Psoriasis, cutaneous sarcoidosis, seronegative spondyloarthritis.

Epidermolysis Bullosa

Laryngo-onycho-cutaneous syndrome.[11]
Epidermolysis bullosa simplex.

---

the first 6 months in a newborn. The pedunculated lesions have a collarette of scale around the base, which is a characteristic of the disease (Figure 6.5a). Established lesions will have an eroded and often prolonged bleeding. The pathological features of a mature lesion show a polypoid exophytic ulcerated mass characterized by newly formed capillaries and venules in edematous stroma.[2]

Pyogenic granuloma can be excised with a cutting loop electrode, providing a specimen for the pathologist while coagulating the base.

The etiology of perionychial pseudo pyogenic granuloma (PPPG) is indicated in Table 6.2.[2–5]

PPPG differs from pyogenic granuloma as the latter presents an excess granulation tissue mainly observed in the distal–lateral ingrowing nail (Figure 6.5b).

Removing the cause or tapering the doses of the anticancer therapies is mandatory. Pathological examination that rules out melanoma reassures the parents of adolescents presenting an isolated lesion.

The local treatment may either use 10% silver nitrate (AgNO3) once a week or 35% trichloroacetic acid twice a month; curettage after topical or local anesthesia shortens the duration of healing. Pulsed dye laser is an effective therapy after failure of surgical excision, especially in multiple PPG (two sessions: 595 nm, 7-mm spot size, 8 J/cm^2, 0.45 ms pulse width with a 1-week interval).[6]

Faulty Attachment of the Nail Plate

Nail shedding following the separation of the nail from the matrix is called *onychomadesis*. The nail plate shows a transverse split but continues growing for some time because there is no disruption in its attachment to the nail bed (latent onychomadesis). Growth ceases when the nail is cast off after losing this connection. Onychomadesis has been associated with infection, autoimmune diseases, critical illness, and medications[7] (Table 6.3).

The process termed *onychoptosis defluvium*, or alopecia unguium, is sometimes a component of alopecia areata even though it is confined to the nails.

Onycholysis refers to the detachment of the nail from its bed at its distal and/or lateral attachment. The pattern of separation of the plate from the nail bed takes many forms (Table 6.4). "Toenail onycholysis is often

TABLE 6.3

Onychomadesis

Association	Causes
Autoimmune	Alopecia areata, pemphigus vulgaris
Major medical illness	Cronkhite–Canada syndrome, Guillain–Barré syndrome, immunodeficiency, Kawasaki disease, major depressive disorder, meningitis, mycosis fungoïdes, peritoneal dialysis, Stevens–Johnson syndrome
Medication induced	Antiepileptics, azithromycin, chemotherapeutic agents, lead, lithium, penicillin, retinoids
Neonatal	Trauma of birth, *Candida albicans*
Infection	*C. albicans*, *Fusarium solani*, hand–foot–mouth disease (Coxackie A6), *Trichophyton tonsurans*, varicella
Idiopathic	Hereditary, idiopathic

TABLE 6.4

Onycholysis in Infants and Adolescents

1   **Idiopathic**
     Leukoonycholysis paradentotica

2   **Systemic**
     Circulatory (lupus erythematosus, Raynaud's syndrome, etc)
     Cytotoxic drugs
     Drug-induced photoonycholysis
     Endocrine (hypothyroidism, thyrotoxicosis, etc)
     Iron deficiency anaemia, pellagra
     Retinoids
     Syphilis
     Yellow nail syndrome.

3   **Congenital and/or hereditary**
     Hereditary ectodermal dysplasia
     Hereditary nail dysplasia of the fifth toe
     Hyperpigmentation and hypohidrosis
     Hypoplastic enamel, onycholysis and hypohidrosis inherited as an autosomal dominant trait
     Malalignment of the big toenail
     Pachyonychia congenita
     Partial hereditary onycholysis
     Periodic shedding, leprechaunism
     Speckled hyperpigmentation, palmoplantar punctate, keratoses and childhood blistering

4   **Cutaneous diseases**
     Atopic dermatitis, contact dermatitis
     Hyperhidrosis
     Psoriasis, vesiculous or bullous disease, lichen planus, alopecia areata, histiocytosis-X
     Tumours of the nail bed

5   **Local causes**
     Traumatic
     Infectious
        Fungal
        Bacterial
        Viral (e.g., warts; herpes simplex)
     Chemical
        Prolonged immersion in (hot) water, alkalies and detergents, sodium hypochlorite etc.
        Paint removers, rust-removing agents
     Thermal injury

mechanical, the result of pressure on the toes from the closed shoes, while walking because of the ubiquitous uneven flat feet producing an asymmetric gait with more pressure on the foot with the flatter sole."[8]

Abnormality of the Proximal Nail Fold

Dorsal pterygium (Figure 6.6a and b), consists of a gradual shortening of the proximal nail groove, leading to progressive thinning of the nail plate and secondary fissuring caused by the fusion of the PNF to the matrix, and subsequently to the nail bed. The portions of the divided nail plate progressively decrease in size as the pterygium widens. After several years, the pathologic process results in total loss of the nail with permanent atrophy and sometimes scarring in the nail area. Pterygium is characteristic of lichen planus. It may also follow severe bullous dermatoses, radiotherapy, trauma, onychomatricoma, or digital ischemia, but is rarely congenital (Table 6.5).

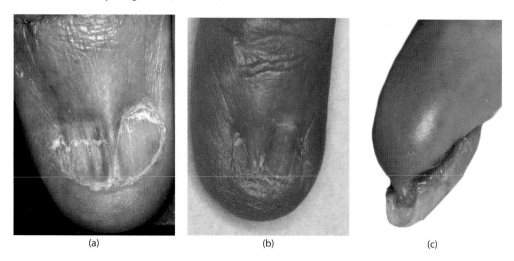

(a)   (b)   (c)

FIGURE 6.6 (a) Median dorsal pterygium (lichen planus). (b) Lateral dorsal pterygium (lichen planus). (c) Ventral pterygium (scleroderma).

TABLE 6.5

Causes of Dorsal Pterygium (Pterygium Inversum Unguis) in Infants and Adults

Atherosclerosis
Burns
Cicatricial pemphigoid
Congenital etiology
Diabetic vasculopathy
Dyskeratosis congenita
Graft-versus-host disease
Idiopathic atrophy of the nails
Inadequate corticosteroid matrix infiltration for *Candidal paronychia*
Lichen planus
Onychotillomania
Pemphigus foliaceus
Radiodermatitis
Raynaud's phenomenon
Sarcoidosis involving the proximal nail fold
Systemic lupus erythematosus
Toxic epidermal necrolysis
Trauma
Type 2 lepra reaction

TABLE 6.6

Causes of Ventral Pterygium (Pterygium Inversum Unguis) in
Infants and Adults

Causalgia of the median nerve
Chronic graft-versus-host disease
Congenital etiology
Family history
Formaldehyde-containing nail hardeners
Lenticular atrophy of the palmar creases
Leprosy
Neurofibromatosis
Paresis
Scarring in the vicinity of the distal nail groove
Subungual exostosis
Systemic connective tissue diseases
Systemic lupus erythematosus
Systemic sclerosis

Abnormalities of Hyponychium

Ventral pterygium (pterygium inversum unguis [PIU]) (Figure 6.6c) is a distal extension of the hyponychial tissue that is anchored to the undersurface of the nail, thereby obliterating the distal groove.[9]

An interesting classification of hyponychium abnormalities based on origin, pathology, and outcome has been proposed (Table 6.6) as described below[10]

- *Congenital, painful, aberrant hyponychium*
  This is caused by the arrested development of the distal surface of the embryo digit between 11 and 20 weeks of age. The distal ridge, normally eliminated, remains located anatomically where the adult hyponychium would be.[11] Pain can be variable.

- *Acquired irreversible PIU*
  This condition is produced by repetitive vascular occlusion episodes that create infarcts, followed by scarring, which leads to reduced and deformed fingertips. These lesions are painful and classically described in scleroderma,[12] but any disease compromising the vascular or nervous system in the area may produce this type of scarring (connective tissue disease, leprosy, stroke, subungual exostosis) and recently severe chronic graft-versus-host disease (GVHD).[13] Pain depends on the underlying cause.

- *Acquired reversible extended hyponychium*
  It is clinically similar to the congenital aberrant hyponychium but caused by a temporary painful inflammatory reaction due to fingertip exposure to some chemical irritant like formaldehyde in nail hardeners and acrylate allergy. This variety is expected to improve completely after removal of the exposure to the cause.

Beside the anecdotal topical treatment of hydroxyl chitosan,[14] the treatment of PIU is surgical and provides relief from pain: after avulsion of the distal 5-mm nail plate, a strip of nail bed and hyponychium 3–4 mm wide is resected and replaced by a split-thickness graft.

Painful Dorsolateral Fissure of the Fingertip

This condition is not uncommon; it can be seen in patients receiving chemotherapy or targeted therapies where the fissures, often painful, are associated with xerosis and become infected. Interestingly, the fissures are distal to and often in line with the lateral nail groove.[15]

Onychotrichia

Ectopic growth of hair follicle under the nail plate is a very rare entity. Two cases were reported in early infancy: one involved the second right toenail without any deformity in a 16-month-old child,[16] and the second affected a 4-year-old girl with a history of an asymptomatic longitudinal dark-brown streak on the second right toenail, evolving for 20–25 days.[17] There was a 0.1-mm-wide straight brownish-black line under the nail, beginning from one-third of the proximal nail plate to the distal end.

Till now one case has been observed in a 37-year-old Caucasian patient with a notch on the nail plate of his right thumb.[18]

Nail Degloving

Nail degloving refers to partial or total avulsion of the nail and surrounding tissue (perionychium). Typically, it appears as a thimble-shaped nail shedding or a partial or total loss of the nail organ with soft tissue. Nail degloving is the end result of a variety of insults to the nail apparatus, including trauma, dermatologic diseases, and drug reactions.[19]

There are several presentations, some are described as follows:

1. *Trauma*

   The etiology of trauma is well-known and may be found anywhere at any age. If proximal and distal nail matrices are necessary to produce a normal nail, nail bed also plays an essential role in the regrowth and size of the nail plate. After disinfection, the avulsed nail plate on the torn nail bed is replaced and sutured on the lateral nail folds. When the nail is unavailable, silicone sheets can be used as a substitute, sutured in place of the nail plate.

2. *Iatrogenic causes*

   They can be responsible for nail degloving. Toxic epidermal necrolysis provides the most typical cases (Figure 6.7). Usually, a normal nail will regrow.

3. *Gangrenous conditions*

   The occurrence of acute peripheral gangrene in newborns is a rare emergency event (Figure 6.8a and b). A few hours after delivery, the newborn develops blisters on the digits. Gangrene appears the following day. The differential diagnosis includes metabolic and genetic (congenital erosive vesicular dermatosis with reticulated supple scarring),[20] drug-induced conditions, vasculitis syndrome, or conditions related to vascular malformations.

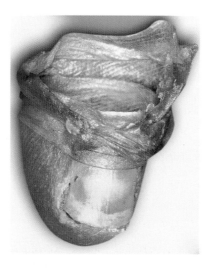

FIGURE 6.7 Nail degloving (carbamazepine). (Courtesy of Souteyrand, P.)

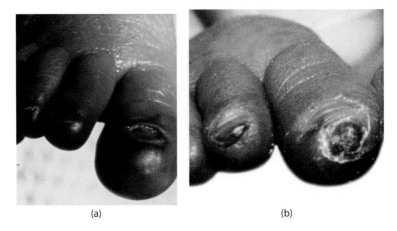

(a)   (b)

FIGURE 6.8   (a) Congenital gangrene. (b) Same patient after spontaneous degloving. ([a] Courtesy of Eschard C.)

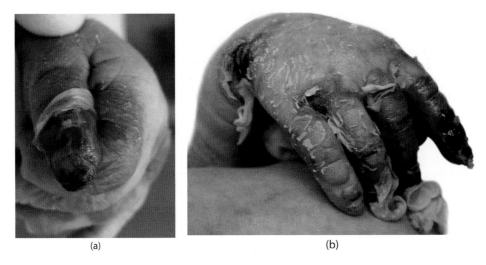

(a)   (b)

FIGURE 6.9   (a) Nail degloving in epidermolysis bullosa. (b) Nail degloving in epidermolysis bullosa. (Courtesy of Cambazard, F.)

4. *Epidermolysis bullosa*

Nail degloving has been observed in autosomal dominant epidermolysis bullosa (Figure 6.9a and b).

5. *Kawasaki disease*

A 5-month-old boy presented with typical signs of Kawasaki disease (KD)[21] associated with an unusual eruption. There was an extensive, papuloverrucous plaque-like eruption most prominent on the hands, feet, and around the nails of all the digits. A progressive extrusion of the entire nail apparatus with nail degloving was limited to the fingers, and occurred after 7 weeks, and lasted for 15 days (Figure 6.10). The cutaneous eruption resolved after 3 months with regrowth of normal nails.

Chilblains (Perniosis)

These localized inflammatory lesions affect mainly children and young women on the dorsal and lateral aspect of the digits. Lesions are usually bilateral and symmetrical, and occur acutely as single or

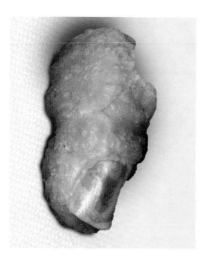

FIGURE 6.10 Nail degloving in Kawasaki disease. (Courtesy of Lacour JP.)

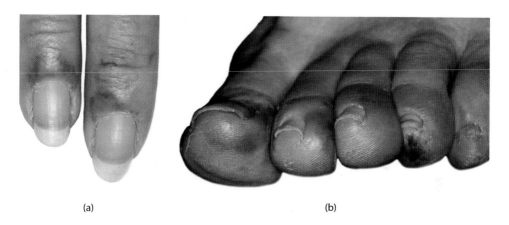

(a)   (b)

FIGURE 6.11 (a) and (b) Chilblain in adolescent.

multiple erythematous or dusky swellings as papules, or plaques that may ulcerate or blister. They are accompanied by a pruritic or burning sensation highly suggestive of chilblain (Figure 6.11a and b). Often, this condition is associated with Raynaud's phenomenon, acrorhigosis, and above all acrocyanosis. Chilblains are caused by exposure to cold, ambient temperatures above freezing point. High humidity and wind play a significant part as well.

A case of chilblains associated with interleukin-1 receptor-associated kinase 4 (IRAK-4) deficiency has been reported in an 11-year-old girl with recurrent pyogenic bacterial infections.[22]

Chiblains may also reveal in adolescents the presence of antiphospholipid antibodies, which should be part of the initial screening of this condition. Some patients will eventually develop systemic lupus erythematosus and/or antiphospholipid antibody syndrome[23] (Table 6.7).

The treatment encompasses avoidance of cold injury, calcium channel blockers (nifedipine), topical high-potency corticosteroids, and applying minoxidil 5% lotion three times a day.[24]

Nail and Type 1 Interferonopathies

The type 1 interferonopathies comprise a group of Mendelian diseases, characterized by an upregulation of type 1 interferon signaling. These monogenic phenotypes include classical Aicardi–Goutières

TABLE 6.7

Diseases Associated with Chilblains[23]

Type of Disease	Example
Hemoproliferative disease/solid carcinoma	Chronic myelomonocytic leukemia
	Metastatic breast carcinoma
Connective tissue disease	Lupus erythematosus
	Behçet disease
Cryopathies	Cryoglobulinaemia
	Cryofibrinogenaemia
	Cold agglutinin disease
Hyperviscosity syndrome	Macroglobulinaemia
Genetic disease	Aicardi–Goutières syndrome
	IRAK-4 deficiency
Miscellaneous	Anorexia nervosa

Source: Adapted from Lutz V et al., *Br J Dermatol*, 163, 645–646, 2010.

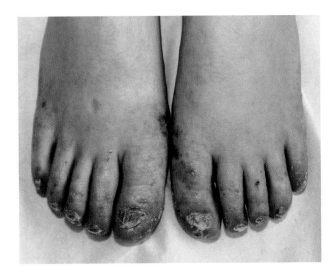

FIGURE 6.12 Type 1 interferonopathies. (Courtesy of Bessis D.)

syndrome, familial chilblain lupus, and STING-associated vasculopathy with onset in infancy (SAVI). Among clinical characteristics of each of these affections, marked dermatological phenotypic overlap is described, particularly with regards to the chilblains and the nail abnormalities. The latter consists, in ascending order of severity, of the fragile nail with longitudinal striations,[25] clubbing,[26] subungual petechial lesions,[27] onychodystrophy including onycholysis, nail plate crumbling, and partial or complete destruction of the nail plates[28,29] (Figure 6.12). All these nail abnormalities seem to be related to severe inflammation and does not appear to be specific.

Several clinical features can help to distinguish chilblain lupus associated with type 1 interferonopathies from idiopathic chilblain or sporadic chilblain lupus: early-onset typically during the neonatal period or shortly after (<6 months of age), as opposed to idiopathic chilblain, which usually begins at around 13 years; atypical locations of chilblain on the trunk and/or the limbs, and risk of skin ulcerations, eschars, and digital gangrene, which can lead to surgical amputation during type 1 interferonopathies (Table 6.8) is seen.

TABLE 6.8

Main Characteristics of Interferonopathies

IFNpath	Gene Mutation/ Transmission	Dermatologic Lesions	Extracutaneous Involvement	Biology and Images
Aicardi–Goutières syndrome	*TREX1*/AR or AD, *RNASEH2A, 2B* and *2C*/AR *SAMHD1*/AR; *ADAR*/AR or AD, *IFIH1*/AD	Frequent chilbain ulcerations, necrosis, possible amputation, rare panniculities	Encephalopathy, spastic tetraplegia, variable mental retardation, microcephaly, RCSP, repetitive febrile episodes	Inflammatory syndrome, autoimmunity signs, intracranial calcifications
Familial chilblain lupus	*TREX1*/AD, *SAMHD1*/AD	Characteristic chilbains identical to SAG		Inflammatory syndrome, autoimmunity signs
STING-associated vasculopathy with onset in infancy	*TMEM173*/AD	Chilbains and severe vasculitis, diffuse pustulosis, telangiectatic surfaces, livedo, buccal ulceratous, nail dystrophies, atrophic scars	RCSP, repetitive febrile episodes, recurrent infections, and interstitial lung disease.	Inflammatory syndrome, autoimmunity signs, leucopenia, anemia, thrombocytosis
SPENCD	*ACP5*/AR	Cutaneous manifestations associated with autoimmune diseases possible chilblains	Osseous dysplasia combined with enchondromas, autoimmune disorders	Inflammatory syndrome, anemia, thrombopenia, leucopenia, autoimmune disorders, possible intracranial calcifications
PRAAS	*PSMB8*/AR	Annular erythematous, papular rash, erythema nodosum, eylid, purple edema, digital clubbing, lipodystrophies, possible chilblains	Upper trunk lipodystrophy, severe arthropathy, amyotrophy	Inflammatory syndrome, leucopenia, anemia, autoimmune disorders and possible intracranial calcifications
Singleton–Merten syndrome	*IFIH1* and *DDX58*/AD	Psoriasis	Vascular calcifications (aorta, cardiac valves), dental, and osseous abnormalities	

Source: Munoz J et al., *Ann Dermatol Venereol*, 142, 652–663, 2015.
Abbreviations: AR, autosomal recessive; AD, autosomal dominant.

REFERENCES

1. Witkowski JA and Parish LC. Scabies. Subungual areas harbor mites. *JAMA*. 1984; 252: 1318–1319.
2. Piraccini BM, Bellavista S, Misciali C et al. Periungual and subungual pyogenic granuloma. *Br J Dermatol*. 2010; 163: 941–953.
3. High WA. Gefinitb: A cause of pyogenic granulomalike lesions of the nail. *Arch Dermatol*. 2006; 146: 930.
4. Williams LH and Fleckman P. Painless pyogenic granulomata associated with reverse transcriptase inhibitor therapy in a patient with human immune-deficiency virus infection. *Br J Dermatol*. 2007; 156: 163–164.

5. Barzegar M, Mozafari N, Kariminejad A et al. A new homozygous nonsense mutation in *LAMA3A* underlying laryngo-onycho-cutaneous syndrome. *Br J Dermatol.* 2013; 169(6): 1353–1356.

6. Miller PK and Levitt J. Treatment of multiple periungal pyogenic granulomata from pincer nails with pulsed dye laser. *Dermatol Surg.* 2011; 37: 1176–1178.

7. Hardin J and Haber RM. Onychomadesis: Literature review. *Br J Dermatol.* 2015; 172: S92–S96.

8. Zaias N, Escovar SX, Zaiac MN. Finger and toenail onycholysis. JEADV. 2015; 29(5): 848–53.

9. Caputo R and Prandi G. Pterygium inversum unguis. *Arch Dermatol.* 1973; 108: 817–818.

10. Zaias N, Escovar SX, Zaiac MN et al. Hyponychium abnormalities. Congenital aberrant hyponychium vs. acquired pterygium inversum unguis vs. acquired reversible extended hyponychium: A proposed classification based on origin, pathology and outcome. *J Eur Acad Dermatol Venereol.* 2015; 29: 1427–1431.

11. Odom RB, Stein KM, and Maibach HI. Congenital, painful, aberrant hyponychium. *Arch Dermatol.* 1974; 110: 89–90.

12. Patterson JW. Pterygium inversum unguis-like changes in scleroderma. Report of four cases. *Arch Dermatol.* 1977; 113: 1429–1430.

13. Huang JT, Lehmann L, and Duncan C. Eosinophilia, edema and nail dystrophy: Harbingers of severe chronic graft versus host disease of the skin in children. *Bone Marrow Transplant.* 2014; 49: 1521–1527.

14. Gondim RMF, Neto PBT, and Baran R. Pterygium inversum unguis: Report of an extensive case with good therapeutic response to hydroxyl chitosan and review of the literature. *J Drugs Dermatol.* 2013; 12: 344–346.

15. Dawber RPR and Baran R. Painful dorso-lateral fissure of the fingertip: An extension of the lateral nail groove. *Clin Exp Dermatol.* 1984; 9: 419–420.

16. Emeksiz MC and Uzar Kocak M. Subungual ectopic hair. *J Eur Acad Dermatol Venereol.* 201; 28: 1263–1264.

17. Cerman AA. Subungual ectopic hair. *J Eur Acad Dermatol Venereol.* 2011; 25: 1115–1116.

18. Ferreira O, Baudrier T, Mota A et al. Onychotrichia?: Subungual hair follicle as another cause of longitudinal melanonychia or pigmentation-hair follicle as a cause of melanonychia. *J Eur Acad Dermatol Venereol.* 2010; 24: 1238–1240.

19. Baran R and Perrin C. Nail degloving a polyetiologic condition with 3 main patterns: A new syndrome. *J Am Acad Dermatol.* 2008; 58: 232–237.

20. Cohen BA, Esterly NB, and Nelson PF. Congenital erosive and vesicular dermatosis healing with reticulated supple scarring. *Arch Dermatol.* 1985; 121: 361–367.

21. Passeron T, Olivier V, Sirvent N et al. Kawasaki disease with exceptional cutaneous manifestations. *Eur J Pediatr.* 2002; 161(4): 228–230.

22. Gurung P, Lee A, Armon K et al. A case of chilblains associated with interleukin-1 receptor-associated kinase-4 deficiency. *Br J Dermatol.* 2015; 173(Suppl S1): 215–216.

23. Lutz V, Cribier B, and Lipsker D. Chilblains and antiphospholipid antibodies: Report of 4 cases and review of the literature. *Br J Dermatol.* 2010; 163: 645–646.

24. Kanelleas A and Berth-Jones J. Chilblains. In Lebwohl M, Heymann WR, Berth-Jones J, and Coulson I (eds.), *Treatment of Skin Diseases*, Third Edition. London: Saunders; 2010. pp. 137–138.

25. Bursztejn AC, Briggs TA, Del Toro Duany Y et al. Unusual cutaneous features associated with a heterozygous gain-of-function mutation in IFIH1: Aicardi–Goutières–Singleton–Merten overlapping syndrome. *Br J Dermatol.* 2015; 173: 1505–1513.

26. Liu Y, Jesus AA, Marrero B et al. Activated STING in a vascular and pulmonary syndrome. *N Engl J Med.* 2014; 371: 507–518.

27. Günther C, Hillebrand M, Brunk J, and Lee-Kirsch MA. Systemic involvement in *TREX1*-associated familial chilblain lupus. *J Am Acad Dermatol.* 2013; 69: e179–e181.

28. Günther C, Berndt N, Wolf C, and Lee-Kirsch MA. Familial chilblain lupus due to a novel mutation in the exonuclease III domain of 3′ repair exonuclease 1 (TREX1). *JAMA Dermatol.* 2015; 151: 426–431.

29. Munoz J, Rodière M, Jeremiah N et al. Stimulator of interferon genes-associated vasculopathy with onset in infancy: A mimic of childhood granulomatosis with polyangiitis. *JAMA Dermatol.* 2015; 151: 872–877.

7

Onychomycosis in Children

Robert Baran and Roderick Hay

Onychomycosis (OM) in children resembles that in adults to a great extent. The cross-section of patterns is slightly different in superficial onychomycosis (SO) that it is more common, and it rarely involves multiple digits.[1]

In contrast to adults, OM in children is relatively uncommon, with a prevalence of approximately 0.44%[2] and extremely rare in children younger than 2 years old.

Several hypotheses have been advanced to explain this: the nail surface is smaller, nails are thinner, athlete's foot is rare, cumulative trauma is less, and above all, there is an increase in the linear nail growth compared to that of adults. However, this practical explanation has been considered debatable by some authors[3] and genetic predisposition has been reported in some cases of distal subungual OM caused by *Trichophyton rubrum*.[4] In fact, OM is no longer a rare finding in children. In one study, fingernail OM was recognized in 52 (10.4%) out of 99 cases.[5] Children under 3 years of age were predominantly involved. *Candida albicans* was the most common pathogen isolated. Toenails were involved in 47 (9.4%) patients. The incidence increased steadily with increasing age. *Trichophyton rubrum* was the most common etiological agent in toenail infection followed by *Trichophyton mentagrophytes* and *Trichophyton interdigitale*. The majority of fungal nail infections presented with distal and lateral subungual OM.

In 100 Mexican children with nail problems, the prevalence of OM was found to be 23%.[6] Belgian authors reported that fungal infections accounted for 30.74% of nail diseases sampled in childhood.[7]

Dermatophyte OM in 16 children under 2 years of age have been reported in Mexico City, where parents and relatives who interacted with children were also studied.[8] Toenail OM was predominant (12/6). The most important predisposing factor was Down's syndrome in 7/16 cases. A common association of tinea pedis and OM was found among parents and siblings. The youngest patient with distal and lateral superficial onychomycosis (DLSO) reported in the literature is an 8-week-old neonate.[9] Severe OM in children should alert the clinician for the possibility of human immunodeficiency virus (HIV), chronic mucocutaneous candidiasis (CMCC), or other forms of immunosuppressions.[1] Interestingly, the first case of congenital OM caused by *Fusarium oxysporum* acquired in utero has been described in a newborn whose mother was immunosuppressed.[10]

Diagnostic Approach

Four main portals of entry for fungi can be identified on the nail (see Table 7.1),[11,12] each resulting in different clinical patterns of infections (Figure 7.1).

1. *Via the distal subungual area and the lateral nail groove* leading to DLSO. The fungus invades the horny layer of the hyponychium and/or the nail bed and then the undersurface of the nail plate, which becomes opaque (Figure 7.2a through g). Endonyx onychomycosis (EO) is a variant of this type sparing the nail bed.

TABLE 7.1

Updated Classification of Onychomycosis

1.	Distal Lateral Subungual Onychomycosis (DLSO)
1.a	With hyperkeratosis
1.b	With onycholysis
1.c	With paronychia
1.d	With melanonychia
2.	Endonyx Onychomycosis (EO)
3.	Superficial Onychomycosis (SO)
3.1	Classical superficial type
3.1.a	With leukonychia
3.1.b	With melanonychia
3.2	Originating from beneath the proximal nail fold
3.2.a	Patchy, mono- or polydactylous
3.2.b	Striate transverse, mono- or polydactylous
3.2.c	SO with deep penetration
4.	Proximal Subungual Onychomycosis (PSO)
4.1	Without Paronychia
4.1.a	Patchy, mono- or polydactylous
4.1.b	Striate transverse, mono- or polydactylous
4.1.c	Striate longitudinal
4.2	With Paronychia
4.2.a	Secondary to chronic paronychia
4.2.b	True *Candida* paronychia
4.2.c	Paronychia due to molds
4.2.d	Dermatophyte paronychia
5.	Mixed Pattern Types
6.	Totally Dystrophic Onychomycosis (TDO)
6.1	Primary type TDO
6.2	Infection progression culminating in TDO
7.	Onychomycosis Associated with Other Conditions

Sources: Hay RJ, Baran R, *J Am Acad Dermatol*, 65, 1219–1227, 2011; Baran R, Hay RJ *J Myc Med*, 24, 247–260, 2014.

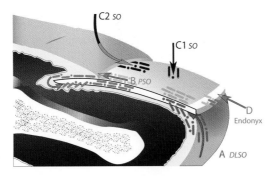

FIGURE 7.1 Routes of entry of infection in onychomycosis: SO, superficial onychomycosis; PSO, proximal subungual onychomycosis; DLSO, distal lateral superficial onychomycosis; C1, classic superficial onychomycosis; C2, superficial onychomycosis emerging from under the proximal nail fold.

2. *Via the visible dorsal surface of the nail plate*, producing SO. This is normally confined to the toenails (Figure 7.3a). There is a rare variety of SO, recently described that emerges from

beneath the proximal nail fold (PNF) (Figure 7.3b) as patchy or more commonly transverse striate discoloration. A rare type presents with deep fungal penetration into nail keratin.

3. *Via the undersurface of the PNF*, which usually appears clinically normal in proximal subungual onychomycosis (PSO) (Figure 7.4a). Sometimes, however, paronychia can be observed, mainly with molds or yeasts (Figure 7.4b) especially in patients with acquired immunodeficiency syndrome (AIDS); "simultaneous polydactylous acute proximal OM" might be the appropriate wording for this type of infection. Of note, the nail bed infection in DLSO caused by *T. rubrum, T. interdigitale, Epidermatophyton floccosum,* and *Neoscytalidium* is the result of the fungus spreading from the plantar to the palmar surface of the feet and hands, a pattern seen in the one-hand-two-foot syndrome (Figure 7.2h).

4. *Totally dystrophic onychomycosis (TDO)*, represents *the most advanced form* of all the types described above (Figure 7.5). In contrast to this more common form, *primary* TDO (Figure 7.6) is observed only in patients suffering from CMCC or other immunodeficiency states.

Patients with OM may present with mixed forms of the above patterns of the nail plate infection. Tinea pedis generally affects adolescent and adults with one of the five possible distinct clinical patterns: interdigital type, moccasin type, vesicular type, acute ulcerative type, and occult infection.

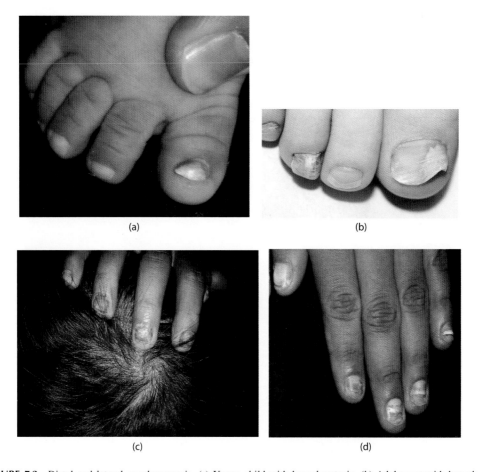

(a)

(b)

(c)

(d)

FIGURE 7.2 Distal and lateral onychomycosis. (a) Young child with hyperkeratosis. (b) Adolescent with hyperkeratosis. (c) Adolescent with *Trichophyton tonsurans* associated with tinea capitis. (d) Adolescent with onycholysis due to *Trichophyton rubrum*. ([a,c,d] Courtesy of Bonifaz A; [b] courtesy of Duvert-Lehembre S.)

(Continued)

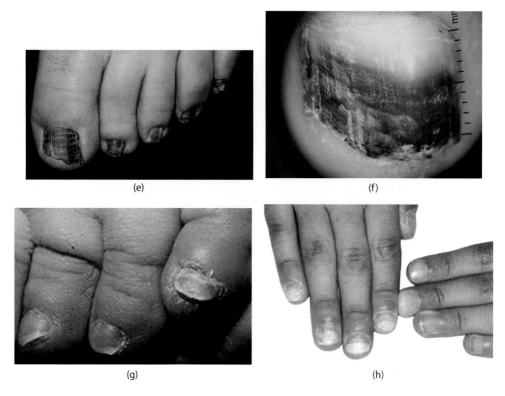

FIGURE 7.2 (*Continued*) Distal and lateral onychomycosis. (e) Fungal melanonychia due *T. rubrum* in adolescent. (f) Fungal melanonychia due to *Cladosporium* in adolescent (dermoscopy). (g) *Trichophyton rubrum* with paronychia in a 1-year-old girl. (h) A 15-year-old adolescent with one-hand-two-foot syndrome *(T. rubrum)*. ([e,f,g] Courtesy of Bonifaz A.)

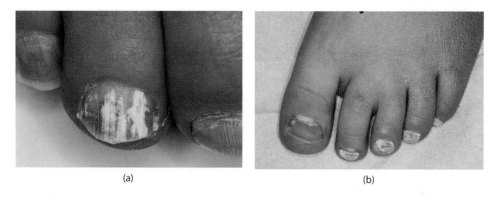

FIGURE 7.3 Superficial onychomycosis (SO). (a) Classical type. (b) SO originating from beneath the proximal nail fold (PNF). (Courtesy of Bonifaz A.)

Update on the Diagnosis of OM

OM is so frequently encountered in daily practice that any nail dystrophy, especially in isolation, may lead to a mistake in clinical diagnosis. Many nail disorders are labeled as fungal infections when they may be caused by a totally different pathology.

The diagnosis of OM always requires laboratory confirmation. After proper cleaning the nail plate with 70% isopropyl alcohol, mycological diagnosis is based on the detection of fungal elements in

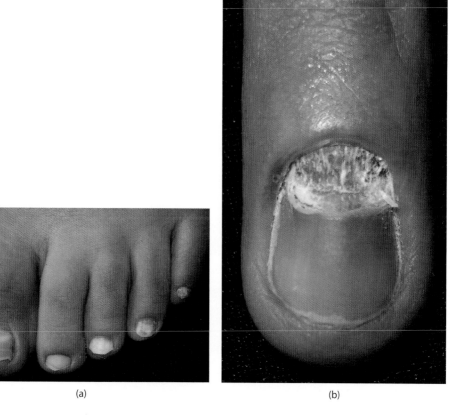

(a)   (b)

FIGURE 7.4 Proximal subungual onychomycosis (PSO). (a) Striated transverse PSO involving the big toe. Patchy involvement of the other digits. (b) PSO with dermatophyte paronychia. ([a,b] Courtesy of Bonifaz A.)

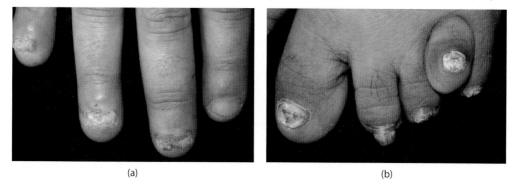

(a)   (b)

FIGURE 7.5 Totally dystrophic onychomycosis (TDO). (a) Involving all the fingernails, resulting from DLSO. (b) Severe hyperkeratosis resulting from DLSO in an adolescent with Down's syndrome. ([a,b] Courtesy of Bonifaz A.)

direct microscopy preparations and identification of the responsible fungus by culture: molecular diagnostic methods are also available in some laboratories. When there are repeated false negative mycological results, histopathological examination of nail keratin, as well as reflectance confocal microscopy can be helpful.

Of note, a single pathogen can give rise to more than one clinical pattern of nail involvement.

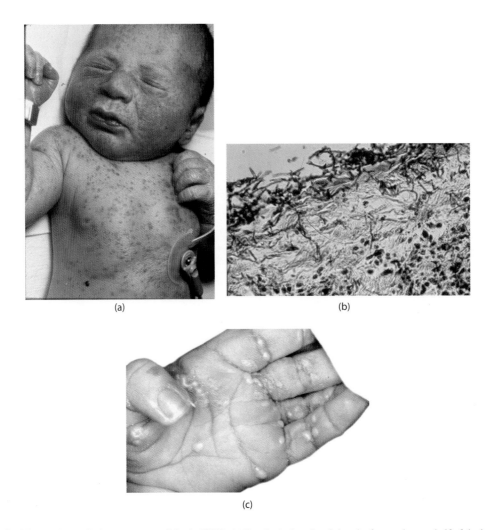

(a)

(b)

(c)

FIGURE 7.6 Congenital cutaneous candidiasis (CCC). (a) Papular lesions involving the face and upper half of the body. (b) Mycology of the same patient. (c) Pustular lesions of the palm. (d) Paronychia present at birth on several fingers. (e) Onychomadesis. ([a,b] Courtesy of Dupont B; [c] courtesy of Malleville J; [d] courtesy of Cambazard F.)

(Continued)

Diagnosis of Dermatophytosis

The diagnosis of dermatomycoses comprises the microscopic detection of fungi using potassium hydroxide preparation or alternatively the optical fluorescence Blankophor or Calcoflor preparations together with culture. Histological fungal detection with periodic acid–Schiff (PAS) staining has a high sensitivity, and it plays an important role in the diagnosis of OM.

Molecular biological methods, based on the amplification of fungal DNA with use of specific primers for the distinct causative agents are being used increasingly. With polymerase chain reaction (PCR), such as dermatophyte-PCR-enzyme-linked immunosorbent assay (ELISA), fungi can be detected directly in clinical material in a highly specific and sensitive manner without prior culture. Molecular methods like matrix-assisted laser desorption/ionization time-of-flight, mass spectrometry (MALDI-TOF-MS) as culture confirmation assay complete the range of potential mycological diagnostics.

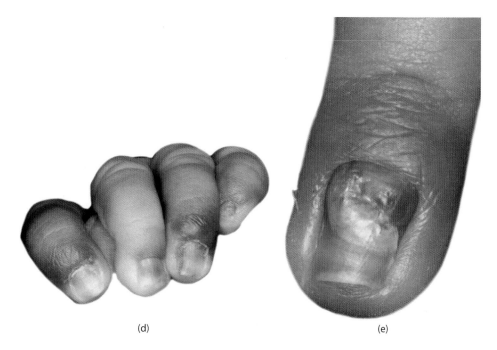

(d) (e)

FIGURE 7.6 Congenital cutaneous candidiasis (CCC). (a) Papular lesions involving the face and upper half of the body. (b) Mycology of the same patient. (c) Pustular lesions of the palm. (d) Paronychia present at birth on several fingers. (e) Onychomadesis. ([a,b] Courtesy of Dupont B; [c] courtesy of Malleville J; [d] courtesy of Cambazard F.)

Rational Scheme for the Treatment of Pediatric Dermatophyte OM

A rationale for a stepped therapeutic approach to the treatment of pediatric OM takes into account the risk of failure caused by the fungal involvement of the lunula, the lateral edge of the nail, or the subungual area. Infection of the subungual area may lead to extensive onycholysis or to *dermatophytoma* presenting either as a soft subungual mass or as a distal to proximal yellow spike, in both of which the penetration of the antifungals into the diseased areas is suboptimal.

The first line of therapy for mild or moderate fungal involvement, which spares the proximal half of the nail plate is topical monotherapy with the nail lacquers or chemicals formulated as transungual drug delivery systems (amorolfine, ciclopirox water-soluble nail lacquer, efinoconazole, luliconazole, and tavabarole). In SO, topical antifungal lacquers should be preceded by nail scraping. Oral therapy with terbinafine or itraconazole should be considered if there is no treatment response (Table 7.2). OM in children is surprisingly unresponsive to topical antifungal therapy and oral treatment should not be delayed.

If single drug therapy is ineffective after 6 months, this is an indication to proceed to the second therapeutic stage, a combination of treatments. However, when the proximal portion of the nail is involved, a combined approach in therapy should be considered as the first step, and an antifungal nail lacquer like amorolfine or ciclopirox should be combined with systemic medications like itraconazole, terbinafine, or fluconazole. This will, additionally, provide effective oral therapy against tinea pedis, which often precedes OM.

When there is a risk of failure, because of interruption in the transport of the drug from the nail into the nail bed or from the nail bed into the ventral nail plate, physical removal of the infected area is indicated. In this triple therapy, mechanical or chemical removal of all the diseased portion of the nail is combined with systemic therapy; the antifungal nail lacquer should be maintained on the normal looking part of the nail keratin, as some fungi may be left beneath its lateral margin. It may be tempting to propose laser treatment for OM in childhood as an alternative to traditional pharmacotherapy. Although

TABLE 7.2

Treatment of Onychomycosis in Children

Dosage Regimens of Itraconazole, Terbinafine, and Fluconazole for Children		
Antifungal Agents	**Dosage**	**One Pulse = 1 Week Therapy/3 Weeks Off**
Itraconazole (capsules)	Pulse therapy	TN: three pulses; FN: two pulses
	10–20 kg	5 mg/kg/day
	20–40 kg	100 mg/kg/day
	40–50 kg	200 mg/kg/day
	>50 kg	200 mg/kg twice a day
Itraconazole (oral solution)	Pulse therapy	TN: three pulses; FN: two pulses
		3–5 mg/kg/day
Terbinafine	Continuous therapy	TN: 3 months; FN: 6 weeks
		1 tablet/day
	Intermittent therapy	Once a day, 1 week monthly as long as needed
	<20 kg	62.5 mg/day
	20–40 kg	125 mg/day
	>40 kg	250 mg/day
Fluconazole	Intermittent therapy	TN: 26 weeks; FN: 12 weeks

Abbreviations: TN, toenail; FN, fingernail.

Note: None of these antifungals is approved for use in dermatophyte onychomycosis in children in all countries. Consequently blood tests and liver function should be performed regularly.

many laser systems are on the market and despite the fact that the Food and Drug Administration has partially approved several of them, there is still some lack of evidence concerning long-term eradication of fungal infection. Moreover, there are neither studies with sufficiently extended follow-up periods nor studies comparing the efficacy of laser systems with oral drugs. This is also true for photodynamic therapy.

Nail Avulsion: The Therapeutic Adjuvant of OM

Chemicals like 40% urea or bifonazole-urea (both under occlusion) or surgical avulsion can be very useful in the treatment of OM. Partial nail avulsion is helpful but only as an adjunct to oral or topical antifungal agents. It is a logical way to eradicate the pathogen. In addition to dermatophyte nail infections, nail plate avulsion is very helpful in treating OM, caused by mold fungi, which is difficult to treat.

Nevertheless total surgical removal has to be discouraged: the distal nail bed may shrink and become dislocated dorsally. In addition, the loss of counterpressure produced by the removal of the nail plate allows expansion of the distal soft tissue and the distal edge of the regrowing nail then embeds itself. This can be largely overcome by using partial nail avulsion, which can be performed under local anesthesia in a selected group of patients in whom the fungal infection is of limited extent. It permits removal of the affected portion of the nail plate in one session, even when the disease has reached the buried region of the subungual tissue, beneath the PNF.

In DLSO, partial surgical avulsion consists of removal of the lateral or medial segment of the nail plate. Therefore, enough normal nail is left to counteract the upward force exerted on the distal soft tissue when walking, and this will prevent the appearance of a deep distal nail groove. However in a small percentage of cases, when total surgical removal has been proposed, the patient should use a prosthetic nail (preformed plastic nail daily fixed with a tape) so that the width of the nail is maintained and subsequent distal or lateral ingrowth is avoided.

In *Candida* onycholysis, a thorough clipping away of as much of the detached nail as possible facilitates the daily application of antifungal drug until nail growth is achieved.

In PSO, removal of the nonadherent base of the nail plate when cut transversely leaves the distal portion of the nail in place, which decreases discomfort and shortens the length of the treatment. In any type of OM treated surgically, the avulsed segment must always include a margin of the normal nail. Recalcitrant *Candida* paronychia with secondary nail plate invasion may sometimes be treated by surgical excision of a crescent of the thickened nail fold.

Ingrowing Toenails as an adverse Consequence of Effective Treatment of OM

Clinically, the therapeutic response is a proximal clearing of the nail plate with resolution of the distal subungual debris.

As the healthy nail plate advances, it may adhere to the nail bed, cutting into the lateral nail folds. This could explain the emergence of onychocryptosis, and clinicians should be aware that this may be a potential complication of effective oral treatment for OM. Acrylic gel reshaping the nail may act as a preventive measure.

Treatment of Nondermatophyte Mold OM

Three patterns of infection should be considered as follows:

- SO caused by *Acremonium*, *Aspergillus*, or *Fusarium* spp. are able to grow and invade healthy human nails as a single source of nutrients, involving the visible portion of the nail plate or emerging from beneath the PNF.
- DLSO caused by *Scopulariopsis brevicaulis*, *Pyrenochaeta unguium hominis*, *Neoscytalidium dimidiatum* and *Neoscytalidium hyalium*.
- PSO due to *Fusarium* spp.

In localized superficial nail plate invasion, abrasion of the dorsum of the nail plate should be associated with one of the effective nail lacquers.

If the molds emerge from under the PNF, or if the fungus presents with a proximal or subungual pattern, partial or total nail avulsion may be useful associated with any of the three main systemic antifungals combined with 3% salicylic acid ointment for 1 week, then followed by nail lacquer applications or topical amphotericine B (Ampho-Moronal suspension®).

In addition, good response on *Aspergillus* spp. has been observed with terbinafine 500 mg daily, 1 week monthly for 3 months in adolescents.

Prevention of Recurrence of Dermatophyte OM

- Check the nails of the family's child and treat them, if they are affected.
- Amorolfine twice a month[13] as well as ciclopirox may be used.

True *Candida* OM

In children, true *Candida* OM may be mainly seen in three instances: as perinatal candidiasis, congenital cutaneous candidiasis, and in children with iatrogenic immunodepression.[14]

Perinatal Candidiasis

The clinical manifestations of perinatal candidiasis and the light which this may shed on some currently poorly understood nail disorders are particularly interesting.

Candida infections contracted in utero present clinically at birth, and congenital cutaneous candidiasis (CCC) is extremely rare. On the other hand, neonatal acquired candidiasis (NAC) contracted during passage through the vagina and the onset of the eruption during the first 2 weeks of life is more common. Consequently these main types are described.

Congenital Cutaneous Candidiasis

The clinical features of CCC are well described. Skin lesions are present at birth (Figure 7.6a and b) or within the first 12 hours of life but sometimes later, up to the sixth day of life. Nail involvement is often seen later. Maculopapular lesions are the first to appear, followed by the more typical vesiculopustular rash and secondary desquamation. Involvement of the face and upper half of the body is frequent. Interestingly, palm and sole pustules are almost invariably seen (Figure 7.6c). Oral, periungual, and conjunctival lesions are rare.

Different clinical presentations of the nail appearance have been observed.

Paronychia may be present at birth on several fingers and toes[15] (Figure 7.6d), and inflammation of the periungual area has been observed in a 2-week-old male infant.[16] In these types, paronychia is almost invariable after birth.

The nails of these affected digits may be thickened and discolored[1]; CCC may be restricted to finger and toenails, first noted within 5 days from birth as a slight yellow discoloration on all toenails and all or two fingernails,[17] or all 20 nails.[18]

Deformity, thickening associated with discoloration of most fingernails may be found during the fifth week or the sixth week of life with mild paronychia.[19,20] Onychomadesis (Figure 7.6e) may follow paronychia.[21] Nail loss is observed in 2–4 months.[22]

In most cases, healing occurs within 10 days of topical treatment using either nystatin or imidazole derivatives. Rarely (2/22), systemic candidiasis may be associated and may progress to death because of lung or meningeal involvement.[23] The risks factors for congenital systemic candidiasis include the use of indwelling catheters, prematurity, antibiotic therapy, intravenous hyperalimentation, intrauterine device, cervical sutures, and use of diagnostic amniocentesis.

Differential diagnosis includes postnatal acquired candidiasis, infectious pustulosis—impetigo, herpes simplex, varicella—and syphilis. Beside infantile acropustulosis, eosinophilic pustulosis, transient neonatal pustular melanosis, tinea, dyshidrotic eczema, and pustular palmoplantar psoriasis, pustular *erythema toxicum* is the most difficult diagnosis to rule out, and the value of the direct smear must be emphasized.

The clinical picture of CCC corresponds to intrauterine infection due to *Candida* chorioamniotitis, for the following reasons: (1) the rash may occur at birth; (2) experimental cutaneous candidiasis requires from 2 to 7 days of incubation; (3) *C. albicans* has been demonstrated in the adnexae, even in cases with late onset; and (4) culture of *C. albicans* in multiple sites favors intrauterine infection. Ascending infection of the fetal skin by *C. albicans* via the birth canal occurs probably through intact membranes, but membrane breaches or late amniocentesis may create a portal of entry. CCC is very rare compared with the frequent maternal carriage of *C. albicans*.

Neonatal Acquired Candidiasis

NAC is characterized by a triad that makes the differential diagnosis with CCC easy: delay in appearance of the cutaneous lesions, initial location of the rash, and absence of chorioamniotitis.[24]

Contamination is perinatal or postnatal if the mother is infected by *Candida,* and often it occurs after passage through the infected birth canal. The risk of developing NAC increases with the length of time between rupture of the membranes before delivery.

In contrast to CCC, NAC starts from the second week, and presents with oral thrush, followed by involvement of the anal and the groin regions (Figure 7.7a and b), after colonization in the gastrointestinal (GI) tract and other skin sites.

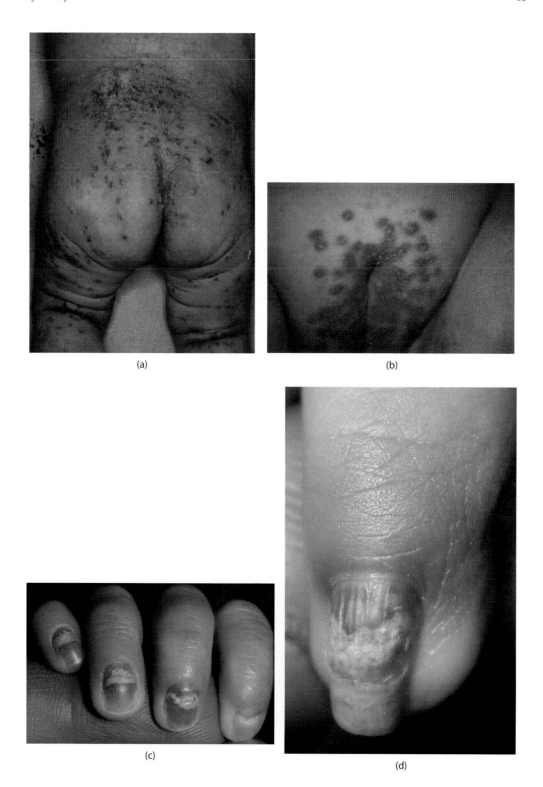

FIGURE 7.7   Neonatal acquired candidiasis (NAC). (a) Papular lesions involving the buttocks. (b) Maculopapular lesions involving the genital groin regions. (c) Onychomadesis that appeared after 4 weeks. (d) Affected by onychomadesis ([a] Courtesy of Taieb A; [b] courtesy of Arenas R; [c] courtesy of Lyon C; [d] courtesy of Silverman RA.)

However, it is difficult to prove that *Candida* paronychia observed from the 15th day of life with secondary colonization of the nail plate belongs to CCC or to NAC following perinatal contamination during the labor or the first days of life. Onychomadesis (Figure 7.7c and d) appears 4–8 weeks due to a functional interruption of the growth of the matrix, and some authors[25,26] have compared cases of onychomades, due to CCC and NAC to onychomadesis observed in a preterm baby of 30 weeks who had developed this dystrophy on all the nails attributed to intrauterine stress responsible for a total but temporary interruption of nail growth.[27] As short duration growth disruption leading to Beau's lines that grow out to the distal edge can occur in up to 92% of normal infants between the ages of 4 and 12 weeks,[28] it is important to exclude an inflammatory or infectious etiology concerning onychomadesis because neonatal cases may be the sole manifestation of congenital candidiasis.[25,29]

Chronic Mucocutaneous Candidiasis

This is a rare syndrome characterized by chronic and recurrent *Candida* infections of the nails, mucous membranes, and skin.

A rash may appear at birth or within a few hours, and if it occurs early is almost always present by 12 hours following birth as erythematous, macular, or papular; the vesicular, and pustular lesions affecting the face trunk, and the lower limbs. The palms and soles are involved, while the back or the buttocks are spared.

Rare at birth nail involvement is often delayed until a few years of age.

Candida invasion rapidly involves all the tissues of the nail apparatus (Figure 7.8a), and produces chronic paronychia (Figure 7.8b). The thickening of the soft tissues results in a swollen distal phalanx more bulbous than clubbed (Figure 7.8c through e). The nail plate is thickened, crumbly, opaque, and sometimes yellow-brown in color. Hyperkeratotic areas secondary to *Candida* invasion may develop on skin adjacent to the nail. Primary TDO is observed only in patients suffering from CMCC or other immunodeficiency states. Oral candidiasis is generally present in these patients.

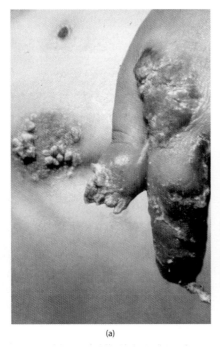 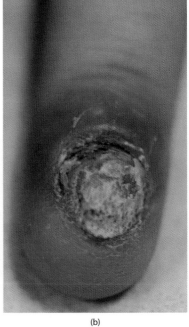

(a)   (b)

FIGURE 7.8 Chronic mucocutaneous candidiasis (CMCC). (a) Hyperkeratotic areas secondary to *Candida* invasion developed on body, Hands, and digits, showing a primary totally dystrophic onychomycosis. (b) Chronic paronychia involving some digits with TDO.

(Continued)

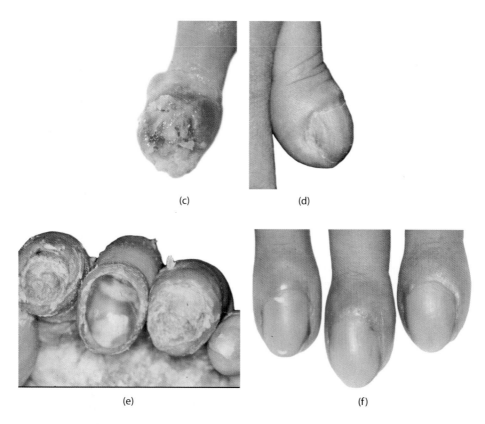

(c)   (d)

(e)   (f)

FIGURE 7.8 (*Continued*)   Chronic mucocutaneous candidiasis (CMCC). (c) The thumb is treated with 40% urea and systemic drug. (d) Cured thumb with thickening of the soft tissues resulting in a pseudoclubbing. (e) Primary TDO, one before cure and (f) two after cure, presenting with bulbous appearance. ([b] Courtesy of Ribeaudeau F.)

Most infections are caused by *C. albicans*, and many patients are unable to develop effective cell-mediated immune response against *Candida*. Dual nail infection with dermatophytes or dermatophyte OM alone may occur in patients with CMCC. The main genetic abnormalities described are mutations in the autoimmune regulator (AIRE1) or signal transducer and activator of transcription 1 (STAT1) genes. Isolated nail candidiasis has also been associated with genetically determined intercellular adhesion molecule 1 deficiency.[30] Table 7.3 provides the list of the subtypes of CMCC.[31]

Differential diagnosis should rule out other infections, such as neonatal pustulosis (see CCC). Infective pustulosis, especially neonatal herpes simplex usually presents with lesions on the face or on the buttocks as vesicles grouped on an inflammatory skin. Tzanck's smear shows the balloon cells and electronic microscopy or immunofluorescence on a smear confirms the diagnosis in a few hours.

Congenital listeriosis is severe with multiple visceral and in 15%–20% of the cases with cutaneous and sometimes pustular involvement. Discovery of *Listeria monocytogenes* in bacteriological samples is diagnostic. In fact, the only problem is to rule out CCC although this is very rare, whereas NAC occurs in 4–5% of newborns, presenting first with thrush acquired during the delivery if the mother is affected by candidiasis or shortly after delivery following handling of the newborn baby.

Treatment of Perinatal Candidiasis

There are a number of different scenarios that have been describe as follows:

- No treatment is administered, and the nails continue to grow out with complete normalization within 3 months.

TABLE 7.3

Subtypes of chronic mucocutaneous candidiasis (CMCC)

Type	Pattern of Inheritance	Special Clinical Immunological Features
CMCC		
Without indocrinopathy (212,050)	Recessive	Childhood onset
With endocrinopathy (240,300)	Recessive	Childhood onset. Patients have the polyendocrinopathy syndrome
Without endocrinopathy (114,580)	Dominant	Childhood onset
With endocrinopathy	Dominant	Childhood onset. Associated with hypothyroidism
Sporadic CMCC	None known	Childhood onset
CMCC with keratitis	None known	Childhood onset. Associated with keratitis
Late-onset CMCC	None known	Onset in adult life. Associated with thymoma

Source: Coleman R, Hay RJ, *Br J Dermatol*, 136, 24–29, 1997.

[a] It is possible that CMCC cases classified under these headings may have to be reassigned to one of the other groups including those with known gene mutations.

- Systemic or topical nail antifungal therapy is not given, and all the 20 nails return to their normal appearance by 5 months of age.[17] In most cases, healing occurs within 10 days of topical treatment using either nystatin or imidazole derivatives. Rarely (2/22) systemic candidiasis may be associated and may progress to death because of lung or meningeal involvement.[32]
- The risks factors for congenital systemic candidiasis include the use of indwelling catheters. These should be removed or changed, and this alone may be followed by the resolution of the *Candida* infection.

These anecdotal reports show that the course of the disease is benign in otherwise, full-term normal newborns, and the benefit of a topical or oral antifungal therapy is not really established in the benign form of perinatal candidiasis involving the newborn. However, if laboratory testing (blood, urine, and cerebrospinal fluid) is positive by systemic treatment with an antifungal like fluconazole, there is no other manifestation.[23]

On contrary, in the severe forms seen in premature infants (<1000 g) with congenital candidiasis, intravenous fluconazole (4 mg/kg) should be administered promptly. If there is no response, liposomal amphotericin B should be prescribed. *Candida glabrata* that can cause this rare infection is resistant to fluconazole.

Clotrimazole may also be used to treat the skin lesions.[33]

Treatment of CMCC

Topical antifungal therapy plays no role in the treatment of CMCC. It is important though to confirm the diagnosis of *Candida* infection. The best approach is to use fluconazole or itraconazole orally, and daily treatment is best as there are no data on the use of intermittent or pulse treatment. Normally, if treatment is continued until laboratory proven clinical and mycological recovery, the relapse rate of OM is low; by contrast, relapse of oral *Candida* infection is very frequent. If there is a relapse of nail infection, it is important to confirm that the infection is still due to *Candida*, as dermatophytoses can intervene particularly if the infection has spread to the soles or dorsum of the foot.

REFERENCES

1. De Berker DAR. Childhood nail diseases. *Dermatologic Clinics.* 2006; 24: 355–363.
2. Gupta AK, Skinner AR. Onychomycosis in children: A brief overview with treatment strategies. *Pediatr Dermatol.* 2004; 21: 74–79.
3. Yu G, Kwon HM, Oh DH et al. Is slow nail growth a risk factor for onychomycosis? *Clin Exp Dermatol.* 2004; 29: 415–418.
4. Zaias N. Onychomycosis. *Arch Dermatol.* 1972; 105: 263: 74.
5. Lange H, Roszkiewicz J, Szczerkowska-Dobosz E et al. Onychomycosis is no longer a rare finding in children. *Mycoses.* 2006; 49: 55–59.
6. Iglesias A, Tamayo L, Sosa-de-Martinez C et al. Prevalence and nature of nail alterations in pediatric patients. *Pediatr Dermatol.* 2001; 18: 107–109.
7. Lateur N, Mortaki A, André J. Two hundred ninety-six cases of onychomycoses in children and teenagers: A 10-year laboratory survey. *Pediatr Dermatol.* 2003; 20: 385–388.
8. Bonifaz A, Saůl A, Mena C et al. Dermatophyte onychomycosis in children under 2 years of age: Experience of 16 cases. *J Eur Acad Dermatol Venereol.* 2007; 21: 115–117.
9. Borbujo-Martinez JM, Fonseca Capdevila E, Gonzalez Martinez A. Onychomicosis por *T. rubrum* en recien nacido. *Acta Dermo-Sif.*1987; 78: 207–208.
10. Carvalho VO, Vicente VA, Werner B et al. Onychomycosis by *Fusarium oxysporum* probably acquired in utero. *Med Mycol Case Rep.* 2014; 6: 58–61.
11. Hay RJ, Baran R. Onychomycosis: A proposed revision of the clinical classification. *J Am Acad Dermatol.* 2011; 65: 1219–1227.
12. Baran R, Hay RJ. Nouvelle classification Clinique des onychomycoses. *J Myc Med.* 2014; 24: 247–260.
13. Sigurgeirsson B. Efficacy of amorolfine nail lacquer for the prophylaxis of onychomycosis over 3 years. *J Eur Acad Dermatol Venereol.* 2010; 24: 910–915.
14. Piraccini BM, Patrizi A, Sisti A et al. Onychomycosis in children. *Expert Rev Dermatol.* 2009; 4: 177–184.
15. Sonnenschein H, Tasehdjian CL, Clark DH. Congenital cutaneous candidiasis. *Am J Dis Child.* 1964; 107: 260–266.
16. Sardana K, Garg VK, Manchanda V et al. Congenital candidal onychomycosis: Effective cure with ciclopiroxolamine 8% nail lacquer. *Br J Dermatol.* 2006; 154: 573–575.
17. Arbegast KD, Lamberty LF, Koh JK et al. Congenital candidiasis limited to the nail plates. *Pediatr Dermatol.* 1990; 7: 310–312.
18. Lim MK, Kwon KS, Jang HS et al. A case of congenital cutaneous candidiasis with nail involvement in a premature baby. *Ann Dermatol.* 1996; 8: 129–134.
19. Abraham Z, Sujov P, Blazer S et al. Candida onychomycosis in a preterm infant. *Mykosen.* 1986; 29: 357–359.
20. Jahn CL, Cherry JD. Congenital cutaneous candidiasis. Experiences and reason. Briefly recorded. *Pediatrics.* 1964; 3: 440–441.
21. See G, Guillaumin JP, Mingasson F. Erythrodermie vésiculeuse néonatale à *Candida albicans. Arch Fr Pediatr.* 1960; 17: 1242–1249.
22. Gaudelus J, Vinas A, Nathanson M et al. Candidose cutanée congénitale. *Med Infantile.* 1984; 91: 659–663.
23. Perel Y, Taieb A, Fontan I et al. Candidose cutanée congénitale: Une observation avec revue de la littérature. *Ann Dermatol Vénéréol.* 1986; 113: 125–130.
24. Roger H, Barroux M, Souteyrand P et al. Congenital cutaneous candidiasis. *Ann Pediatr.* 1986; 33: 521–529.
25. Patel NC, Silverman RA. Neonatal onychomadesis with candidiasis limited to affected nails. *Pediatr Dermatol.* 2008; 25: 641–642.
26. Ameline M, Oillic H, Misery L et al. Onychomadèse secondaire à une candidose congénitale cutanée. *Ann Dermatol Venereol.* 2011; 138: A146. Poster 44.
27. Wolf D, Wolf R, Goldberg MD. Beau's lines: A case report. *Cutis.* 1982; 29: 191–194.
28. Turano AF. Transverse nail ridging in early infancy. *Pediatrics.* 1968; 41: 996–997.

29. Plantin P, Jonan N, Calligaris C et al. Onychomadèse du nourrisson à *Candida albicans* contamination néonatale. *Ann Dermatol Vénéréol.* 1992; 119: 213–215.

30. Mangino M, Salpietro DC, Zuccarello D et al. A gene for familial isolated chronic nail candidiasis maps to chromosome 11p12-q12.1. *Eur J Hum Genet.* 2003; 11: 433–436.

31. Coleman R, Hay RJ. Chronic mucocutaneous candidiasis associated with hypothyroidism: A distinct syndrome? *Br J Dermatol.* 1997; 136: 24–29.

32. Clegg HG, Prose NS, Greenberg DN. Nail dystrophy in congenital cutaneous candidiasis. *Pediatr Dermatol.* 2003; 20: 342–344.

33. Taieb A, Enjoiras O, Vabres P et al. *Dermatologie Néonatale.* Paris, France: Maloine; 2009.

8

Nails in Primary Skin Disease

Robert Silverman

The nail unit is secondarily affected in many primary skin diseases, regardless of the age of the patient. As with adults, the appearance of the nail depends on the extent and severity of the disorder and the location of the primary pathology in the nail bed, matrix, or supporting periungual tissues.

Atopic Dermatitis

Atopic dermatitis is the most prevalent among primary skin diseases in children. Pruritus, a major criterion for diagnosis and infection with *Staphylococcus aureus*, a major complication, are directly responsible for nail disease in this disorder. Fingernail plates of atopic children with chronic disease may be shiny and buffed from constant rubbing. Disruption of the cuticle and inflammation of the matrix during intense atopic flares may result in wavy irregular repetitive transverse grooves of varying size or length (Figure 8.1). Controlling disease flares along with twice-daily application of a high potency topical steroid lotion or solution to the nail folds of the affected nails for several weeks may improve nail contour. In patients with darker skin types, hyperpigmentation of the proximal nail folds and associated faint longitudinal pigmented bands are not uncommon (Figure 8.2). This inflammatory melanocyte activation should not be confused with Addison disease or other causes of multiple plates with longitudinal melanonychia. Bacterial paronychia can develop from overt infection or heavy colonization with *S. aureus* or *Streptococcus pyogenes* (Figure 8.3). One should also be alert for a distinctive presentation of Staph infection that may be associated with underlying osteomyelitis of the distal phalanx (Figure 8.4). These patients have one or more black, triangular-shaped infarct-like macules under the distal-free edge of the nail plate. These may be associated with painful dactylitis. In those cases, an X-ray examination of the digit demonstrates destruction of bone, but inflammatory markers (erythrocyte sedimentation rate [ESR]) are normal.[1] After culture and sensitivities are performed, if osteomyelitis is present, a course of appropriate antibiotic for 3 or more weeks is necessary. If there is no underlying bone infection present, antiseptic washes with chlorhexidine or 0.006% dilute sodium hypochlorite (bleach) along with topical antimicrobial therapy may be sufficient to treat this problem.

Psoriasis

Approximately one-third of patients with psoriasis will develop this autoimmune-driven hyperproliferative disease during the first 2 decades of their life. The nails are affected in 30%–40% of affected children. The severity of nail disease in children is neither correlated with HLA-Cw6 that is more common in children with inherited disease[2] nor with the presence of symptomatic psoriatic arthritis. However, nail involvement is slightly more prevalent in boys (55% vs. 29%).[3] Nail disease may be the first or only sign of psoriasis and may precede skin involvement with the passage of years.

The clinical appearance of psoriatic nail disease is not different than that seen in adults. Pitting is most common (Figure 8.5). The pits vary in size, shape, and are a reflection of involvement of the proximal nail matrix. Trachyonychia (vertical striated sandpaper nails) can be a sign of the presence

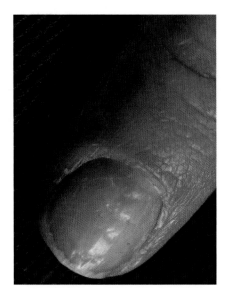

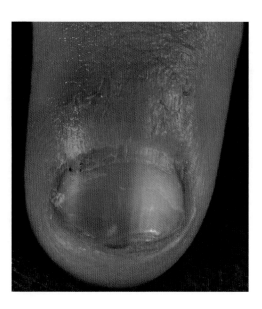

FIGURE 8.1   A shiny, buffed appearance and transverse grooves from chronic scratching and repetitive flares of atopic dermatitis is observed.

FIGURE 8.2   Broad longitudinal melanonychia from melanocyte activation in a patient with atopic dermatitis.

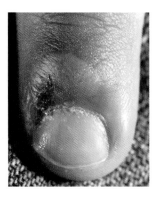

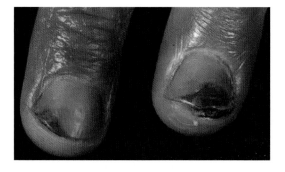

FIGURE 8.3   Bullous impetigo of the proximal nail fold in a patient with atopic dermatitis.

FIGURE 8.4   A wedge-shaped subungal eschar of the distal-free edge of the nail plate may indicate underlying staphylococcal osteomyelitis in patients with atopic dermatitis.

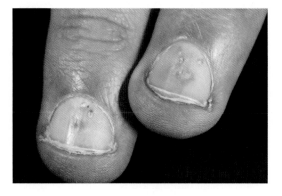

FIGURE 8.5   Variably sized pits and an oiled drop sign, and only cholysis are commonly observed in children with psoriasis vulgaris.

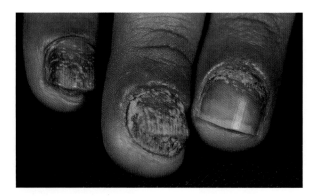

FIGURE 8.6 Isolated psoriasis of the nails can present itself as regular pits of the dorsal nail plate, onychauxis, distal subungual debris, and dyschromia.

of psoriasis in children too. A yellowish discoloration, leukonychia, oil spot sign, distal onycholysis, subungual debris, onychauxis, and ridging that are all due to nail bed involvement (Figure 8.6) are all common as well.

Treatment of psoriatic nail disease should be guided by the presence of pain and quality of life issues faced by the patient that could include chipping, catching on clothing, or being socially ostracized. Combinations of topical medications that include solutions of high potency topical steroids and calcipotriene or tazarotene could be applied daily for 3 or more months. Intralesional triamcinolone in specific circumstances would be acceptable for individual nails. Concentrations as low as 1 mg/mL mixed in saline or local anesthetic delivered after ice anesthesia through a 30-gage needle can be performed in children with good distraction techniques. Oral or topically compounded cyclosporine should be efficacious as with adults, but biologic agents such as the tumor necrosis factor alpha (TNF-α) inhibitors are probably most beneficial. Oral janus kinase (JAK) inhibitors (e.g., Otezla™) have also been successful in improving nail diseases. Oral methotrexate, retinoids, and narrowband UV-B laser are not as successful as the biologics.

Parakeratosis Pustulosa

Parakeratosis pustulosa is a noninfectious inflammatory distal dactylitis seen almost exclusively in young children from 3 to 10 years of age (Figures 8.7 and 8.8).[4] Girls are affected more than boys by this disease. Usually one finger is involved, but on occasions, multiple distal digits may be inflamed.[5] The presence of this disease on toes and multiple digits should make the clinician suspect psoriasis, eczema, or contact dermatitis. Clearly, a diagnosis of the latter two diseases should be entertained if there is a positive family history of either condition. Some clinicians believe that all patients with parakeratosis pustulosa have a form of psoriasis, acrodermatitis continua of Hallopeau; however, long-term studies do not support this opinion. Fungal disease should be ruled out and if the child is diagnosed at the onset of the disease, and when a rare pustule is present, then a bacterial etiology can be sought as well. This is especially true if the patient is sucking on the digit.

Examination demonstrates bright erythema and induration of the distal phalanx with a distinct cutoff border at the distal interphalangeal joint. The nail folds are swollen and cuticle may be absent. Very early in the course of the disease, a subungual or periungual pustule may be transiently observed. The nail plate becomes brittle and chipped when subungual debris accumulates and causes onychauxis.

Parakeratosis pustulosa may persist from months to years, but resolution is common. A 3-month trial of twice-daily application of fluocinonide topical solution in combination with clindamycin solution may be partially effective. There are no reports of oral antibiotics (erythromycin or dapsone) or nonsteroidal anti-inflammatory agents being beneficial.

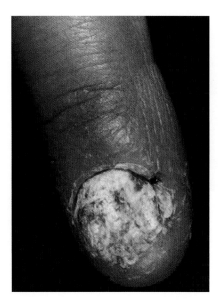

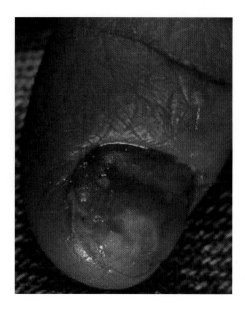

FIGURE 8.7 Unidigital well-demarcated distal dactylitis associated with a chipped, brittle, crumbling nail
plate is characteristic of parakeratosis pustulosa.

FIGURE 8.8 Early subungual pustule of parakeratosis
pustulosa.

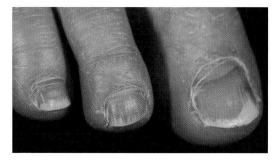

FIGURE 8.9 Onycholysis, distal subungual hyperkeratosis and a yellow-brown discoloration of the toenails is evident in
this patient with Griffith type IV focal well-circumscribed pityriasis rubra pilaris (PRP).

Juvenile Pityriasis Rubra Pilaris

Juvenile pityriasis rubra pilaris (juvenile PRP) is a rare reactive papulosquamous disorder characterized by an abrupt onset, papules, and plaques of the elbows, knees, scalp, and face. Micaceous scale is
not prominent as in psoriasis (Figure 8.9). The palms and soles of these patients are characteristically
thick, leather-like, and display an orange to salmon pink color. The nails may be affected in 10%–40%
of patients with focal circumscribed disease.[6,7] There is hard distal subungual hyperkeratosis that may
be difficult to trim, splinter hemorrhages, onychorrhexis, or a distal yellow-brown discoloration. Pitting
has also been described.

Lichen Striatus

Lichen striatus is a self-limited inflammatory dermatitis that develops in linear bands that extend over
1–3 months and conforms to Blaschko's lines (Figure 8.10). It is usually seen as an extreme condition

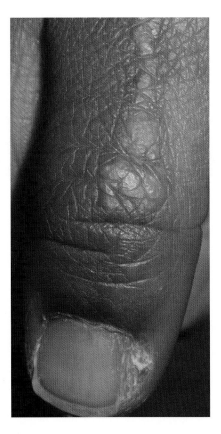

FIGURE 8.10 Longitudinal fissures and furrows of a portion of the nail plate are evidence of Blaschkoid mosaicism as seen in this case of lichen striatus.

and on rare occasions it can involve the nail matrix.[8] In the latter cases, lichen striatus can manifest as a longitudinal fissure or furrow that extends from the proximal nail fold. The severity of the deformity depends on the width of the band. Treatment is generally not needed since the disorder resolves on its own in 1–2 years. Many other inflammatory or genetic mosaic conditions can involve the nail unit. These include psoriasis, lichen planus (LP) and lichen niditus, linear porokeratosis and epidermal nevi, and Goltz syndrome, to name a few.

Alopecia Areata

Alopecia areata (AA) is a common autoimmune disease characterized by the abrupt onset of circumscribed patches of hair loss that may be single, few in number, or widespread enough to encompass the entire scalp. Nail changes are not as common in children with AA than in adults. They may precede the effluvium or be noticed at the time of hair loss. They are usually observed with more severe cases. Nail disease in AA may be associated with other autoimmune diseases such as concomitant vitiligo, LP, or psoriasis. Because of this, it is the author's belief that the association or AA with nail disease is an autoimmune epiphenomenon.

Clinical findings of nail disease in AA may include random pits (Figure 8.11), uniform superficial grid-like pits, trachyonychia, Beau's lines, punctate erythronychia of the lunula, longitudinal erythronychia, or leukonychia (punctate, transverse, or total). When inflammatory activity in the scalp subsides and hair regrows, nails usually revert to normal within another 6 months.

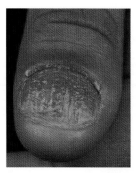

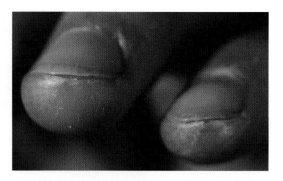

FIGURE 8.11   Small, superficial, relatively uniform pits cover the nail plate of a teenager with extensive alopecia areata.

FIGURE 8.12   Separation of the palmar digital skin from the hyponychium occurs several days after resolution of the non-pitting edema of the hands and feet in a case of Kawasaki disease.

Kawasaki Disease

Kawasaki disease (KD) is a distinctive form of medium arteriolar vessel vasculitis that occurs sporadically, seasonally, or in epidemics. It primarily affects children from 2 to 8 years of age and is more common among Japanese or children of Asian descent. KD is defined by five clinical criteria that include fever of 39.5°C or above unresponsive to antipyretics for 5 or more days; mucositis that includes nonpurulent conjunctivitis, cracked red lips, and nonulcerated oral erythema; varying degrees of lymphadenopathy; a polymorphous rash; and peripheral extremity changes. It is this inflammatory erythema and non-pitting edema of the hands and feet along with high, prolonged fever that result in the characteristic nail changes of KD. These include desquamation of the palmar and plantar skin that begins with separation at the distal-free edges of the nails (Figure 8.12), Beau's lines, and rarely, latent onychomadesis several weeks after the acute illness. A golden brown chromonychia of the nail plates is rarely observed within a few weeks after the onset of the illness.[9] It is the author's opinion that this color change is a result of closely spaced small splinter hemorrhages that can be identified by dermoscopy.

Stevens–Johnson Syndrome

Stevens–Johnson syndrome and toxic epidermal necrolysis (TEN) are severe generalized immunologically mediated reactive disorders to medications or microbes. Some investigators believe that these conditions differ in their pathophysiology while others contend that they are the same disease on a spectrum of extent and severity. Destruction of the skin in this disease is by cytokine-driven apoptosis. The nails can be affected by Beau's lines, latent onychomadesis, pterygium, or total anonychia (Figures 8.13 and 8.14).[10,11] If acute nail loss occurs, it is paramount to protect the nail unit from infection and reduce inflammation so as to minimize scarring with application of topical steroid ointment.

Photo-onycholysis

Phototoxicity from ingestion of medications is a distinctive, frightening, and painful condition that rarely occurs in children. It is most commonly seen in teenagers being treated with doxycycline for acne (Figure 8.15). It has also been reported in immunosuppressed children on voriconizole[12] and in one patient on griseofulvin.[13] Initially, nails are painful when pressure is applied. There may or may not be evidence of sunburn on the dorsum of the fingers and hands. The toes are usually spared. Pain may be followed by subungual ecchymoses and then separation of the nail plate from the nail bed. The condition is transient and nails grow out normally once the offending agent is discontinued.

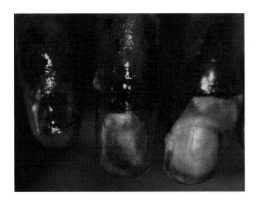

FIGURE 8.13 Anonychia during the acute phase of toxic epidermal necrolysis.

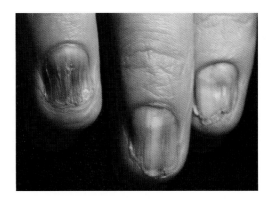

FIGURE 8.14 Pterygium and onychoatrophy secondary to toxic epidermal necrolysis.

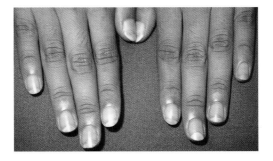

FIGURE 8.15 Photo-onycholysis in a teenager taking doxycycline.

Lichen Planus

Lichen planus (LP) is an inflammatory dermatosis that may involve the nails in combination with generalized skin disease, in association with mucosal disease, linear or Blaschkoid presentation or with only ungual involvement.[14] Most of the time, in children, the profusion of purple to violaceous, flat-topped, polygonal papules with occasional scale and the classic Wickham striae arise de novo, but viral triggers (hepatitis C) and immunizations with hepatitis B vaccine and medications have been reported. Some investigators consider LP to be an autoimmune disorder since it has been described to be associated with a number of other autoimmune diseases such as vitiligo, Hashimoto thyroiditis, and lichen sclerosis among others.

The appearance of ungual LP depends on the location of the band like lymphocytic infiltrate, lymphocytic exocytosis and saw-toothed acanthosis. It may involve all or a portion of the nail matrix, the nail bed, or the entire nail unit. When the proximal nail matrix is solely involved, the nails have the appearance of trachyonychia (Figure 8.16). This is more common in children than in adults. The plates have a dull, lusterless color from small confluent pits or longitudinal striations that result in a sandpaper-like texture. The distal-free edges are chipped and brittle which result in painful fissures. As more of the nail matrix is involved, the plates become thinner and more ridged. Pterygium of the proximal nail fold is a sign of atrophy and may progress to total anonychia. Longitudinal erythronychia can be observed with distal matrix and nail bed involvement. This can also result in onycholysis and nail shedding. Lontitudinal melanonychia in children with dark pigmentation can also result from LP.[15] Nails that appear as yellow nail syndrome can also result from LP.[16]

LP-like nail disease can be observed in the setting of graft vs. host disease, drug eruptions, and dyskeratosis congenita.

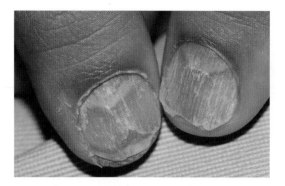

FIGURE 8.16   Trachyonychia, onychoschizia from thinning of the nail plate and erythronychia of the lunula are observed in this 12-year-old girl with lichen planus.

Treatment of LP of the nails in children depends on the extent and severity of the disease.[17] Trachyonychia need not be treated as most of the cases resolve within a decade. However, if distal chipping is a problem, several coats of clear nail hardener may be applied as needed. An attempt should be made to treat LP more aggressively with the slightest sign of atrophy. In young children, a 6- to 12-week trial of high potency topical steroid can be tried first. However, prednisone alone or prednisone followed by methotrexate, hydroxychloroquine, acetretin, and phototherapy with a narrowband UV-B laser may be needed.

Lichen Niditus

Lichen niditus is a widespread patchy dermatosis characterized by pinhead-sized uniform 1–2 mm^2 round, skin-colored papules that may be distributed on the torso, arms, legs, and genitals. It is quite pruritic and Koebner phenomenon is usually present. The "claw clutching the ball" mixed papillary dermal infiltrate of macrophages and helper T-lymphocytes distinguishes it from LP. Nail involvement may be an early sign of lichen niditus. Fortunately, it is non-scarring and gradually resolves along with the self-limited skin rash.[18] Topical antipruritic agents and narrowband UV-B may improve symptoms.

Darier–White Disease

Darier–White disease, also known as Darier disease or keratosis follicularis, is an autosomal-dominant genodermatosis first described almost simultaneously in 1889 by doctors Darier in France and White in Boston. Penetrance is complete, but expressivity is variable. There is also a high spontaneous mutation rate and mosaic or localized forms are reported. It is characterized by histologic acantholytic dyskeratosis and genetically by defective *ATP2A2*. Acral involvement including nail disease may be the first manifestation during childhood. The nails display longitudinal red and white bands that extend through the nail bed from the distal matrix. The plates are thin and will frequently be fissured with "v" shaped notches at the distal-free edge (Figure 8.17). Greasy flat-topped warty papules are seen on the dorsum of the hands, but they become much more confluent in the seborrhea areas of the chest and back in older teens and adults. One should be vigilant of complications of disseminated herpes simplex or *S. aureus* infections.

Differential diagnosis of Darier disease includes acrokeratosis verucifomis of Hopf, Hailey–Hailey disease, and an acatholytic dyskeratotic epidermal nevus all of which have similar histology, genetics and may have similar ungual characteristics as well.

Hailey–Hailey disease (chronic benign familial pemphigus) is due to mutations in *ATP2C1*, which is important in epidermal desmosomal assembly. Most desquamating vesicular lesions are in the flexures and can spread by a positive Nikolsky sign. Longitudinal white bands of the fingernails may occur initially before the disease is fully expressed. Unlike Darier disease, these changes in the nail are not usually symptomatic.[19]

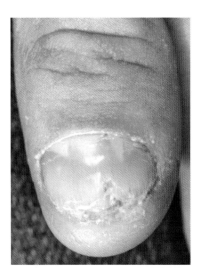

FIGURE 8.17 A "v" shaped notch at the distal-free edge of the nail plate is mirrored by a red, notched lunula in this teenaged patient with Darier disease.

Juvenile Xanthogranuloma

Juvenile xanthogranuloma is a benign proliferative (non-Langerhan cell) histiocytic disorder that may be present at birth or develops in the first 6 months of life. These lesions have a characteristic yellow color and may be single, giant, agminated, or widely disseminated. There are a few case reports of involvement of the nail unit.[20,21] When this occurs in or adjacent to the matrix, the nail plate may have longitudinal grooves or furrows and if the nail bed is involved, the plate may be uplifted and onychogryposis may result. If the diagnosis is doubtful, a small biopsy will demonstrate lipid-laden macrophages and Touton giant cells. There is a rare association with neurofibromatosis type I (NF-1), so the patient should be examined for café au lait macules. Fortunately, spontaneous regression of these lesions occurs in 5–8 years and surgical removal is rarely indicated.

Granuloma Annulare

Granuloma annulare is a common, self-limited asymptomatic skin disorder characterized by small dermal inflammatory papules that are usually arranged in "ring-like" configurations distributed over the hands, feet, digits, arms, and legs. The lesions may be skin-colored, violaceous, or hyperpigmented. There are subcutaneous, papular, and perforating variants. In addition, there are no systemic associations in children who are frequently affected with this presumed reactive, hypersensitivity disorder. The nail unit may be secondarily affected and is reported in one case of disseminated perforating disease.[22]

SAVI Syndrome

STING associated vasculopathy of infancy (SAVI) is a newly described autoinflammatory disease.[23] The functionally abnormal stimulator of interferon genes (STING) is critical for proper innate immune function. Clinically, the disorder is characterized by fevers and scaly violaceous cheeks, nose, ears, fingers, and toes that reflect a leukocytoclasitic vasculitis and a microthrombotic angiopathy. One of the earliest signs of this condition is nail fold capillary loop tortuosity and loss. Dystrophic nail changes precede gangrene and auto-amputation and are present in all children described till date. Pulmonary fibrosis is a major cause of morbidity for these patients. Treatment with JAK inhibitors to reduce interferon production is promising.

Self-Inflicted Bullous Lesions Occurring In Utero

Sucking blisters are lesions that may appear on the dorsum of the thumb or along the dorsal aspect of the index finger at birth or in the immediate postnatal period. They are commonly restricted to one extremity; however, bilateral involvement of fingers on both hands is possible. The bullae measures 0.5–1.5 cm in diameter and the fluid is of a serous, straw color. Bacterial and viral cultures show no growth.[24] There are a few other conditions that are ordinarily associated with bullae in the delivery room period. These may be generalized and single, or focal. They may involve the digits and nail unit and include herpes simplex, epidermolysis bullosa (EB) incontinentia pigmenti (IP), and congenital syphilis. Vesicles and bullae of IP and lues may involve the toes, but those of EB are more likely to be on multiple fingers.

Veillonella Infection of the Newborn

Forty-two epidemics of subungual infection were described by Sinniah et al.[25] among infants in postnatal wards and special care baby units. The number of fingers affected in per patient ranged from 1 to 10; the thumbs were less frequently involved than other digits, and the toenails were spared altogether. Three stages were identified: in the first stage, a small amount of clear fluid appears under the center of the nail along with mild inflammation at the distal end of the finger. This initial vesicle lasts approximately 24 h; it sometimes enlarges but never to the edge of the nail. Some small lesions bypass the second, pustular stage, going directly into the third stage. As a rule, the fluid becomes yellow after 24 h, the pus remaining for 24–48 h before gradually turning brown, and being absorbed. This color fades progressively over a period of 2–6 weeks, leaving the nail and nail bed apparently completely normal. Subungual pus obtained by aseptic puncture of the nails showed tiny, gram-negative cocci about 0.4 μm in diameter. These organisms resembled *Veillonella*, bacteria of dubious pathogenicity and the most common anaerobes to be found in saliva of adults. In neonates, *Veillonella* is more common in the bowel of bottle-fed than breast-fed children, and this is compatible with those in intensive care units. It is also found in the vagina and respiratory tract.

Impetigo

The dorsal aspect of the distal phalanx may be involved by impetigo. It comes in two forms:

1. Vesiculopustular with its familiar honey-crusted lesions, usually due to β-hemolytic streptococci.
2. Bullous, usually due to phage type 71 staphylococci (develops on intact skin).

The latter is characterized by the appearance of large, localized, intraepidermal bullae that persist for longer periods than the transient vesicles of streptococcal impetigo, which subsequently rupture spontaneously to form very thin crusts. The lesions of bullous impetigo may mimic the noninfectious bullous diseases such as drug-induced bullae or bullous pemphigoid.

Oral therapy of bullous impetigo with cloxacillin should be instituted and continued until the lesions resolve. Cefprozil and clarithromycin are acceptable substitutes. The lesions should be cleansed several times daily and topical mupirocin ointment applied to all the affected areas.

Blistering Distal Dactylitis

Blistering distal dactylitis (BDD) is a distinct clinical entity manifested by a superficial blistering lesion over the anterior fat pad of the distal portion of a finger or thumb (Figure 8.18).[26] BDD presents itself as tense, non-tender bullae due to β-hemolytic streptococcal skin infection. This disease appears almost exclusively in 2- to 16-year-olds, but cases in adults have been reported as well. The increasing incidence in isolation of *Staphylococcus* from cases of BDD suggests a change in pathogenic patterns. These

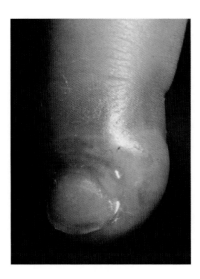

FIGURE 8.18   Blistering distal dactylitis.

bacterial pathogens can be distinguished only by Gram stain and culture. Patients with staphylococcal infections have responded well to a 10-day course of dicloxacillin, a penicillinase-resistant antibiotic that is well absorbed orally and well tolerated.[27]

Differential diagnosis includes traumatic, thermal, or chemical burns; herpes simplex virus (HSV) infections; and staphylococcal bullous impetigo. Except for bullous impetigo, all these conditions can usually be distinguished by history alone. The blisters of impetigo, however, are extremely superficial compared with those of BDD. Differentiation of BDD and herpetic whitlow involves using a Tzanck test, a Gram stain, and bacterial and viral cultures to evaluate the lesions. If lesions of both infections show up clinically, confirmation of which infection is present is needed to select appropriate treatment, but coexistent infections on a child's distal phalanx has been reported.[28]

For local care, incision of the bullae, drainage, and soaking are indicated and facilitate a more rapid response to systemic antibiotic therapy. The latter seems to be justified since prompt treatments of streptococcal skin infections decreases the reservoir of streptococci by preventing spread to family and community contact.

Recurrent blistering distal dactylitis of the great toe has been reported in a 10-year-old boy with a 3-month history of a painful ingrowing toenail and a 6-day history of blistering of the periungual skin of the same digit.[29]

Herpetic Paronychia (Synonym: Herpetic Whitlow)

This uncommon condition is due to primary inoculation of the HSV and presents itself as single or grouped blisters close to the nail; it may give a honeycomb appearance (Figure 8.19). Clear at first, the blisters, soon become turbid, may break, and be replaced by crusts. It is usually very painful and takes about 3 weeks to resolve, with pain setting in half that time. Lymphangitis sometimes occurs and may precede vesiculation. The diagnosis is established by recovering the virus from a recent blister, by cytological examination of the blister floor (Tzanck smear), or by polymerase chain reaction (PCR) of blister fluid. Transmission to contacts may occur, which explains the appearance of herpetic whitlow associated with herpes labialis. Herpetic paronychia may cause complete destruction of the nail, bacterial superinfection, and systemic spread that may cause meningitis. Kaposi varicelliform eruption or HSV superinfection of preexisting skin lesions may complicate atopic dermatitis and Darier disease. Longstanding cases, particularly in patients with HIV infection, may have an atypical, often verrucous appearance.

Fatal infection of the newborn with HSV may be acquired from the mother by transplacental infection, or from the birth canal of a mother with primary herpetic vulvovaginitis.[30,31]

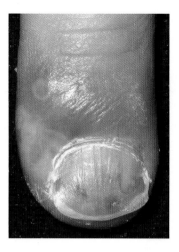

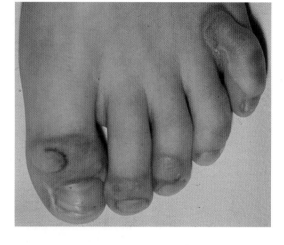

FIGURE 8.19 Herpes.   **FIGURE 8.20** Periungual bullous lesions due to zinc deficiency.

Treatment early in the course of the illness with oral or systemic acyclovir (20 mg/kg/dose Q6h) may shorten the course of the disorder, and gentle cleansing with chlorhexidine followed by application of a bland cream is recommended. Relapse may occur as with other primary herpetic infections. The value of long-term treatment with thymidine analogues, such as oral acyclovir, famciclovir, and valacyclovir, when recurrences are frequent, might be useful.

Early Congenital Syphilis

Vesiculobullous lesions and eroded lesions which are sometimes hemorrhagic can be seen especially on the distal parts of arms and legs. In other cases, a dry desquamation can be seen either as a generalized phenomenon, or as a localized change in the acral periungual areas. This dry, desquamating eruption may occur as a major feature or as sequela of the vesiculobullous phase.[32]

Zinc Deficiency

Periungual bullous lesions may be isolated or associated with the other signs of this condition (Figure 8.20).

Neonatal Frostbite

It is unusual to encounter severe neonatal cold injury. An abandoned neonate with marked hypothermia presented with purplish to blackish discoloration with edema and blister formation of the toes. Despite the treatment, the toes develop gangrene and are autoamputated after 2 weeks of discoloration.[10]

Juvenile Pemphigus Vulgaris

This condition is very rare. Its clinical atypical presentation can result in delayed diagnosis and management occasionally. Besides multiple buccal erosions, intradermal bullae of the skin cheilitis, and bilateral conjunctivitis, the nail unit may be involved as paronychial inflammation and subungual hemorrhages or subungual pus and Beau's lines.[33] Immunofluorescence rules out bullous pemphigoid. Systemic corticosteroids are the first-line treatment. In nonresponder, intravenous immunoglobulin (IVIG), or rituximab should be used.

Onychotillomania

The term *onychotillomania* implies a destructive irrational preoccupation with one's nails. However, in a broad sense, it is used to describe a number of behaviors that are self-inflicted and are associated with a wide range of mental stability issues. Nail-biting (onychophagia), nail picking, cuticle picking, and habit-tics are all included under this heading.

Nail-Biting

It is interesting to note that in some cultures, nail-biting is not only an accepted way of self-grooming, but the first way a neonate's nails are trimmed. In these cultures, nail-biting is a learned behavior and proper technique can actually prevent damage. In western cultures, the practice of mother's biting their newborn's nails is controversial and generally frowned upon because of fears of secondary infection.

The frequency of onychophagia increases from preschool ages through adolescence. It has been estimated that nearly 25% of normal young children and 50% of teens will episodically bite their nails in response to some anxiety-provoking situation.[34] These include parental disharmony, sibling rivalry, problems in school, peer rejection, loneliness or boredom, and overcrowded living conditions. Sometimes onychophagia is accompanied by some other body focused repetitive behavior such as hair-twisting or skin picking. These children may also have obsessive–compulsive disorder, depression, or attention-deficit hyperactivity disorder (ADHD).[35] Many ADHD medications (e.g., methylphenidate) actually accentuate this problem. Some nail biters will choose one nail while others may chew all but one nail. Onychophagia may be familial and is more common in identical twins. In toddlers, nail-biting may be an extension of the oral stage of development. However, it may also be one of the earlier signs of psychopathology or developmental delay if it is chronic, unremitting and is not extinguished by pain and other complications. Children with Lesch–Nyhan syndrome, familial dysautonomia and congenital insensitivity to pain, or hereditary sensory neuropathies may go as far as to produce anonychia and total destruction of the distal phalanges.

Complications of onychophagia include pain, onychocryptosis (ingrown nails), paronychia, pyogenic granulomas, dactylitis, osteomyelitis,[36] the spread of verrucae (Figure 8.21), and herpetic whitlow.

Treatment of onychophagia in children can be frustrating. An individual approach is necessary. For young children, sometimes all that is necessary is to point out the triggering situation and give the child a substitute means of expression or activity such as drawing or a squeeze ball. Positive reinforcement for a reminder of not biting at the time of the behavior with help of stickers or a visual calendar or record may be beneficial too. Painting on a bitter-tasting substance (e.g., clindamycin 1% solution, Control-IT™) has been recommended by some practitioners, but success depends on additional positive reinforcement techniques. In practice, continued exposure to a bitter substance produces tolerance and may actually reinforce the behavior. Snapping a rubber band in the palm of the hand is perhaps the only negative noxious stimulus that may replace biting. In girls, application of colored nail polish highlights the damage caused by biting and may serve to heighten awareness of the activity, thus, making it consciously unpleasant for the patient to perform the behavior.

Nail picking is always pathologic. Usually some sharp instrument is used to damage the plate and results in pits, gouges, onychoschizia or total anonychia, and pterygium formation (Figure 8.22).

Cuticle picking is not uncommon in children with dry cuticles. Low environmental humidity, chronic exposure to surfactants or solvents, and preexisting conditions with poor barrier function (e.g., atopic dermatitis) can predispose this habit. Cuticle picking may be reduced by careful trimming and frequent application of humectants such as urea-containing moisturizers and products that restore barrier function (e.g., ceramides).

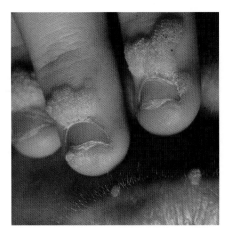

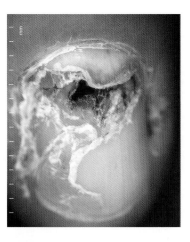

FIGURE 8.21   Onychophagia has resulted in the spread of verrucae from the nail folds to the lips.

FIGURE 8.22   Obsessive picking of the nail plate with a pointed nail file has resulted in destruction of the nail unit.

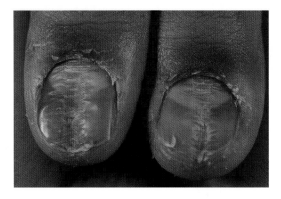

FIGURE 8.23   Habit-tic of pushing back the cuticle.

Habit-tic deformities result from repeatedly pushing back or down on the cuticle of the proximal nail fold (Figure 8.23). It produces closely spaced depressions of varying width in the median portion of the nail plate that are reminiscent of a longitudinal groove. The lunula may be elongated as well. If the matrix is scarred, then this may produce a longitudinal fissure similar to Heller's median nail dystrophy.

Although thumb sucking and mouthing of digits in toddlers are a persistent form of oral gratification or pacification that may result in damage to the nails,[37] they are not primarily behaviors that are directed at the nails themselves, and resulting dystrophy is a secondary phenomenon. An undulating nail dystrophy and severe dactylitis and dental malocclusion can result if the primary dentition has erupted. Sequelae are more common in children with atopic dermatitis. Approaches to extinguishing this behavior in older children are not unlike those used for onychophagia.

REFERENCES

1. Boiko S, Kaufman RA, Lucky AW. Osteomyelitis of the distal phalanges in three children with severe atopic dermatitis. *Arch Dermatol.* 1988; 124(3): 418–423.
2. Gudjonsson JE, Karason A, Antonsdottir A et al. Psoriasis patients who are homozygous for the HLA-Cw*0602 allele have a 2.5-fold increased risk of developing psoriasis compared with Cw6 heterozygotes. *Br J Dermatol.* 2003; 148(2): 233–235.
3. Mercy K, Kwasny M, Cordoro KM et al. Clinical manifestations of pediatric psoriasis: Results of a multicenter study in the United States. *Pediatr Dermatol.* 2013; 30(4): 424–428.
4. Hjorth N, Thomsen K. Parakeratosis pustulosa. *Br J Dermatol.* 1967; 79(10): 527–532.

5. Tosti A, Peluso AM, Zucchelli V. Clinical features and long-term follow-up of 20 cases of parakeratosis pustulosa. *Pediatr Dermatol.* 1998; 15(4): 259–263.
6. Allison DS, El-Azhary RA, Calobrisi SD, Dicken CH. Pityriasis rubra pilaris in children. *J Am Acad of Dermatol.* 2002; 47: 386–389.
7. Gelmetti C, Schiuma AA, Cerri D, Gianoti, F. Rityriasis rubra pilaris in childhood: A long-term study of 29 cases. *Pediatr Dermatol.* 1986; 3: 446–451.
8. Tosti A, Peluso AM, Misciali C, Cameli N. Nail lichen striatus: Clinical features and long-term follow-up of five patients. *J Am Acad Dermatol.* 1997; 36(6 Pt 1): 908–913.
9. James R, Burgner D. Orange-brown chromonychia in Kawasaki disease. *Arch Dis Child.* 2015; 100: 872.
10. Sheridan RL, Schulz JT, Ryan CM et al. Long-term consequences of toxic epidermal necrolysis in children. *Pediatrics.* 2002; 109(1): 74–78.
11. Hansen RC. Blindness, anonychia, and oral mucosal scarring as sequelae of the Stevens-Johnson syndrome. *Pediatr Dermatol.* 1984; 1(4): 298–300.
12. Willis ZI, Boyd AS, Di Pentima MCJ. Phototoxicity, pseudoporphyria, and photo-onycholysis due to voriconazole in a pediatric patient with leukemia and invasive aspergillosis. *Pediatric Infect Dis Soc.* 2015; 4(2): e22–e24.
13. Bentabet Dorbani I, Badri T, Benmously R et al. Griseofulvin-induced photo-onycholysis. *Presse Med.* 2012; 41(9 Pt 1): 879–881.
14. Price HN, Zaenglein AL. Lichen planus and lichen niditus. In Irvine AD, Hoeger PH, Yan AC (eds.), *Harper's Textbook of Pediatric Dermatology*, Third Edition. Oxford, United Kingdom: Wiley-Blackwell; 2011. pp. 1–85.
15. Juhlin L, Baran R. Longitudinal melanonychia after healing of lichen planus. *Acta Derm Venereol.* 1989; 69(4): 338–339.
16. Baran R. Lichen planus of the nails mimicking the yellow nail syndrome. *Br J Dermatol.* 2000; 143(5): 1117–1118.
17. Piraccini BM, Saccani E, Starace M et al. Nail lichen planus: Response to treatment and long term follow-up. *Eur J Dermatol.* 2010; 20(4): 489–496.
18. Tay EY, Ho MS, Chandran NS et al. Lichen nitidus presenting with nail changes—Case report and review of the literature. *Pediatr Dermatol.* 2015; 32(3): 386–388.
19. Kirtschig G, Effendy I, Happle R. Leukonychia longitudinalis als ein leitsymptom des morbus Hailey-Hailey. *Hautarzt.* 1992; 43: 451–452.
20. Piraccini BM, Fanti PA, Iorizzo M, Tosti A. Juvenile xanthogranuloma of the proximal nail fold. *Pediatr Dermatol.* 2003; 20(4): 307–308.
21. Chang P, Baran R, Villanueva C et al. Juvenile xanthogranuloma beneath a fingernail. *Cutis.* 1996; 58(2): 173–174.
22. Samlaska CP, Sandberg GD, Maggio KL, Sakas EL. Generalized perforating granuloma annulare. *J Am Acad Dermatol.* 1992; 27(2 Pt 2): 319–322.
23. Liu Y, Kastner DL, Paller AS et al. Activated STING in a vascular and pulmonary syndrome. *New Eng J Med.* 2014; 371: 507–518.
24. Murphy WF, Langley AL. Common bullous lesions—presumably self-inflicted—occurring in utero in the newborn infant. *Pediatrics.* 1963; 32: 1099–1101.
25. Sinniah D, Sandiford BR, Dudgate AE. Subungual infection in the newborn. An institutional outbreak of unknown etiology, possibly due to Veillonella. *Clin Pediatr.* 1972; 11: 690.
26. Hays GC, Mullard JE. Blistering distal dactylitis: Clinically recognizable streptococcal infection. *Pediatrics.* 1975; 56: 129.
27. McCray MK, Esterly NB. Blistering distal dactylitis. *J Am Acad Dermatol.* 1981; 5: 592–594.
28. Ney AC, English III JC, Greer KE. Coexistent infections on a child's distal phalanx: Blistering dactylitis and herpetic whitlow. *Cutis.* 2002; 69: 46–48.
29. Telfer NR, Barth JH, Dawber RPR. Recurrent blistering distal dactylitis of the great toe associated with an ingrowing toenail. *Clin Exp Dermatol.* 1989; 14: 380–381.
30. Mitchell JE, Mc Call FC. Transplacental infection by herpes simplex. *Amer J Dis Child.* 1963; 106: 207–209.
31. Wheeler CE, Huffiness WD. Primary disseminated herpes simplex of the newborn. *J Amer Med Assoc.* 1965; 191: 55–60.
32. Cohen B, Todd G, Fischer G. Sexually transmitted diseases. In Schachner LA, Hansen RC (eds.), *Pediatric Dermatology*, Fourth Edition. The Netherlands: Mosby Elsevier; 2011. p. 1592.

33. Abil S, Benzekri L, Bourra H et al. Pemphigus vulgaire juvénile. Trois observations marocaines. *Nouv Dermatol.* 2013; 32: 522–524.

34. Pacan P, Grzesiak M, Reich A et al. Onychophagia and onychotillomania: Prevalence, clinical picture and comorbidities. *Acta Derm Venereol.* 2014; 94(1): 67–71.

35. Ghanizadeh A. Association of nail biting and psychiatric disorders in children and their parents in a psychiatrically referred sample of children. *Child Adolesc Psychiatry Ment Health.* 2008; 2(1): 13.

36. Waldman BA, Frieden IJ. Osteomyelitis caused by nail biting. *Pediatr Dermatol.* 1990; 7(3): 189–190.

37. Lubitz L. Nail biting, thumb sucking and other irritating behaviors in childhood. *Australian Fam Physician.* 1992; 21: 1090–1094.

9

Nail Hamartomas

Gerard Lorette and Annabel Maruani

Hamartomas result from an abnormal formation of tissue, sometimes with a tumor-like appearance. They are composed of an excess of tissue normally present in the affected site of origin with an overgrowth of mature cells. The proliferation may result from epidermis, soft tissue, bone (exostosis), and nail tissue. Hamartomas differ from choristomas, which are an excess of tissue in an abnormal situation.

Many early changes of the nail plate may be considered hamartomas, whereby the naturally occurring stratum corneum is changed without being linked to a tumor or infection.

Nail Plate Changes

Pigmentation (or Melanonychia)

One or more hyperpigmented bands are longitudinally arranged in the nail plate. The area up to the nail can be fully hyperpigmented. These bands are due to melanin deposits; they can be early and benign and more frequent in subjects with hyperpigmented skin naturally or related to melanocyte activation. Differential diagnoses include a lentigo; nevus (Figure 9.1), which can be congenital[1] or very early onset[2]; melanoma; and drug pigmentation.

Leukonychia

A family-pachyleukonychia form of longitudinal strips has been described[3] (Figure 9.2a and b). The strips measure 1.25-mm wide. The number of ribs (one to four per nail) and intensity vary among patients. The white appearance is due to a thickening of the ventral part of the nail plate; a few outbreaks of sebaceous glands have been observed. The lesions are acquired, and the transmission is autosomal dominant.

An inherited subtotal leukonychia of 20 nails was observed in one family. These nails were soft with slow growth. Histology revealed a thickened granular layer. A lamellar appearance and dissociated keratinocytes were seen through electron microscopy. The white, milky color was attributed to disruption of intracytoplasmic vacuoles and tonofilaments.[4]

Yellow Nails (Xanthonychia)

Yellow nails and lymphedema syndrome were described in 1964 by Samman and White. Nails may be yellow from childhood[5] or exceptionally congenital but are most often seen in adults. The nails are hard, with accentuated curvature and slow growth. The yellow color can be intense or pale or greenish yellow. Nails can be pigmented in full or only distally. The nails are opaque. There may be an inflammatory aspect of the proximal nail fold and side folds. The nails of the feet and hands are affected, sometimes only some nails. The condition is associated with a moderate lymphedema of the lower limbs and pulmonary manifestations, particularly pleural effusions. Several nails are thickened, curved, yellow or greenish in color. The clinical picture is more or less complete. The exact cause of these nail changes remains unknown. Pathological associations have been described, in particular arthritis and neoplasia.[6] The condition is autosomal-dominant inherited.

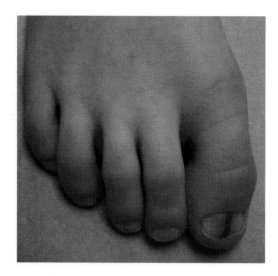

FIGURE 9.1 Longitudinal melanonychia: nevus.

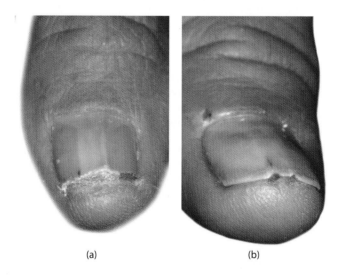

(a)   (b)

FIGURE 9.2 (a) Double longitudinal pachyleukonychia congenita. (b) Same patient showing the thickening of the affected ventral keratin, distally (Copyright R Baran).

Pachyonychia

Congenital pachyonychia (Figure 9.3a through c) is an inherited autosomal-dominant disease. In the early stages, patients show a thickening of the nail tablets, which have a rough surface. The crescents are absent. Subungual hyperkeratosis is evident. The nails have a brown color. Other events are related: palmoplantar keratoderma, neonatal teeth, etc.

Congenital malalignment of the big toenail is a lateral deviation of the nail plate of both big toenails (Figure 9.4). The nails are thickened, with oyster-shell-like transverse grooves. The nails have a gray-brown discoloration. The disease is sporadic or familial, autosomal dominant. If spontaneous recovery does not occur, surgical intervention may be proposed to realign the nails.

A pachyonychia, especially of the big toenails, is characteristic of several congenital forms of epidermolysis bullosa (Figure 9.5).

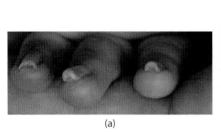
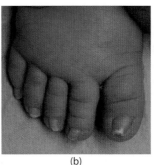
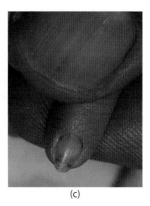

(a) (b) (c)

FIGURE 9.3 (a) Early pachyonychia congenita. (b) Pachyonychia congenita in infancy. **(c)** Neonatal pachyonychia.

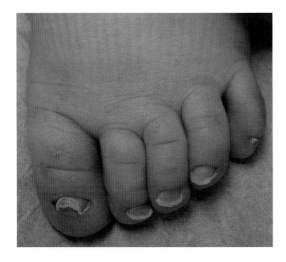
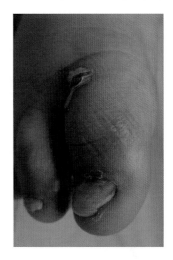

FIGURE 9.4 Congenital malalignment of the big toenail.   **FIGURE 9.5** Pachyonychia in epidermolysis bullosa.

Anonychia

Several genetic diseases feature anonychia.

Nail–patella syndrome combines anonychia or congenital hyponychium, median fissure, thin nail plate, and triangular, or absent lunula. Aplasia or absence of patellae suggests renal disease.

Hyponychia, Macronychia, and Racket Thumb

Onset of these symptoms occurs before puberty by welding premature epiphyseal growth plates of the distal phalanx, which causes a shortening of the phalanx. A plurality of fingers can be seen. Transmission is usually inherited, autosomal dominant.

Supernumerary or Ectopic Nails (Onychoheterotopia)

A nail is not in its usual location. The palmar nail syndrome was described by Ridder in 1992 and features a palmar nail, lack of finger flexion, and brevity of the third phalanx. These are sporadic cases, but two familial cases have been reported; some are associated with chromosomal abnormalities. The malformation can be bilateral.[7] Two nails can be located on the same finger: one on the ventral side, the other on the dorsal side of both small fingers.[8] Ectopic nail may also be not always associated with a finger or toe; for example, it was reported on the heel.[9]

Tumour Appearance

Multiple Ungual Fibromas (Koenen's Tumors)

Tuberous sclerosis is an autosomal-dominant disorder characterized by multiple hamartomas. It is evident in the first few years of life as white spots, achromia, and oval and elongated nails (leaf rowan). The diagnosis can be made clinically, or by genetic analysis: mutation of tumor suppressor tuberous sclerosis 1 (*TSC1*), or tuberous sclerosis 2 (*TSC2*) genes. The condition may be associated with spasms during the first month for a newborn. Then, from approximately two years of age, angiofibroma papules appear on the face, with hypomelanotic macules or shagreen patches. Cardiac problems and renal tumors can be associated with this condition as well as mental retardation. Firm masses, ovoid, white or pinkish, that may appear from the nail folds are Koenen tumors. They can appear after puberty, never before the age of 5 years. They appear under the proximal nail fold or under a side fold on the fingers or toes. Particularly, globoid or fusiform aspects may be associated. Distal hyperkeratosis is common. Koenen tumors may be alone or multiple. Over the years, they can become large if not treated. They usually result in a longitudinal leuconychia, splinter hemorrhage, canaliform depression, or groove of the nail plate (Figure 9.6a and b), sometimes without visible periungual fibroma, or large nail dystrophies or complete destruction of the nail. The tuberous sclerosis may be responsible for longitudinal leukonychias, splinter hemorrhages, sometimes "red comets."[10] Koenen tumors may not produce nail color abnormalities or subungual hyperkeratosis. A macrodactyly is possible.[11] Koenen tumors may be the only cutaneous manifestation of tuberous sclerosis.[12] Histologically, they are seen composed of fibroblast cells, collagen fibers, and blood vessels.

Glomangioma (or Glomus Tumor)

Glomus tumours are uncommon benign hamartomas. Most are developed from myo-arterial glomus of the distal phalanges of the fingers or toes. Adults are most commonly affected,[13] but there are cases found in children[14] predominantly among the female population. Lesions are a few millimeters in diameter. They are painful spontaneously when pressure is applied (sign of love) or when they come in contact with cold. Sometimes, there is a deformation of the nail, a ridge, fissure, distal nail plate splitting, longitudinal erythronychia, or subungual keratosis. In most cases, there is only a bluish or a red discoloration, which is limited and visible through the nail plate. The diagnosis is often made late, sometimes after years. Diagnostic confirmation is by X-ray or magnetic resonance imaging (MRI), which can show a notch of the phalanx, ultrasound showing a round or oval mass. Treatment consists of surgical removal of the lesion. No nail deformity occurs after excising the tumor after total removal of the nail temporarily.[14] Glomus tumors are more common than previously recognized and associated with neurofibromatosis type I.[15] Diagnostic problems concern the origin of pain.

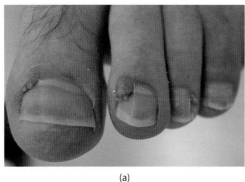
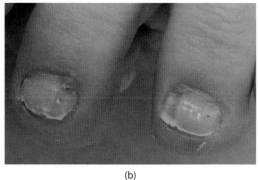

(a)   (b)

FIGURE 9.6   (a) Koenen's tumor in adolescent. (b) Koenen's tumor in early infancy.

Subungual Exostosis

A bone exostosis is a benign solitary lesion. It is characterized by a growing mass of hyaline cartilage, then lamellate trabecular bone (Figure 9.7a) occurring from the distal phalanx, most often of the great toe. On a long bone, it may particularly appear as a hand fingernail. There is often painful onycholysis (Figure 9.7b). The diagnosis is confirmed radiologically (Figure 9.7c). The treatment is complete surgical resection of the bone protrusion. Multiple exostosis syndrome[16] is rare, familial, with autosomal-dominant inheritance. The condition often occurs early, in the first few years of life. Other bones may be also concerned by exostosis.

Painful Subungual Tumor in Incontinentia Pigmenti

The condition is very rare and found late in life. Tumors can appear after the age of 15. They are more frequent on the fingers than toes.[17] The lesions are hyperkeratotic under the nails. They can cause onychodystrophy or onycholysis. Histologically, the epidermis is hyperplastic, made of glassy keratinized keratinocytes.[17] The best treatment is surgical excision.

Peripheral Nerve Hamartoma with Macrodactyly of the Hand (Peripheral Lipofibromatous Hamartoma of the Median Nerve)

Hamartomas of the median nerve or its branches cause congenital macrodactyly, called nerve territory-oriented macrodactyly, also called lipofibromatous hamartoma.[18,19] There is an enlargement of the nerve with large quantities of fat in the lesions of one or two fingers. The nails of the affected fingers can be enlarged.[20]

Angiomatous Hamartoma

Vascular malformations, described in another chapter, are defined as hamartomas. We describe only some specific aspects. Eccrine angiomatous hamartoma of the fingers is very rare. It is congenital or occurs in infancy. The lesions are nodules or plaques, located on the limbs. A woman presented asymptomatic nodules on the hand and foot, first developed around the age of 12 years. It presented itself with almost total destruction of several nails.[21] Clinically, there were firm nodules, elastic, of about 1 cm in diameter. Osteolytic lesions were seen through radiographs. Histologically, proliferation of eccrine sweat glands and capillaries in close association was observed.

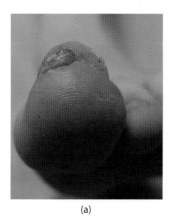 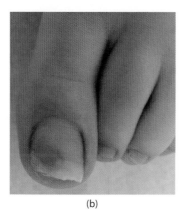 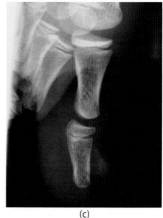

(a) (b) (c)

FIGURE 9.7 (a) Subungueal exostosis. (b) Exostosis presenting with onycholysis. (c) X-ray in subungual exostosis.

Epidermal Nevus

Epidermal nevi are hamartomas with generally a configuration along the lines of Blaschko that reflect a cutaneous mosaicism. The epidermal nevus is named verrucous if it is formed only of keratinocytes, epidermolytic or not, and organoid if associated with sebaceous or follicular cells. Epidermal nevus syndrome is considered when extracutaneous lesions are associated with an epidermal nevus. Some of the lesions are congenital, but a number on the lines of Blaschko occur secondarily. If the fingernail is reached, onychodystrophy is recognized. It features a thinned nail, breaking on a ridge, split longitudinally, transverse, or leukonychia punctuated with onycholysis, and a longitudinal red band. Nail involvement may be isolated.[22] The term may be used for destruction of the nail. It may precede rash. The tissue changes may be visible only after the action of cofactors.

Such nevi can be considered as a variant of potential hamartomas. In children or infants, the terms lichen striatus (Figure 9.8) and inflammatory linear verrucous epidermal nevus (ILVEN) are frequently used for lesions along the lines of Blaschko. Healing usually occurs within a few months to 2 years of duration with lichen striatus. Nail involvement is rare; lateral longitudinal ridges and splitting have been described though.[23] In adults, we use the term *blaschkite* to describe this situation. Many dermatoses may appear in genetically modified tissues—lichen planus, Darier disease, Mibelli syndrome—with the nail modifications of those dermatoses.

Epidermal nevi may be isolated or be part of many complex syndromes: segmental overgrowth, lipomatosis, arteriovenous malformation, epidermal nevus (SOLAMEN), congenital lipomatous overgrowth, vascular malformations, epidermal nevus (CLOVES), and Proteus syndrome.

Complex Hamartomas

Proteus Syndrome

This syndrome overlaps with Klippel–Trenaunay, CLOVES syndrome, etc. It is caused by a somatic mutation of PTEN. Manifestations include cerebriform connective tissue nevus, epidermal nevus, vascular malformations, lipomas, disproportionate asymmetric overgrowth with skeletal abnormalities. The nails may be incorrectly positioned; peri-nail infections are related to friction on the shoe.

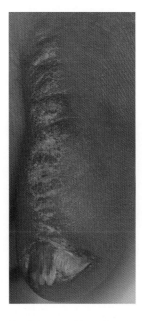

FIGURE 9.8   Lichen striatus involving the fifth left toe and its nail plate. Spontaneous cure has been obtained 2 years later (Copyright R Baran).

Neurofibromatosis

Subungual neurofibromas can occur as isolated elements or associated with a known neurofibromatosis. The condition represents painless swelling, which can cause subungual hyperkeratosis, an accentuation of the curvature of the tablet, a bluish coloration of the proximal part of the nail.[17] The treatment is surgical.

Congenital Hemidysplasia with Ichtyosiform Nevus and Limb Defects (CHILD) Syndrome

CHILD is a hereditary syndrome, usually dominant X-linked (Figure 9.9). The mutation concerns NS DHL. Ipsilateral skin lesions involve the bones, lungs, kidney, heart, and brain. There may be an onychodystrophy paronychia with one or more nails. A characteristic feature is a papillomatous lesion partially covering one to several toes and nails.[24]

Darier–White Disease

This is a rare genodermatosis characterized by keratotic papules of skin. The onset occurs generally after 6 years of age or later. Many ungual lesions are described.

Goltz Syndrome (or Focal Dermal Hypoplasia)

This is a hereditary X-linked dominant genodermatosis. However, most cases are of sporadic occurrence, corresponding to a new mutation. Patients have cutaneous, bone, dental, ocular, and nail disorders. Some nails are dystrophic, striated, or absent (Figure 9.10). Two unilateral cases have been reported.[25]

Ectodermal Dysplasia

This term is used for a large and heterogeneous group of genetic disorders affecting the structures of ectodermal origin: skin, teeth, nails, and glands. Currently, there are about 200 types of ectodermal dysplasias and the causative genes were identified in about 30 types of ectodermal dysplasias. The group of condition combines thick and thin hair; dental anomalies, especially hypodontia; the possibility of anhidrosis. A cleft lip is a particular aspect. The most common diseases are X-linked hypohidrotic ectodermal dysplasia (Christ–Siemens–Touraine syndrome), hidrotic ectodermal dysplasia (Clouston

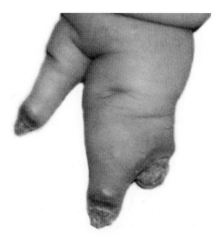

FIGURE 9.9 CHILD syndrome (Copyright Happle R) dysplastic right hand with only three fingers and dystrophic nails.

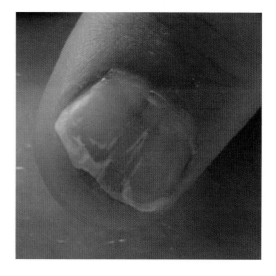

FIGURE 9.10 Goltz syndrome with a dystrophic nail.

syndrome), ectrodactyly–ectodermal dysplasia–cleft lip/palate syndrome (EEC syndrome). Some have a recognizable facial appearance as in Rapp–Hodgkin syndrome.[26]

Many nail dystrophies are described in these syndromes: micronychia, thick nails, pitted nails, scaling of the nail plate, irregular distal edge, anonychia, subungual hyperkeratosis, color changes, and onycholysis.

Oro-Facio Digital Syndromes

This group of congenital disorders involves the mouth, face, and fingers. Type II features a frontal bossing, cleft lip, polydactyly, and a duplication of the first toe; the nail itself is duplicated.[27] There may also be some nail hypoplasia.

Tricho-Rhino-Phalangeal Syndrome

The main features are bright and sparse hair, a bulbous nose, an elongated philtrum, and abnormalities of the fingers. Nails are short and thick, with spatula depression.[28]

Dyskeratosis Congenita (or Zinsser–Cole–Engman Disease)

This is an inherited disorder. The characteristic signs are oral leukoplakia, poikiloderma of the sides of the neck, dystrophic nails with cracked to irregular surface, resulting in an almost complete atrophy of the nails. Systemic manifestations are possible, especially anemia with bone marrow aplasia.

Lethal Hamartoma Syndromes

Aplasia or hypoplasia of the nails is part of the array of several genetic diseases exceptionally observed, which generally include abnormalities of the fingers. An example is Pallister–Hall syndrome.[29] The delineation of these syndromes can be difficult clinically. These cases may be grouped by the acronym for cerebro-acro-visceral-early lethality: CAVE.[29]

REFERENCES

1. Agusti-Mejias A, Messeguer F, Febrer I et al. Congenital subungual and peri ungual melanocytic nevus. *Actas Dermosifiliogr.* 2013; 104: 446–448.
2. Tosti A, Baran R, Piraccini BM et al. Nail matrix nevi: A clinical and histopathologic study of twenty two patients. *J Am Acad Dermatol.* 1996; 34: 765–771.
3. Moulin G, Baran R, Perrin C et al. Epidermal hamartoma presenting as longitudinal pachyleukonychia: A new nail genodermatosis. *J Am Acad Dermatol.* 1996; 35: 675–677.
4. Marcilly MC, Balme B, Haftek M et al. Leuconychie héréditaire subtotale. Etude histopathologique et ultrastructurale des ongles (laiteux). *Ann Dermatol Venereol.* 2003; 130: 50–54.
5. Dessart P, Deries X, Guerin-Moreau M et al. Syndrome des ongles jaunes: Deux cas pédiatriques. *Ann Dermatol Venereol.* 2014; 141: 611–619.
6. Fayol J. Le syndrome des ongles jaunes. *Ann Dermatol Venereol.* 2000; 127: 93–96.
7. Schoofs M, Robert G. Le syndrome de l'ongle palmaire congénital. A propos d'un cas. *Ann Chir Plast Esth.* 2005; 50: 320–322.
8. Keret D, Ger E. Double fingernails on the small fingers. *J Hand Surg.* 1987; 12A: 608–610.
9. Kopera D, Soyer HP, Kerl H. Ectopic calcaneal nail. *J Am Acad Dermatol.* 1996; 35: 484–485.
10. Aldrich S, Hong C-H, Groves L et al. Acral lesions in tuberous sclerosis complex: Insights into pathogenesis. *J Am Acad Dermatol.* 2010; 63: 244–251.
11. Norman-Taylor F, Mayou BJ. Macrodactyly in tuberous sclerosis. *J R Soc Med.* 1994; 87: 419–450.
12. Unlu E, Balta I, Unlu S. Multiple ungueal fibromas as an only cutaneous manifestation of tuberous sclerosis complex. *Ind J Dermatol Venereol Leprol.* 2014; 80: 464–465.
13. Marchadier A, Cohen M, Legre R. Tumeurs glomiques sous-unguéales des doigts: Diagnostic échographique. *Chir Main.* 2006; 25: 16–21.

14. Bayram H, Herdem M, Bicer S et al. Evaluation of the nail changes after surgical excision through the nail bed for subungual glomus tumor. *Journal of Hand Surgery* (European volume). 2007; 32: 87.

15. Stewart DR, Sloan JL. Diagnosis, management, and complications of glomus tumors of the digits in neurofibromatosis type 1. *J Med Genet.* 2010; 47: 525–532.

16. Schmitt AM, Bories A, Baran R. Exostoses sous-unguéales des doigts au cours de la maladie exostosante héréditaire. *Ann Dermatol Venereol.* 1997; 124: 233–236.

17. Willard KJ, Cappel MA, Hozin SH et al. Benign subungual tumors. *J Hand Surg.* 2012; 37A: 1276–1286.

18. Tahiri Y, Xu L, Kanevsky J et al. Lipofibromatous hamartoma of the median nerve: A comprehensive review and systematic approach to evaluation, diagnosis, and treatment. *J Hand Surg.* 2013; 38A: 2055–2067.

19. Agarwal S, Haase SC. Lipofibromatous hamartoma of the median nerve. *J Hand Surg.* 2013; 38A: 392–397.

20. Frykman GK, Wood VE. Peripheral nerve hamartoma with macrodactyly in the hand: Report of three cases and review of the literature. *J Hand Surg.* 1978; 3: 307–312.

21. Sezer E, Kosoglu RD, Filiz N. Eccrine angiomatous hamartoma of the fingers with nail destruction. *Br J Dermatol.* 2006; 154: 998–1023.

22. Markouch I, Clérici T, Saiag P, Mahé E. Lichen striatus avec dystrophie unguéale chez un nourrisson. *Ann Dermatol Venereol.* 2009; 136: 883–886.

23. Michel JL, Wolf F, Fond L et al. Lichen striatus de l'enfant et blaschkites de l'adulte. *Ann Dermatol Venereol.* 1997; 124: 187–191.

24. Happle R. The group of epidermal nevus syndromes Part 1. Well defined phenotypes. *J Am Acad Dermatol.* 2010; 63: 1–22.

25. Denis-Thely L, Cordier MP, Cambazard F et al. Syndrome de Goltz unilatéral. *Ann Dermatol Venereol.* 2002; 129: 161–163.

26. Crawford PJM, Aldred MJ, Clarke A et al. Rapp-Hodgkin syndrome: An ectodermal dysplasia involving the teeth, hair nails, and palate. *Oral Surg Oral Med Oral Pathol.* 1989; 67: 50–62.

27. Shawky RM, Elsayed SM, Abd-Elkhalek HS et al. Oral-facial-digital syndrome type II: Transitional type between More and Varadi. *Egypt J Med Hum Genet.* 2013; 14: 311–315.

28. Carrington PR, Chen H, Altick JA. Trichorhinophalangeal syndrome, type 1. *J Am Acad Dermatol Venereol.* 1994; 31: 331–336.

29. Verloes A, David A, Ngo L et al. Stringent delineation of Pallister-Hall syndrome in two long surviving patients: Importance of radiological anomalies of the hands. *J Med Genet.* 1995; 32: 605611.

10

Vascular Anomalies of Nail and Finger Extremities

Jean-Philippe Lacour

Vascular anomalies (VAs) can localize on extremities, thus possibly inducing subsequent nail involvement. Despite a somewhat frequent occurrence of VAs in childhood, specific nail alterations are rarely described in the literature, probably because they have few consequences for benign vascular lesions and because the prognosis is not conditioned by ungual involvement in severe VAs. Furthermore, VAs are not always symptomatic in childhood and may progress later on, at puberty or during pregnancy. In addition, genetic syndromes can have incomplete penetrance in childhood. However, the discovery of nail involvement in the context of VA may have functional or therapeutic consequences. On the other hand, some VAs have a specific location on digital extremities.

Classification of VAs

The accurate denomination of VAs is mandatory to allow greater consistency with nomenclature and precise communication between specialists. In 1996, the International Society for the Study of Vascular Anomalies (ISSVA) adopted a classification system that was expanded in 2014.[1] This new system keeps separating VAs into tumors and malformations but provides much greater detail, including newly named anomalies and identified genes. Vascular tumors are divided into benign, locally aggressive, and malignant entities, hemangiomas being the most frequent benign vascular tumor in childhood. Vascular malformations are divided into simple and combined. Their classification is based on vessel types that are involved (capillary, venous, lymphatic, lymphedema, and arteriovenous). Vascular malformations that are associated with other anomalies such as overgrowth in Klippel–Trenaunay syndrome (KTS) are also categorized separately.

Vascular Tumors

Infantile Hemangiomas

Infantile hemangiomas (IHs), also named hemangiomas of infancy, are the most common soft tissue tumors of infancy with an incidence estimated between 4% and 10% among all infants and children. They are more frequent among females and premature babies. They appear within the first few days or weeks of birth as a solitary cutaneous lesion that progressively enlarges over months and then slowly regresses. IHs are mainly composed of proliferating endothelial cells, which possess unique immunohistochemical markers, and pericytes. IHs are very rare in the fingernails, the favored site of their development being the head (60%) and the trunk (25%).

Acral IH patterns have rarely been studied. In a retrospective multicenter cohort study, Weitz et al.[2] described the morphologic subtypes, distribution, complications, and indications for treatment of 73 segmental IHs on the hands and feet. They were more likely to be segmental and to be of minimal arrested growth type, more than half of them having a predominantly reticular morphology. The authors described a "biker-glove" distribution, which means IH extending onto the digits, sparing the distal tips, and often maintaining a contiguous border across digits when the fingers or toes are approximated (Figure 10.1). This pattern, sparing nails, was noted in nearly three-quarters of patients. Acral extension onto the distal digits was noted in a minority of cases (13%) and was associated with larger segmental IH, often extending beyond the extremity onto the neck and torso. In only 5% of cases, there was an involvement of some fingertips or toes and sparing of others. Overall, IH affected radial/medial surfaces more often than ulnar/lateral surfaces. Most segmental IH involved both the medial and lateral surfaces (86%), whereas a medial predominance of indeterminate and localized IH was observed. Dorsal surfaces were involved more commonly than ventral on both the upper and lower extremities. The authors do not comment on nail involvement and none of the published figures shows involvement of the nails, even when IH extends close to the finger extremity. Indeed, hemangiomas of the nail bed and tip of the digit are extremely rare. Localization under the proximal nail fold has very rarely been reported in the available literature.

In rare cases, IHs can induce nail abnormalities (Figure 10.2). Piraccini et al.[3] reported three cases of congenital pseudoclubbing of a fingernail caused by subungual hemangioma. In two of the described children, the IHs were superficial and produced nail pseudoclubbing caused by the capillary vessel proliferation in the soft tissues of the subungual region. The small size probably resulted from compression of the IH by the nail matrix and the bone of the distal finger, blocking its increase in size. The third child had a deeper IH, which possibly involved the dermis and the subcutaneous fat of the digit, producing distal swelling and a drumstick appearance. This proliferation produced an uplifting and an overcurvature of the nail in both the longitudinal and transverse axes, giving it a pseudoclubbing appearance. The nail matrix was only uplifted and not damaged by the vascular tumor and the nail plate was completely normal. The vascular proliferation produced a reddish discoloration of the nail, which typically faded with compression. The diagnosis of IH in their three children was based on the clinical examination and ultrasonography showing a superficial hypoechogenic mass under the proximal nail fold. One of the IHs showed a tendency to early spontaneous involution suggesting the diagnosis of a rapidly involuting congenital hemangioma (RICH). Al Buainian et al.[4] reported one case of total regression of an IH of the fingernail with pulsed dye laser therapy in a 12-week-old girl. However, because of the rapid tendency to regress spontaneously and the lack of matrix damage, proximal nail fold IHs in children are not at risk to become big masses with tissue damage. For this reason, a regular monitoring of the spontaneous regression is probably a better approach than any other treatment. Propranolol is now considered the most effective, well-tolerated, and safe first-line treatment for IH, but no case of ungual IH treated by propranolol has been reported so far.

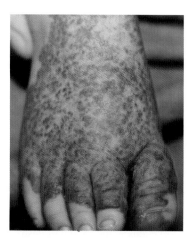

FIGURE 10.1 A "biker glove pattern" of a superficial infantile hemangioma. Note that the infantile hemangioma spares the extremities of four of the digits but involves the nail matrix as well as the nail bed of the great toe. (Courtesy of Labreze C.)

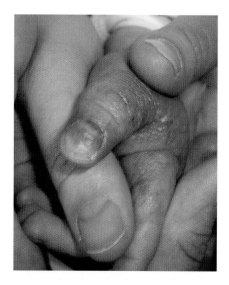

FIGURE 10.2 Infantile hemangioma with nail deformity. (Courtesy of Bocccara O.)

Other Vascular Tumors

Tufted Angioma and Kaposiform Hemangioendothelioma

Tufted angioma (TA) is a relatively rare vascular tumor manifesting clinically as pink, red, purple, or red-brown patches and plaques with superimposed papules or nodules. Most TAs appear during child-hood in the first 5 years. They are most frequently found on the abdomen, lower limbs, trunk, head, and neck and less frequently on the upper limb. Their typical growth pattern is a slow extension over several months to years. Histologically, it shows many lobules or "tufts" of capillaries in the mid or lower der-mis. They are composed of benign spindle cells, which may protrude into the lumen of larger vessels.

The features of a TA may overlap with kaposiform hemangioendothelioma (KHE), a similar endothe-lium derived spindle cell neoplasm, and it has been suggested that these two disease entities may exist on a continuum, TA being a milder, more superficial form of KHE. Although histologically benign, KHE can display local extension, including deep soft tissues and even the retroperitoneum. Clinically, it has a violaceous color, with a nodular growth pattern mimicking a malignant tumor.

Both KHE and TA can be associated with Kasabach–Merritt phenomenon (KMP) characterized by profound thrombocytopenia due to platelet trapping within the tumor, sometimes accompanied by microangiopathic hemolytic anemia, and secondary consumption of coagulation factors. KHE and TA account for the vast majority of KMS cases.

The location and hematological effects of the lesion may determine whether the treatment is medical or surgical. Several treatment regimens for TA/KHE with or without KMS have been reported, including abstention, compression therapy, surgery, laser, topical, or systemic corticosteroids, interferon, proprano-lol, vincristine, and sirolimus.

When affecting the limbs, TA and KHE usually have a proximal location. There is only one reported case of TA/KHE affecting the finger (but sparing the nail) described in the available literature. Collins et al.[5] described a 3-year-old male presenting since the age of 16 months with a slow enlarging lesion on the dorsal aspect of the left middle finger. The lesion was excised but recurred 2 months later. Histopathology showed aspects of TA with some overlap features with KHE. The lesion increased in size, resulting in a 2 × 1.5 cm nodule over the dorsal aspect of the distal phalanx, extending toward the interphalangeal joint but sparing the nail. Because of the effect on function of the finger and the potential for progressive growth of the lesion, a second surgical excision was performed and the deficit was covered with a mini free vascularized groin flap. Surgical outcome was uncomplicated with a return to full use of the digit.

Multifocal Lymphangioendotheliomatosis

Multifocal lymphangioendotheliomatosis (MLT) is a rare disorder involving the skin and the gastroin-testinal system, characterized by a proliferation of multiple congenital and progressive vascular lesions usually associated with mild-to-moderate thrombocytopenia.[6] Gastrointestinal bleeding is usually pres-ent and may cause mortality. Cutaneous lesions are violaceous to brown-red papules or plaques ranging from a few millimeters to 5 cm. Although lesions of MLT can localize on feet and hands (Figure 10.3), no case of ungual involvement has been reported so far.

Hemangioendotheliomas

The hemangioendothelioma group includes papillary intralymphatic angioendothelioma (PILA), reti-form hemangioendothemioma (RHE), and epithelioid hemangioendothelioma (EH). They are borderline between benign hemangiomas and angiosarcomas, having a tendency to recur but a limited capacity to metastasis. PILA (or Dabska tumor) and RHE usually appear during childhood, but no case involving the nails have been reported so far. A case of EH with a scar-like appearance and nail destruction on a finger has been described in an adult, and there is a unique case described on the extremities in child-hood. Kitagawa et al.[7] reported a 12-year-old girl with mild pain and firm swelling on the dorsal surface of the middle portion of the right index finger for 8 months. The aspect of the nail was not described. Radiographs showed a combination of lytic destruction and irregular sclerotic changes. Magnetic

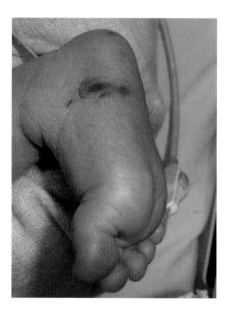

FIGURE 10.3 Lymphangioendotheliomatosis.

resonance images showed a mass involving the middle phalanx and the extensor tendon, extending to the dorsal subcutaneous tissue with destruction of the phalangeal cortex. Angiogram showed staining of the tumor, early venous filling, and an arteriovenous shunt, suggesting that the tumor was hypervascular. Curettage and grafting of the tumor using autogenous bone from the iliac crest were performed. Microscopically the tumor consisted of atypical epithelioid cells forming a nest in a hyalinized background and vascular channels. Immunohistochemical staining was positive for endothelial markers. The tumor recurred 16 months later, and a second surgery was performed. The resection of the entire middle phalanx with surrounding soft tissues including the flexor tendon sheath was performed. Ten years after there was neither local recurrence nor metastasis.

Pyogenic Granuloma

Pyogenic granuloma (PG), also referred to as "lobular capillary hemangioma," is a relatively common acquired benign vascular tumor that frequently involves the nail, including the periungual tissues and the nail bed. It starts around the nail with a tiny red papule, which rapidly grows to reach the size of a few to 10 mm in diameter. Its surface may become eroded, and crusted. Tenderness and a ready tendency to bleed are characteristic features of this tumor. A collarette can be seen. It can be present as a solitary nodule or as multiple lesions of several digits. PG is commonly located at the proximal nail fold but may develop distally in the hyponychium region with onycholysis in the nail bed or even in the matrix after a penetrating wound of the nail plate.

There are several causes of PG.[8] If it involves only one finger, the possible causes are local trauma (foreign body, acute trauma, nail manipulation, paronychia) or peripheral nerve injury (bone fracture treated with immobilization more often than peripheral nerve diseases in childhood). If PG involves only one toe, the most frequent causes are ingrown nail, retronychia, frictional trauma, or a peripheral nerve injury. The location of PG and the history of the patient help to identify the right cause. When PG is single, histological examination is necessary to rule out malignant tumors, especially amelanotic melanoma. If periungual PGs are multiple, both in hands and feet, they may be due to drugs such as retinoids, particularly systemic isotretinoin in adolescents. Other drug-induced cases such as systemic etretinate, systemic acitretin, antiretrovirals (indinavir, lamivudine), or antineoplastic drugs (epidermal growth factor receptor inhibitors, capecitabine, cyclosporin, docetaxel, mitoxantrone) are rarely seen in childhood. Guhl et al.[9] reported the case of a child who developed multiple Beau's lines and periungueal PGs after a long stay in an intensive care unit. Immobilization, hypoxia, and drugs might have acted as potential causative factors.

Therapy should be as simple as possible to avoid disfiguring scars or nail deformity. PG may be removed by excision at its base or curettage followed by electrodesiccation. The use of lasers, particularly pulsed dye laser, is also curative. If PG is due to local repeated trauma, the removal of the trauma is necessary. PG can also be treated by cryotherapy. If PGs are due to drugs, topical medication or curettage may be effective, but a decrease in the drug dose may be necessary.

Vascular Malformations

Vascular malformations are divided into four groups: simple malformations, combined malformations, malformations of major named vessels, and malformations associated with other anomalies.[1] The classification is based on vessel types that are involved. Thus, simple malformations are divided in capillary, venous, lymphatic, lymphedema, and arteriovenous malformations (AVMs). The combined vascular malformations are named specifically for the vessels involved in the malformation. Most simple malformations are composed mainly of only one type of vessel (capillaries, lymphatics, or veins), with the exception of AVMs, which contains arteries, veins, and capillaries.

Capillary Malformations

Cutaneous Capillary Malformations ("Port Wine" Stain)

Capillary malformations (CMs), often referred to as "port wine" stains, mainly affect the skin and mucosa, appearing as pink to red macules. They consist of dilated capillaries and/or postcapillary venules. They are present at birth and they are caused by a somatic activating mutation in *GNAQ* gene. They can sometimes partially lighten during the first weeks of birth, the darker aspect at birth being probably due to physiological polyglobulia and relative neonatal cyanosis. However, they generally persist throughout life and they may even thicken and darken with time. They may be associated with soft tissue or bone overgrowth and with other vascular and nonvascular anomalies and syndromes.

When they are located on the extremities, CMs usually have a segmental pattern, involving a whole limb, extending from the shoulder to the fingers on the upper limb and from the buttocks to the toes on the lower limb. When they involve a whole limb, they are usually darker in acral location such as the hands and feet. They may look violet through the nail. Paradoxically, normal color (Figure 10.4) or true leukonychia can be observed.[10]

CM with Bone and/or Soft Tissue Overgrowth

CMs can be associated with hypertrophy, even when they do not belong to complex malformations such as KTS or other overgrowth syndromes.

In a study of 73 patients with diffuse CMs with overgrowth, Lee et al.[11] reported that digital anomalies were noted in 30% of patients: soft tissue syndactyly, especially involving the second and third toes; a widened first pedal web space (i.e., "sandal gap"); and macrodactyly (fingers or toes). There was an association between extent of staining (number of regions involved) and soft tissue syndactyly.

CM of Capillary Malformation–Arteriovenous Malformation Syndrome

Capillary malformation–arteriovenous malformation (CM–AVM) is a recently recognized autosomal-dominant disorder due to inactivating mutations of the *RASA1* gene characterized by multifocal CMs and high risk for fast-flow lesions.[12] Multiple CMs are often the first sign in children. They are localized on the head and neck, trunk, or extremities (Figure 10.5). Involvement of the tips of the fingers or nails has not been specifically described in the literature but can occur. Their color varies from pale pink to red or brown,

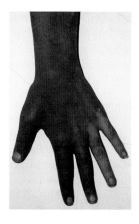

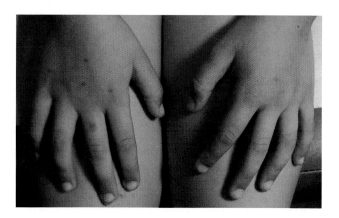

FIGURE 10.4 Capillary malformation with minimal change in the color of the nail. (Courtesy of Dompmartin A.)

FIGURE 10.5 Capillary malformations of the capillary malformation–arteriovenous malformation (CM–AVM) syndrome due to *RASA1* mutations.

and their size from a few millimeters to several centimeters in diameter. They are round, oval, or with irregular borders and are often surrounded by a pale halo. Patients also have zones of numerous punctuate red spots surrounded by a white halo, located mainly on the extremities. Associated fast-flow lesions can be cutaneous, subcutaneous, intramuscular, intraosseous, intracerebral, or intraspinal. Evaluation of the neuroaxis for fast-flow lesions is usually recommended, but further studies are needed to examine the optimal approach to screening patients and family members for internal arteriovenous lesions.

CM of Microcephaly–Capillary Malformation Syndrome

The microcephaly–capillary malformation (MIC–CAP) syndrome is characterized by microcephaly, generalized cutaneous CMs, hypoplastic distal phalanges of the hands and/or feet, epilepsy, and profound developmental delay. The CMs are usually multiple, involving the face, trunk, and extremities and ranging in size from 2 to 15 mm. This pattern resembles the CM–AVM syndrome. The distal phalanges are hypoplastic with hypoplasia or aplasia of one or several toenails.

MIC–CAP syndrome results from biallelic *STAMBP* gene pathogenic variants, most often autosomal recessive inheritance and rarely from uniparental isodisomy.

CM of Megalencephaly–Capillary Malformation–Polymicrogyria

Megalencephaly–capillary malformation-polymicrogyria (MCAP) is a sporadic overgrowth syndrome characterized by megalencephaly, CMs, asymmetric growth, polymicrogyria, finger or toe syndactyly, postaxial polydactyly, among other features.

MCAP overlaps with megalencephaly–polymicrogyriapolydactyly–hydrocephalus (MPPH) syndrome, which lacks consistent vascular or somatic manifestations besides postaxial polydactyly in almost half of the reported individuals. Both are due to *PIK3CA* mutations.[13]

Hereditary Hemorrhagic Telangiectasia

Hereditary hemorrhagic telangiectasia (HHT) or Osler–Weber–Rendu syndrome is characterized by mucocutaneous telangiectases that bleed easily, recurrent epistaxis, and AVMs occurring most commonly in the liver, lung, or brain. Mutations in two genes (*ENG* and *ACVRL1/ALK1*) cause approximately 85% of cases.

One of the most common features of the disorder is telangiectases. They frequently appear early in life but may be subtle during childhood necessitating careful examination. They are most evident on the lips, tongue, face, and fingers, and the nasal and buccal mucosa. They appear as pink to red, pinpoint-to pinhead-size lesions, or occasionally as larger, even raised purple lesions. Capillary microscopy of the fingernail folds can be a valuable tool in diagnosing HHT showing giant capillaries and giant loops between capillaries of normal shape and size.[14] HHT can also induce morphological changes detectable by capillaroscopy on the dorsum of the hands.[15]

Cutis Marmorata Telangiectatica Congenita

Cutis marmorata telangiectatica congenita (CMTC) is a congenital capillary and venous vascular malformation of unknown origin. The major clinical features of CMTC are congenital presence of persistent cutis marmorata, phlebectasia, telangiectasia, and occasional ulceration and atrophy of the involved skin. The lesions are usually present at birth and preferentially involve the lower limbs, followed by the trunk and face. CMTC is often localized but may be segmental or widespread in distribution. The cutaneous changes have a tendency to spontaneously resolve over time. Various associated congenital anomalies have been reported, and among these, hypertrophy or atrophy of affected limb is one. CMTC has been described in Adams–Oliver syndrome, which associate also congenital scalp defects and terminal transverse limb defects. The defects involve more often the lower limbs and characteristically affect the distal phalanges or entire digits. The described anomalies include shortened fingers and toes, loss of terminal phalanges, syndactyly, clubfoot, absence of toes or limbs, and hypoplastic nails.[16]

Venous Malformations

Common and Familial Venous Malformations

Venous malformations (VMs) are slow-flow VA that generally manifest as a blue skin discoloration when superficial or as a soft subcutaneous mass and may affect every tissue or viscera. They are usually present at birth and grow proportionately with the child, but in many cases, particularly those with predominantly intramuscular disease, these are often present later in life with pain provoked by physical activity. They can become extensive causing chronic complications such as pain, bleeding, functional impairment, and local thrombosis. Common VMs are soft and compressible and tend to increase in volume with an increase in venous pressure (e.g., Valsalva maneuver or straining), exercise, or when the affected segment is in a dependent position. Because of slow flow of blood into the malformed vessels, thrombosis may occur, resulting in pain and formation of phleboliths that may be palpable or visible on imaging when calcified. VMs may be focal, multifocal, or diffuse, the latter typically involving an entire muscle or limb.

Common VMs are generally sporadic. VMs limited to the nail apparatus are rare and should be left untreated (Figure 10.6). The shape of the nail may remain normal, but the nail bed becomes blue.[10] When VMs are more extensive, involving a whole limb, the extremities may be severely affected, causing deformation of the digital extremities and nails (Figures 10.7 and 10.8).

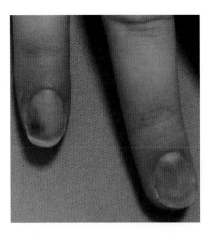

FIGURE 10.6 Venous malformation involving the nail plate. (Courtesy of Delaporte E.)

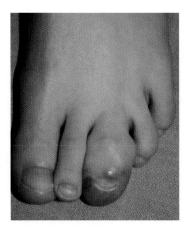

FIGURE 10.7 Venous malformation of a toe involving the nail matrix. (Courtesy of Dompmartin A.)

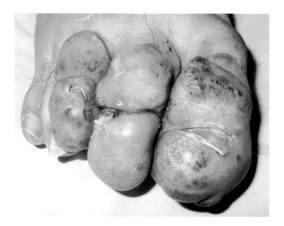

FIGURE 10.8 Severe venous malformation with nail involvement. (Courtesy of Blaise S.)

Familial VMs present generally as small multiple lesions affecting the skin and mucosa. They are caused by germ line autosomal-dominant mutations in the tyrosine kinase with immunoglobulin-like and EGF-like domain 2 (*Tie2*) gene. Sporadic VMs are also caused by somatic mutations in the same *Tie2* gene or in *PIK3CA* gene.[17] Both common and familial VMs are composed of a network of veins with thin walls, defective in smooth muscle cell media, dissecting the host tissue.

The imaging of VMs is mainly performed with Doppler ultrasonography (US) and magnetic resonance imaging (MRI). MRI best demonstrates VMs and their extent and relationship to adjacent structures as well as digital collateral vessels. In general, VMs show an increased signal on T2 sequences in a lobular or serpiginous pattern. Decreased T2 signal can be seen within areas of thrombosis and phleboliths. Characteristic delayed and heterogeneous enhancement within the VMs is seen with the administration of gadolinium.

Available therapies are sclerotherapy and surgical resection. However, both are invasive and often ineffective as lesions tend to recur. Conservative management is recommended in the initial care of VM of the hand, but many cases require radical resection, including amputation, because of pain, bleeding, nerve compression, and functional impairment. Gu et al. reported the case of a 15-year-old girl with a VM of the pulp, distal phalanx, and nail bed on her left third finger. The VM was treated by radical excision including skin, distal phalanx, and nail bed, followed by reconstruction with free medial plantar artery perforator flap and split thickness nail bed graft from the great toe.[18]

Blue Rubber Bleb Nevus Syndrome

Patients affected by the blue rubber bleb syndrome (Bean syndrome) present multiple VMs affecting the skin, soft tissue, and gastrointestinal tract, the latter responsible for chronic bleeding and anemia. Some of the skin VMs, especially on the soles and palms, present as small, round, dark hyperkeratotic bleb-like or nipple-like lesions.They are often present from birth or early childhood. No case of blue rubber bleb nevus of the finger extremities or nail has been specifically reported in the literature, but blue rubber bleb nevus of the hand and fingers may be accompanied by leukonychia.[10]

Glomuvenous Malformations

Glomuvenous malformations (GVMs), formerly known as glomangioma or glomangiomatosis, are usually raised, nodular with a pink to purplish-dark blue color. They are present at birth and slowly expand during childhood. They are often multifocal and hyperkeratotic. Their number varies from a few to hundreds. Most are located on the extremities. Plaque-like GVM, which is less frequent, is flat and purple in the newborn but darkens with time. They are generally of darker blue to purple color; they cannot be emptied by compression compared to common VMs and are usually painful to palpation. Their histologic appearance is similar to common VMs except for the presence, at least focally, in the vein walls of rounded "glomus" cells corresponding to modified smooth muscle cells. GVM are related to an inactivating mutation in the glomulin gene. Most cases with multiple GVMs are familial, and autosomal-dominant inheritance has been demonstrated. Histologically, GVM is characterized by the presence of a variable number of mural glomus cells in distended venous channels. Similar cells are present in solitary glomus tumors. The glomus cell component may vary widely between regions, and some microscopic fields may show only veins devoid of glomus cells, leading to a misdiagnosis of VMs. They differ from solitary glomus tumors that are subungual, painful lesions exclusively composed of glomus cells without a major vascular component.

The best therapy for GVM is surgical resection. Pulsed dye laser is ineffective, due to its limited depth of penetration, but neodymium-doped yttrium aluminum garnet (Nd:YAG) laser therapy seems to be efficient.

Although GVM is frequently located on the extremities, there are no reports or specific studies in the literature on nail involvement. Hill et al. reported a 13-year-old girl with GVM presenting multiple painless nodules mostly located subungually and laterally on her fingers and toes, interfering with her ability to write. The nodules had been present since birth, and they had increased in size during childhood. In addition, she had temporal triangular alopecia, heterochromia irides, epidermal nevus, and lipoblastoma.[19]

Arteriovenous Malformations

AVMs are potentially the more aggressive type of VM. They are fast-flow VMs composed of malformed arteries, veins, and capillaries, with direct arteriovenous communications resulting in arteriovenous shunting. They are present at birth or may become evident in infancy or childhood. Puberty and trauma may trigger growth making the fast-flow nature clinically evident. They may present as a pseudo-CM with pulsation at palpation or a bruit, as an enlarging red, warm, painful mass, or as an ulcerated and bleeding lesion due to trophic skin alterations.

AVMs may be sporadic or observed in patients presenting with HHT or CM-AVM. Arteriovenous fistulas (AVFs) may be associated with other vascular and nonvascular anomalies.

Sporadic AVMs

When localized on fingers or toes, AVM may gradually shorten the distal phalanx and cause violaceous skin atrophy due to ischemia of the distal capillary bed and progressive shortening of the nail plate presenting a slight transverse overcurvature. The veins become prominent on the fingers and dorsum of the hand or foot (Figure 10.9). Diagnosis is confirmed by Doppler US, MRI, and digital arteriography.

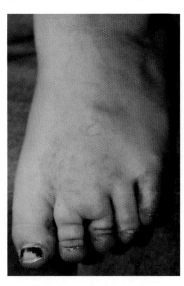

FIGURE 10.9   Arteriovenous malformation of the dorsum of the foot. (Courtesy of Labreze C.)

In the pediatric age, AVMs are frequently in a quiescent stage and require no treatment. Intervention may become necessary when local complications such as ulceration, necrosis, pain, bleeding, diminished function, or a combination of these occur. The therapeutic decision must be taken by a multidisciplinary team. Treatment of the AVM includes conservative treatment, selective embolization, partial excision, and radical excision. However, recurrence due to recruitment of reconstituted arterial flow into the nidus, repeated surgery, and even deformity requiring amputation are common problems. The excision is difficult because there is a risk to damage the normal vascularization of the digit, with subsequent development of ischemia or necrosis. Embolization and partial excision are prone to recurrence as well. Thus, there is a need for long-term observation of these patients, even after apparent remission.

Arteriovenous Fistula

AVF is an AVM having abnormal connection between the feeding arteries and the draining veins, without an intervening capillary bed. They can be congenital or acquired, mainly post traumatic. They have been described in the literature under various different names, cirsoid aneurysm (CA) being one of the most frequently used ones. They may occur in various sites, cutaneous or visceral, but the most common location is the scalp. However, cases have been described on the extremities, and Burge et al.[20] reported five cases occurring in adults located in the subungual or periungual region. Kadono et al.[21] reported six patients with acquired digital AVM. Two of them were children. They had a small patch of AVM localized to the tip of one finger presenting reddish-purple macule consisting of a group of various sized dots and nodules, fading on diascopy and reappearing promptly after release of pressure. Histologically, dilated venous and arterial vessels were present in the dermis. They were mostly related to a previous injury.

Lymphatic Malformations

Common (Cystic) Lymphatic Malformations

Lymphatic malformations (LMs) consist of vesicles or pouches made up of variously dilated lymphatic channels or cysts, lined by endothelial cells with a lymphatic phenotype. They are classified as microcystic, macrocystic, and mixed subtypes. LMs present during infancy or childhood.

Microcystic LM (or lymphangioma circumscriptum) appears as a cluster of clear or blood-filled dark-red vesicles overlying an area of diffuse swelling. They are rarely observed on the distal digit. Oh et al. reported the case of a 16-year-old girl presenting an enlarging, asymptomatic papule on lateral aspect of a distal phalange, recurring after CO_2 laser destruction.[22] A biopsy was performed allowing the diagnosis of lymphangioma circumscriptum.

Common LM develops mainly in the cervicofacial and axillary region, generally under normal-colored skin, except when intralesional hemorrhage occurs. Somatic mutations in the phosphatidylinositol/Akt/mTOR pathway may cause common cystic LMs.[23]

LM in Gorham–Stout Disease

Gorham–Stout disease, also named disappearing or vanishing bone disease, is characterized by LM affecting a single or multiple bones and often neighboring soft tissue, with a progressive osteolysis.[24] Most cases occur in children or in adults aged less than 40. The bones of the upper extremity and the maxillofacial region are the predominant osseous locations of the disease. A few cases have been described with metacarpal or metatarsal involvement, but the phalanges were rarely or minimally affected.

Primary Lymphedemas

Primary lymphedemas are considered a subtype of LM due to a primary dysgenesis of the lymphatic network. They can manifest at birth or later in life by chronic, unilateral or bilateral edema involving the dorsum of the foot, sometimes extending above the knee. Several mutations in lymphatic-specific genes, such as *FOXC2*, *FLT4*, and *SOX18* underlying different types of primary lymphedemas have been associated with inherited forms of lymphedema.

One of the most frequent of them, Milroy disease, is an autosomal-dominant condition due to mutations in the vascular endothelial growth factor receptor 3 (*VEGFR-3*) gene. It is characterized by lower-limb lymphedema, present as pedal edema at (or before) birth, or develops soon after. Swelling is usually bilateral but can be asymmetric and progresses with time. Other features sometimes associated with Milroy disease include hydrocele (37% of males), prominent veins (23%), papillomatosis (10%), and urethral abnormalities in males (4%). Nail abnormalities, described as "upslanting nails," have been observed in 14% of cases.[25]

Nail abnormalities identified by clinical and dermoscopic examination of lymphedematous limbs have been described in adult patients with secondary lymphedema.[26] The most frequent changes are hyperkeratosis of the nail folds, friability of the nail surface, excoriations of the proximal nail fold and of the cuticle, and apparent leukonychia. However, such a detailed ungual examination has never been reported in children with congenital lymphedema.

Yellow nail syndrome (YNS) is characterized by slowly growing, dystrophic, yellow nails, peripheral lymphedema, pleural effusions, rhinosinusitis, and bronchectasias with consecutive recurrent lower respiratory tract infections. Primarily considered to be a syndrome that affects the adult population, YNS is more recently emerging in the pediatric population. Individual manifestations can appear at different times, thus clinical onset varies from birth to late adult life. The diagnosis is made clinically and no specific treatment is known yet.[27]

Lymphedema can be associated with various anomalies. Fatinni et al.[28] reported four offspring of a consanguineous marriage with lower limb edema, dystrophic nails of the lower limbs, and esotropia in two of the children from birth. The lymphedema–dystrophic nails–esotropia combination in this family is consistent with autosomal recessive inheritance. Nail dystrophy observed in both the lymphedematous and the unaffected lower limb in each of the four children constitutes part of the syndrome.

Combined Vascular Malformations

Combined vascular malformations associate two or more vascular malformations in one lesion. Some combined malformations associate a cutaneous CM and an underlying VM, LM, or AVM, or a VM with an LM.

Vascular Malformations Associated with Other Anomalies

Vascular malformations may be associated with anomalies of bone, soft tissue, or viscera. These non-vascular anomalies are often overgrowth of soft tissue and/or bone or, rarely, undergrowth. Most of these associations are eponymous syndromes.

PIK3CA-Related Overgrowth Spectrum

Somatic mutations in the phosphatidylinositol/AKT/mTOR pathway cause segmental overgrowth disorders. The spectrum of diseases with *PIK3CA* mutations include fibroadipose overgrowth (FAO); hemi-hyperplasia multiple lipomatosis (HHML); congenital lipomatous overgrowth, vascular malformations, epidermal nevi, scoliosis/skeletal and spinal (CLOVES) syndrome; macrodactyly; and the MCAP syndrome. These previously described entities have considerable phenotypic overlap.[29] While this spectrum overlaps with Proteus syndrome (PS) (sporadic, mosaic, and progressive), it can be distinguished by the absence of cerebriform connective tissue nevi and a distinct natural history. Unlike PS, most patients with *PIK3CA* mutations have congenital overgrowth, usually asymmetric and disproportionate.

In these syndromes, fingers and nails may be affected by overgrowth or VA that usually do not overlap in the same territory.

Patients with CLOVES syndrome often have triangular-shaped feet with enlarged and dysmorphic toes and display vascular malformations containing lymphatic, venous, and capillary components. Sarici et al.[30] reported the case of a neonate with congenital CLOVES syndrome who had dystrophia in the nail of the first digit of the right foot and bilateral hypertrophy of the first digits of the feet.

Proteus Syndrome

PS is a complex hamartomatous disorder defined by asymmetric somatic overgrowth (macrodactyly or hemihypertrophy), subcutaneous tumors, and various bone, cutaneous, and/or VA including CMs, VMs, and/or LMs. PS is always characterized by lipomatosis, macrocephalia, asymmetry of limbs (with partial gigantism of hands and feet, or both), and plantar cerebriform connective tissue nevi. PS is caused by somatic activating mutations in the *AKT1* gene, which belongs to a class of oncogenes encoding the *AKT1* kinase, an enzyme implicated in several developmental processes including cell proliferation and apoptosis. PS patients can have nail abnormalities, in most cases, localized to a few nails. These abnormalities include thick nails, thin nails, brachyonychia, koilonychia, and bluish nails.[31]

Klippel–Trenaunay Syndrome

Kippel–Trenaunay syndrome (KTS) is a congenital vascular anomaly, originally described as a triad of a CM, asymmetrical hypertrophy of the bones and overlying soft tissue, varicose veins and/or VMs, and/or LMs. KTS has a number of phenotypic features overlapping with those noted in patients with activating mutations in the PI3K-AKT pathway. Mosaic-activating mutations in *PIK3CA* were recently disclosed in patients with KTS, thus it is reasonable to postulate that KTS belongs to the *PIK3CA*-related overgrowth spectrum.[32]

KTS is mostly unilateral, and about 25% of patients with KTS have hand or foot malformations. Anomalies of the extremities such as macrodactyly, clinodactyly, ectrodactyly, camptodactyly, and syndactyly have been described.[33] It has been suggested that the presence of macrodactyly or other hand and foot malformations in children with KTS may be a predictor of deep venous system anomalies that are not always evident at birth and may become more apparent with increasing age.[34] Decreased and increased growth can coexist in the same body area of an individual with KTS. Ruggieri et al. reported a 3-year-old boy with CM extending from the right buttock to the sole of the right foot with clinical and radiological evidence of leg varicosities, and underlying deficiency of the soft tissues and bone. In addition, he had macrodactyly of the first, second, and third toes with small nails, and cutaneous syndactyly of the second and third toes of the ipsilateral foot.[35]

Parkes–Weber Syndrome

Parkes–Weber syndrome (PWS) is characterized by a triad of AVF, varicose veins, and bone and soft tissue hypertrophy leading to limb enlargement. It preferentially involves the lower limbs. It is similar in its presentation to KTS, but the presence of AVF distinguishes PWS from KTS. PWS onset is usually sporadic, but some familial cases have been reported in association with a mutation in *RASA1* gene. The symptoms of PWS are congenital and present at birth. CMs, forming geographic patterns, are typically located on lateral side of the limb, buttocks, or trunk. Local temperature is increased, a pulse or thrill can be palpated, and a murmur is heard on auscultation. The enlargement of a limb is present at birth, and the axial overgrowth can enlarge in postnatal period. Cases of shortened lower extremity have also been described. Arteriovenous shunt may also lead to cardiac system failure or limb ischemia. Toes involvement is frequent, depending on the extent of the lesions, with hypertrophy and secondary trophic changes of toes and nails. The treatment of patients with PWS is mainly symptomatic. Compression therapy is used to reduce symptoms of chronic venous insufficiency and lymphatic edema. In selected cases, invasive procedures are performed. Surgical treatment is difficult and may require several intravascular procedures, such as embolization, sclerotherapy, or classic open operations involving AVF ligation. In severe cases of ischemic extremities, amputation is the only therapy.

Maffucci Syndrome

Maffucci syndrome (MS) is an uncommon disorder characterized by the coexistence of multiple enchondromas and cutaneous exophytic VMs. No familial inheritance has been shown. MS is the result of somatic mosaic mutations in isocitrate dehydrogenase 1 (*IDH1*) and 2 (*IDH2*) genes.[36] MS usually appears in children aged between 4 and 5 years, but 25% of cases are congenital. It manifests before the completion of 1 year in 25% of patients and by puberty in 80%. MS appears in prepubertal years with soft, cutaneous vascular swellings and hard nodules (enchondromas) on the bones of fingers and toes. Skin lesions are blue, noncompressible, subcutaneous or cutaneous nodules, typically occurring on the fingers or feet. The malformation is of venous type, but it is histologically a spindle cell hemangioendothelioma. Some authors do not consider them to be true tumors but rather vascular proliferations within a preexisting VM. MS can be unilateral or bilateral and more frequently involves the upper limbs, but can also affect the lower limbs. Cutaneous and bone lesions may result in gross deformity of the fingers and nail regions. Radiographic signs are nearly pathognomonic, with multiple enchondromas associated with soft tissue swelling and phleboliths. The most frequent location for enchondromas is the small bones of the hands and feet. Involvement of the short tubular bones in the extremities is common; in one-half of patients, bone lesions are unilateral with development of notable malformations. Malignant transformation to chondrosarcoma may occur in 20% to 30% of cases.

Provisionally Unclassified VAs

Verrucous Hemangioma

Verrucous hemangioma (VH) is a rare vascular proliferation that is usually present at birth or appears in early childhood. VH presents solitary or multiple nodules with sometimes a linear distribution. Although usually located on the extremities, no case of VH involving the nail has been described so far. Histopathologically, it is characterized by the proliferation of small vessels in the dermis and subcutaneous tissue; the superficial epidermis usually shows a papillary appearance with ectatic vessels mimicking angiokeratomas. It has been suggested that VH represents a vascular malformation with incomplete lymphatic phenotype.[37]

Angiokeratomas

Angiokeratomas (AKs) are vascular lesions that are defined as one or more dilated vessel(s) lying in the papillary dermis accompanied by an epidermal reaction such as acanthosis and/or hyperkeratosis. The precise mechanism for their development is unknown. AKs are classified into five types: (1) AK of Mibelli, in which acral lesions are associated with cold injury; (2) AK of Fordyce, which are generally genital; (3) AK circumscriptum, which is nevoid with an onset in early life; (4) solitary or multiple AK with an onset in adult life; and (5) AKs in Fabry disease. Despite the possible acral location of some types of AKs, there is no report of nail involvement in childhood. A longitudinal pigmented band in a toenail has been described in an adult due to hemorrhage from an AK arising in the nail matrix. Dolph et al.[38] described a 12-year-old girl with a raised, firm, bluish-purple nodule over the dorsal aspect of the distal index finger. It enlarged with the concomitant appearance of several black dots at the periphery. Histology showed a typical AK.

Acral Pseudolymphomatous Angiokeratoma of Children

Acral pseudolymphomatous angiokeratoma of children (APACHE) is a rare, benign condition that was initially regarded as a benign vascular condition but is now rather considered to be a pseudolymphoma. It generally occurs in children and the majority of patients are females and most lesions are located on the upper or lower extremities. Clinically, lesions are often unilateral. They range from skin-colored papules and nodules to more vesicular and bullous-appearing erythematous and violaceous lesions that can be in groups or arranged in a linear fashion. Involvement of the nail with dystrophy or onycholysis is not rare.[39]

REFERENCES

1. Wassef M, Blei F, Adams D et al.; ISSVA Board and Scientific Committee. Vascular anomalies classification: Recommendations from the International Society for the Study of Vascular Anomalies. *Pediatrics*. 2015; 136: e203–e214.
2. Weitz NA, Bayer ML, Baselga E et al. The "biker-glove" pattern of segmental infantile hemangiomas on the hands and feet. *J Am Acad Dermatol*. 2014; 71: 542–547.
3. Piraccini BM, Antonucci A, Rech G et al. Congenital pseudoclubbing of a fingernail caused by subungual hemangioma. *J Am Acad Dermatol*. 2005; 53: S123–S126.
4. Al Buainian H, Verhaeghe E, Dierckxsens L, Naeyaert JM. Early treatment of hemangiomas with lasers. *Dermatology*. 2003; 206: 370–373.
5. Collins D, Sebire NJ, Barnacle A et al. "Mini" free groin flap for treatment of a tufted angioma of the finger. *J Plast Reconstr Aesthet Surg*. 2011; 64: e128–e131.
6. North PE, Kahn T, Cordisco MR et al. Multifocal lymphangioendotheliomatosis with thrombocytopenia: A newly recognized clinicopathological entity. *Arch Dermatol*. 2004; 140: 599–606.
7. Kitagawa Y, Ito H, Iketani M et al. Epithelioid hemangioendothelioma of the phalanx: A case report. *J Hand Surg Am*. 2005; 30: 615–619.
8. Piraccini BM, Bellavista S, Misciali C et al. Periungual and subungual pyogenic granuloma. *Br J Dermatol*. 2010; 163: 941–953.
9. Guhl G, Torrelo A, Hernández A, Zambrano A. Beau's lines and multiple periungueal pyogenic granulomas after long stay in an intensive care unit. *Pediatr Dermatol*. 2008; 25: 278–279.
10. Baran R, de Berker DAR, Holzberg M, Thomas L (eds). *Baran and Dawber's Diseases of the Nails and their Management*, Fourth Edition. Chichester, UK: Wiley-Blackwell; 2012. pp. 674–675.
11. Lee MS, Liang MG, Mulliken JB. Diffuse capillary malformation with overgrowth: A clinical subtype of vascular anomalies with hypertrophy. *J Am Acad Dermatol*. 2013; 69: 589–594.
12. Revencu N, Boon LM, Mendola A et al. *RASA1* mutations and associated phenotypes in 68 families with capillary malformation-arteriovenous malformation. *Hum Mutat*. 2013; 34: 1632–1641.
13. Rivière JB, Mirzaa GM, O'Roak BJ et al. De novo germline and postzygotic mutations in *AKT3*, *PIK3R2* and *PIK3CA* cause a spectrum of related megalencephaly syndromes. *Nat Genet*. 2012; 44: 934–940.
14. Mager JJ, Westermann CJ. Value of capillary microscopy in the diagnosis of hereditary hemorrhagic telangiectasia. *Arch Dermatol*. 2000; 136: 732–734.
15. Pasculli G, Quaranta D, Lenato GM et al. Capillaroscopy of the dorsal skin of the hands in hereditary hemorrhagic telangiectasia. *QJM*. 2005; 98: 757–763.
16. Mempel M, Abeck D, Lange I et al. The wide spectrum of clinical expression in Adams-Oliver syndrome: A report of two cases. *Br J Dermatol*. 1999; 140: 1157–1160.
17. Limaye N, Kangas J, Mendola A et al. Somatic activating *PIK3CA* mutations cause venous malformation. *Am J Hum Genet*. 2015; 97: 914–921.
18. Gu JH, Jeong SH. Radical resection of a venous malformation in middle finger and immediate reconstruction using medial plantar artery perforator flap: A case report. *Microsurgery*. 2012; 32: 148–152.
19. Hill S, Rademaker MA. Collection of rare anomalies: Multiple digital glomuvenous malformations, epidermal naevus, temporal alopecia, heterochromia and abdominal lipoblastoma. *Clin Exp Dermatol*. 2009; 34: e862–e864.
20. Burge SM, Baran R, Dawber RP, Verret JL. Periungual and subungual arteriovenous tumours. *Br J Dermatol*. 1986; 115: 361–366.
21. Kadono T, Kishi A, Onishi Y, Ohara K. Acquired digital arteriovenous malformation: A report of six cases. *Br J Dermatol*. 2000; 142: 362–365.
22. Oh ST, Kwon HJ, Lee JY, Cho BK. A case of lymphangioma circumscriptum developed on the finger. *Dermatol Surg*. 2007; 33: 648–649.
23. Osborn AJ, Dickie P, Neilson DE et al. Activating *PIK3CA* alleles and lymphangiogenic phenotype of lymphatic endothelial cells isolated from lymphatic malformations. *Hum Mol Genet*. 2015; 24: 926–938.

24. Bruch-Gerharz D, Gerharz CD, Stege H et al.. Cutaneous lymphatic malformations in disappearing bone (Gorham-Stout) disease: A novel clue to the pathogenesis of a rare syndrome. *J Am Acad Dermatol.* 2007; 56: S21–S25.

25. Brice GW, Mansour S, Ostergaard P et al. Milroy disease. In: Pagon RA, Adam MP, Ardinger HH et al (eds.), GeneReviews® http://www.ncbi.nlm.nih.gov/books/NBK1239/. Seattle, WA: University of Washington; 1993–2015. April 27, 2006 [updated September 25, 2014].

26. Le Fourn E, Duhard E, Tauveron V et al. Changes in the nail unit in patients with secondary lymphoedema identified using clinical, dermoscopic, and ultrasound examination. *Br J Dermatol.* 2011; 164: 765–770.

27. Al Hawsawi K, Pope E. Yellow nail syndrome. *Pediatr Dermatol.* 2010; 27: 675–676.

28. Fatinni Y, Asindi A, Al Falki Y et al. Possible new autosomal recessive syndrome of congenital lymphoedema, nail dystrophy and esotropia in a Saudi family. *Acta Pediatr.* 2001; 90: 151–153.

29. Luks VL, Kamitaki N, Vivero MP et al. Lymphatic and other vascular malformative/overgrowth disorders are caused by somatic mutations in *PIK3CA*. *J Pediatr.* 2015; 166: 1048–1054.

30. Sarici D, Akin MA, Kurtoglu S et al. A neonate with CLOVES syndrome. *Case Rep Pediatr.* 2014; 2014: 845074.

31. Nguyen D, Turner JT, Olsen C et al. Cutaneous manifestations of Proteus syndrome: Correlations with general clinical severity. *Arch Dermatol.* 2004; 140: 947–953.

32. McGrory BJ, Amadio PC, Dobyns JH et al. Anomalies of the fingers and toes associated with Klippel-Trenaunay syndrome. *J Bone Joint Surg Am.* 1991; 73: 1537–1546.

33. Vahidnezhad H, Youssefian L, Uitto J. Klippel-Trenaunay syndrome belongs to the *PIK3CA*-related overgrowth spectrum (PROS). *Exp Dermatol.* 2016; 25: 17–19.

34. Redondo P, Bastarrika G, Aguado L et al. Foot or hand malformations related to deep venous system anomalies of the lower limb in Klippel-Trénaunay syndrome. *J Am Acad Dermatol.* 2009; 61: 621–628.

35. Ruggieri M, Pavone V, Polizzi A et al. Klippel-Trenaunay syndrome in a boy with concomitant ipsilateral overgrowth and undergrowth. *Am J Med Genet A.* 2014; 164A: 1262–1267.

36. Amary MF, Damato S, Halai D et al. Ollier disease and Maffucci syndrome are caused by somatic mosaic mutations of *IDH1* and *IDH2*. *Nat Genet.* 2011; 43: 1262–1265.

37. Wang L, Gao T, Wang G. Verrucous hemangioma: A clinicopathological and immunohistochemical analysis of 74 cases. *J Cutan Pathol.* 2014; 41: 823–830.

38. Dolph JL, Demuth RJ, Miller SH. Angiokeratoma circumscriptum of the index finger in a child. *Plast Reconstr Surg.* 1981; 67: 221–223.

39. McFaddin C, Greene J, Parekh P. Linear acral pseudolymphomatous angiokeratoma of children with associated nail dystrophy. *Dermatol Online J.* 2015; 21.

11

Systemic Diseases

Bianca Maria Piraccini, Iria Neri, and Michela Starace

Nail signs associated with systemic disorders in children include nail symptoms that are specific for a disease and well known and also described in adults,[1] i.e., the nails of the yellow nail syndrome, the periungual capillary changes seen in connective tissue disorders, and nail clubbing,[2,3] and nail signs that are nonspecific and occasionally described as single-case reports or in case series not related to a specific disease (Table 11.1).[1,4,5] The latter include symptoms such as nail fragility, Beau's lines, and onychomadesis, which result from the damage to the nail matrix and can be seen in a high number of conditions, as well as nail changes that are very frequent and physiological in children such as toenail koilonychia. In all these cases, assessing the casual relationship with the systemic disease is not easy.

This chapter describes clubbing in association with several disorders in children and then reviews the systemic diseases of children that have been associated with nail lesions.

Clubbing (Watch-Glass Nails, Drumstick Fingers, and Hippocratic Fingers/Nails)

Clubbing is one of the most well-known nail signs of systemic diseases, being described as far back as in the fifth century BC by Hippocrates. It is characterized by a focal bulbous enlargement of the terminal segments of the fingers and/or toes that produce an alteration of the shape of the nail, which resembles a clock glass, being hypercurved both transversally and longitudinally.[6] Characteristics of clubbing include the following: the angle between the proximal nail fold and the nail plate (Lovibond angle) is greater than 180° and the rhomboidal space that is normally seen facing the distal portion of the first two digits disappears (window or Schamroth's sign). On palpation, the enlarged tissues of the proximal nail fold have a spongy sensation. Although the severe clubbing is recognized very easily, the identification of the early stages can be difficult. Two objective measures for diagnosing early clubbing have been proposed: the digital index and the phalangeal depth ratio. The digital index measures the nail bed (NB) circumference and the distal interphalangeal (DIP) joint circumference of all 10 fingernails: the sum of the 10 ratios (NB:DIP) is the digital index, which is indicative of clubbing when it is greater than 10.2. The phalangeal depth ratio, or digital clubbing index (DI), using a caliper, measures the distal phalangeal depth (DPD) and the interphalangeal joint depth (IPD) of the second finger: a DPD/IPD ratio greater than 1 indicates clubbing (Figure 11.1). The phalangeal depth ratio method is best suited for assessing clubbing in children, where the measures can be easily obtained using plaster casts of a finger.[7]

The exact mechanism of the pathogenesis of clubbing is unknown. It results from the accumulation of connective tissues and increased vascularity between the matrix and the periostium. Clubbing may be congenital or acquired, monolateral, or bilateral. It can be isolated or part of the syndrome of hypertrophic osteoarthropathy (HOA), which includes periostosis of long bones, joint pain, and clubbing.

The list of diseases associated with this sign in children is listed in Table 11.2 and includes pulmonary, cardiac (Figure 11.2), gastrointestinal, infectious, and neoplastic diseases. Clubbing may also be idiopathic, when no cause is found. In this case, the patient's parents can be reassured of the benign nature of the condition. Acquired clubbing in children is usually due to lung diseases, and the degree

TABLE 11.1

Nail Signs Associated with Systemic Diseases and Drug Intake in Children

Nail Signs	Associations
Onychomadesis	Partum stress (neonatal onychomadesis)
	Febrile illness
	Infective diseases
	Hand, foot, and mouth disease
	Varicella
	KD
	Drugs:
	Carbamazepine
	Trimethoprim–sulfamethoxazole
	Valproic acid
	Deficiencies
	PEM
Beau's lines	Intrauterine distress (neonatal Beau's lines)
	Chronic urinary tract infections
	Drugs:
	Cancer chemotherapeutic agents
	Deficiencies
	Zinc
	PEM
Leukonychia	Kawasaki disease
	AIDS
	Increased blood strontium levels
	Drugs:
	Cancer chemotherapeutic agents
	Hydroxyurea
	Deficiencies
	Selenium
	Zinc
Nail fragility	Deficiencies
	Selenium
	PEM
	Anorexia nervosa
	Hypothyroidism
Koilonychia	Hemoglobin sickle cell disease
	Deficiencies
	Iron
Onycholysis	Drugs:
	Isotretinoin
Photo-onycholysis	Drugs:
	Doxycycline
Yellow nail syndrome	Nonimmune fetal hydrops
	Respiratory disorders
Melanonychia	Drugs:
	Doxorubicin
	Hydroxyurea
	Zidovudine
	Peutz–Jegher syndrome
Proximal nail fold capillary changes	Connective tissue diseases
	Rheumatic diseases
	Henoch–Schonlein purpura
	Insulin-dependent diabetes
Proximal splinter hemorrhages	Bacterial endocarditis

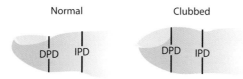

FIGURE 11.1 Determination of the digital clubbing index: distal phalangeal depth (DPD) and interphalangeal joint depth (IPD) of the second finger: a DPD/IPD ratio >1 indicates clubbing.

TABLE 11.2

Systemic Diseases That May Be Associated with Clubbing in Children

Bilateral

Cardiac diseases

  Cyanotic congenital heart diseases (up to 30% of affected children) (Martinez lavin)[a]

  Infective endocarditis

Circulatory diseases

  Abdominal arteriovenous fistula and polysplenia

Pulmonary arteriovenous malformations (up to 10% of affected patients)

Lung diseases

Asthma

Bronchiectasis

Chronic lung infections

Cystic fibrosis

Intrathoracic tumors[a]

  Primary ciliary dyskinesia

  Pulmonary hemangioma

Liver diseases

Biliary atresia[a]

Chronic liver disease

Hepatopulmonary syndrome with or without cirrhosis

Juvenile biliary cirrhosis

Wilson's diseases

Gastrointestinal diseases

Celiac disease

Gastrointestinal tumors

IBD

Polyposis coli

Infective diseases

  Chronic parasite infection (*Trichuris trichiura*, whipworm)

  HIV (cardiac and pulmonary complications secondary to AIDS)

Malignancies

Hodgkin's disease with intrathoracic involvement[a]

Mesothelioma of the pleura[a]

Nasopharyngeal carcinoma[a]

Osteosarcoma[a]

Periosteal sarcoma[a]

(Continued)

TABLE 11.2 (*Continued*)

Systemic Diseases That May Be Associated with Clubbing in
Children

Rabdomyosarcoma[a]

Thymus carcinoma[a]

Hyperthyroidism[a]

Severe malnutrition

Unilateral

Lower limb venous malformation

Klippel–Trenaunay syndrome

[a] May be associated with hypertrophic osteoarthropathy (HPOA).

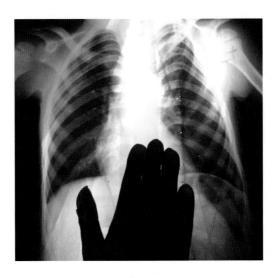

FIGURE 11.2   Clubbing in a child with tetralogy of Fallot. (Courtesy of Bronzetti G.)

of clubbing often parallels that of hypoxia, especially in subjects with cystic fibrosis, possibly reflecting the prolonged duration of hypoxemia.[8–10] The reversal of clubbing has been reported in children with cystic fibrosis, who had undergone lung transplantation, as soon as 3 months after surgery.[11] Clubbing is reported in 8.5% of children with hepatopulmonary syndrome associated with cirrhosis[12] and is less common in children with hepatopulmonary syndrome without cirrhosis. Clubbing is often present in children and adults with infective endocarditis and it has been suggested as a clinical sign to differentiate high-risk patients from low-risk patients on hospital admission.[13]

Digital clubbing is often part of the syndrome of HOA, which is characterized by periostosis of the long bones and occasional painful joint enlargement. HOA may be primary, with familial transmission as an autosomal-dominant trait, or secondary to different diseases. Secondary HOA is very rare in children and is typically considered to be a sign of pulmonary disease, but may also be related to a variety of inflammatory or neoplastic disorders (Figure 11.3).[14–16] When HOA is associated with neoplastic diseases involving the chest, it may precede pulmonary symptoms by 1–18 months and regresses after the successful treatment of the disorder of the chest, both in benign and malignant conditions. Paraneoplastic HOA in childhood accounts for not more than 12% of HOA patients.

In children with clubbing, a complete history and a physical examination will allow the clinician to narrow the differential diagnosis. A review of systems should focus on constitutional, pulmonary, gastrointestinal, and musculoskeletal symptoms for the evidence of malignancy, infection, or inflammation.[17–23]

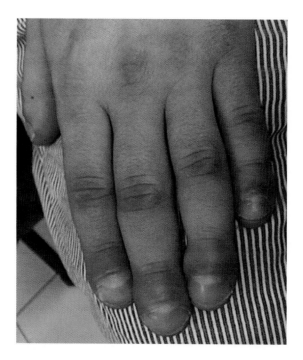

FIGURE 11.3 Clubbing and hypertrophic osteoarthropathy in a 17-year-old boy with Hodgkin's disease with inthrathoracic involvement.

Vasculitic Disorders

Kawasaki Disease

Kawasaki disease (KD) or mucocutaneous lymph node syndrome is an acute febrile systemic vasculitis of unknown etiology that involves small and medium-sized muscular arteries and typically affects young children. Nail changes are common and reversible and vary during the course of the disease. The most typical nail sign is an orange-brown transverse chromonychia of all 20 nails, which is seen in up to 75% of the cases and starts to appear between the fifth and eighth day of the onset of fever, characterizing the subacute phase of KD.[24,25] The discoloration is better appreciated in the fingernails, involves the distal half or third of the nail and migrates distally as the nails grow, disappearing after 2–4 weeks. Dermoscopy shows that the orange color is due to NB erythema and closely spaced splinter hemorrhages,[26] confirming the presence of morphologic alterations in the cutaneous microcirculation reported in KD by laser Doppler flowmetry and dynamic capillaroscopy.[27] Orange-brown chromonychia may be associated with onycholysis and in some cases is replaced by a transient leukonychia. Leukonychia striata has been described independently of orange-brown chromonychia and may be partial, with discoloration localized to the proximal part of the nail.[28] Periungual desquamation of fingers and toes is the most common nail sign: it appears after the chromonychia and may be followed by Beau's lines or onychomadesis (Figure 11.4). Nail degloving is exceptional.[29] Acquired pincer nail deformity, with transverse curling of the nail along the longitudinal axis, is rare.[30] Ischemic necrosis of the extremities is a rare complication due to thrombosed aneurysms that is in turn caused by vasculitis.[31]

Henoch–Schonlein Purpura

Henoch–Schonlein purpura (HSP), also know as anaphylactoid purpura, the most common systemic vasculitis of childhood, primarily affects the skin, gastrointestinal tract, kidneys, and joints. Manifested by a characteristic rash on the buttocks and lower limbs, the course of HSP is typically a benign one but may be accompanied by varying degrees of abdominal pain, arthritis, or arthralgia, gastrointestinal

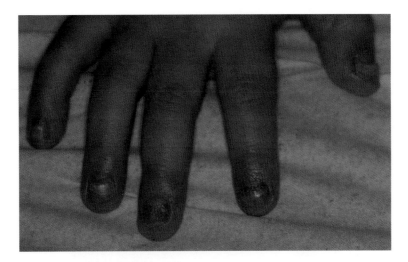

FIGURE 11.4   Onychomadesis following KD.

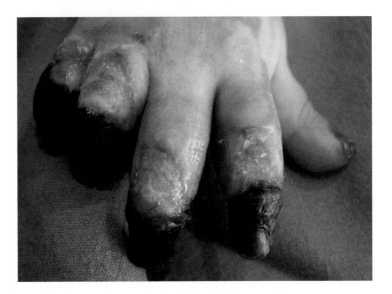

FIGURE 11.5   Gangrene of the distal digits and the nail apparatus in PF following invasive meningococcal disease.

bleeding, and glomerulonephritis. Two studies evaluated the morphology of proximal nail fold capillaries in children with HSP during the acute onset and several months later, and compared them with healthy controls.[32,33] Capillaroscopy features in the acute phase of HSP were statistically significant in comparison with healthy controls, even if they were not specific, consisting of moderate to massive edema and reduced capillary density, with disarranged capillaries of abnormal shape and length. The follow-up results were different in the two series, as capillary changes were still present in the follow-up in one study,[11] whereas they were normalized in the second, with only edema still present after 6 months.[12]

Purpura Fulminans

Purpura fulminans (PF) is a life-threatening hematologic emergency in which there is skin necrosis and disseminated intravascular coagulation. The pathogenesis involves acute transient decreases in proteins C and S or antithrombin III levels. In children, the PF usually follows a bacterial or viral illness (due to meningococci, group A streptococci, pneumococci, and varicella virus) and usually begins 7–10 days after the onset of the infection. The circumscribed ecchymosis of skin and the symmetrical gangrene of the extremities (Figure 11.5) are typical features of the PF, which is associated with a mortality rate of 20%–25%. The treatment of cutaneous necrosis and distal ischemia is difficult and still controversial: antithrombin, protein C, tissue plasminogen activator, and vasodilator infusion have no proven efficacy. Although survival in PF is not dependent on surgery and surgery plays a key role in the early phase of the disease, early surgical consultation to assess if limb perfusion can be improved to achieve limb salvage is still absolutely necessary.[34]

Respiratory Disorders

Yellow Nail Syndrome

Yellow nail syndrome (YNS) is a rare disorder characterized by the triad: yellow nails, respiratory problems, and lymphedema. The three features are not always present together and the diagnosis can be done when two of them are present and even nail changes alone can be enough for diagnosis. The pathogenesis is unknown. The possible hypothesis that anatomic/functional lymphatic abnormalities may be a cause of the disease might explain lymphedema and pleural effusions, but not the other respiratory manifestations. Nail signs diagnostic for YNS are arrested or slowed nail growth rate, nail plate thickening, lack of cuticles, yellow–green discoloration, and increased transverse curvature of the nail plate. The cuticles are absent and the proximal nail fold is swollen, the nail plate is thickened, hard, and opaque, and increased transverse curvature leads to onycholysis, with the possible shedding of the nail (Figure 11.6).

YNS in children is extremely rare and has been described as a congenital or acquired disease. Congenital YNS, transmitted as autosomal dominant or recessive trait, is often associated with other anomalies, including nonimmune fetal hydrops, facial dysmorphism, mental retardation, seizures, inguinal hernia, deafness, cutis marmorata, and eye changes.[35–37] A case of neonatal nail changes suggestive for YNS with no evidence of respiratory manifestations or lymphedema or other abnormalities has also been reported.[38] Congenital YNS has also been reported in siblings, associated[39] or not with mental retardation.[40]

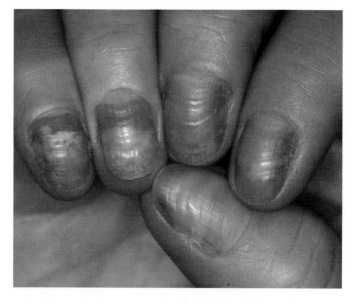

FIGURE 11.6 Yellow nail syndrome in a 15-year-old girl with bronchiectasis and lymphedema. The nails are slow growing, with absent cuticles, yellow discoloration, and transverse hypercurvature that causes onycholysis.

The few cases that received therapy with vitamin E did not achieve success,[40] which was reported in an 8-year-old girl treated with vitamin E associated with fluconazole.[41]

Gastrointestinal Disorders

Celiac Disease (Celiac Sprue)

Celiac disease (CD) or gluten-sensitive enteropathy is an autoimmune chronic disorder of the digestive tract that results in an inability to tolerate gliadin, the alcohol-soluble fraction of gluten. Tissue transglutaminase seems to be the predominant autoantigen both in the intestine and in the skin. Estimates suggest that approximately 1% of the population is affected by CD, with bimodal age distribution: the first at 8–12 months and the second in the third to fourth decades. The mean age at diagnosis is 8.4 years (range, 1–17 years).

Symptoms of classic CD include chronic diarrhea, steatorrhea, abdominal pain, and distension; weight loss, anorexia, and nutritional deficiencies, particularly of iron, folate, calcium, and vitamin D. Children have more severe symptoms than adults. Among extraintestinal manifestations, several cutaneous symptoms are described, the most common presentation being dermatitis herpetiformis, which affects 15%–25% of the patients. Other findings are xerosis, keratosis pilaris, and pallor of skin and mucosae. Nail changes are reported in 10%–20% of children and include the manifestation of iron or zinc deficiencies, such as brittle nails and koilonychia (Figure 11.7), and other symptoms such as leukonychia, the pathogenesis of which is more difficult to explain. Acquired generalized clubbing was seen in 15% of children with CD in a series of 55 cases and was considered indicative of malnutrition.[42]

Inflammatory Bowel Disease

Clubbing has been reported in children with Crohn's disease and ulcerative colitis[43] and may be an indicator of disease activity.[44] Clubbing development was preceded by multiple pyogenic granulomas of the NB in one 17-year-old girl.[45]

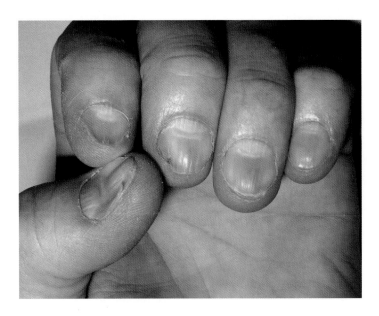

FIGURE 11.7   Koilonychia (spoon nails) in a 17-year-old boy with celiac disease.

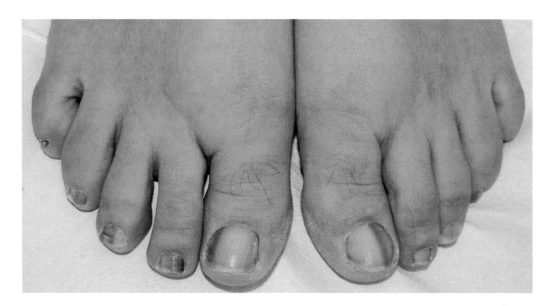

FIGURE 11.8   Longitudinal melanonychia of several nails in a child with Peutz–Jeghers syndrome.

Children with inflammatory bowel diseases (IBDs) have an increased risk of venous and arterial thromboembolism, with a prevalence between 1.3% and 3.3%.[46] Visceral venous thromboses are the most common. Of the 24 reported cases of children with thromboembolism in limbs, all were venous, except for one child with an arterial thromboembolism of a finger, leading to gangrene.[47]

Peutz–Jeghers Syndrome

Peutz–Jeghers syndrome is an autosomal dominant inherited polyposis syndrome, caused by a germline mutation in the *STK11* (LKB1) gene, in which multiple polyps in the gastrointestinal tract are associated with mucocutaneous pigmentation. Mucocutaneous pigmented lesions are seen in around 95% of patients and may be the first clue to diagnosis.[48] Lesions consist of clusters of small, 1–5 mm melanocytic macules around the mouth, nostrils, perianal area, fingers, and toes, and the dorsal and volar aspects of hands and feet. Longitudinal melanonychia of several nails may be seen (Figure 11.8). While cutaneous lesions may fade after puberty, oral–buccal mucosal pigmentation is usually permanent.

Liver Disorders

Cirrhosis

Clubbing of all digits associated with onycholysis, nail plate surface abnormalities, and leukonychia were reported in a 6-year-old girl with cirrhosis. Liver transplantation induced complete regression of nail changes.[49]

Spontaneous Liver Cell Adenoma

Liver tumors are very rare in children, being 1%–4% of all pediatric tumors. Among them, hepatocellular adenoma accounts for about 20% of the benign tumors. The mean age at diagnosis is around 14 years, and type I glycogen storage disease (von Gierke's disease) is a predisposing factor. Generalized osteoporosis, urticaria, and koilonychia were reported as unusual findings in a series of five children with liver cell adenoma.[50]

Wilson's Disease (Hepatolenticular Degeneration)

Wilson's disease (WD) is an autosomal recessive disorder in which copper pathologically accumulates primarily within the liver and subsequently in the neurological system and other tissues. The causative gene, *ATP7B*, encodes a copper-transporting P-type adenosine triphosphatase (ATPase).

Excess copper can damage almost all organs and lead to symptoms of WD. About 70% of children with WD have skin, mucosal, or nail signs, including xerosis, cheilitis, and pigmentation of the palate. A series of 37 children with WD reported nail changes, which was in about 24% of the children, including leukonychia, onychodystrophy, pitting, and clubbing.[51] The most striking nail finding of WD, i.e., blue (azure) lunulae of the fingernails, due to dermal copper deposits, have not been reported in children.

Renal Disorders

Hemodialysis

Nail changes are common in patients in hemodialysis, both in children and in adults, being reported in up to 75% of the patients, independently by age.[52–54] Nail changes are significantly more common in uremic children on hemodialysis than in controls.[54] Half and half nails (Lindsay's nails) are the most typical sign seen in about 20%–30% of the patients, especially in diabetics. Half and half nails are a variety of apparent leukonychia where the proximal area of the nail is dull white and the distal area (20%–60% of the total length) is pink or reddish brown, with a distinct border between the two colors (Figure 11.9). Other nail changes seen in hemodialysis patients include absence of lunulae, koilonychia, nail thinning, nail striation, Beau's lines, onycholysis, subungual hyperkeratosis, Mees' lines, Muehrcke's lines, and splinter hemorrhages. Mees' lines appear as one or several parallel transverse white bands of true leukonychia affecting all nails at the same level and moving distally with the nail growth. Muehrcke's lines are a variety of apparent leukonychia, where the nail has multiple transverse whitish bands, parallel to the lunula (Figure 11.10).

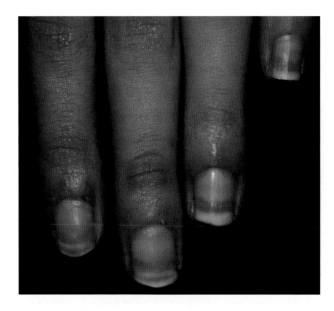

FIGURE 11.9 Half and half nails in a uremic child on hemodialysis: the proximal area of the nail is white and the distal area is red.

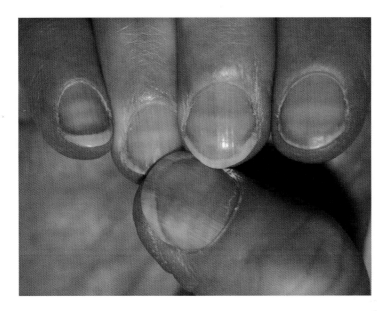

FIGURE 11.10 Muehrcke's lines in a 17-year-old girl who underwent renal transplantation: the nails show two to three transverse whitish bands, parallel to the lunula.

Nail Changes in Renal Transplant Recipients

A study on 302 kidney transplant patients, which included children above the age of 11, found nail changes in about 40% of the patients.[55] Muehrcke's line (seen in 4.3% of the patients) and true leukonychia (punctate or subtotal, seen in 3.6%) had a higher prevalence, compared with the controls, and their presence was independent by age. All patients were not under steroid medication and the presence of Muehrcke's lines was explained by NB edema not decreased by corticosteroids. The presence of true leukonychia was not significantly related to age, sex, duration of transplantation, or immunosuppressive regimens. In another case series, 2 of 32 children presented pigmented transverse bands of the toenails caused by uremia while 34% showed lamellar onychoschizia.[56]

End-Stage Renal Disease

Calciphylaxis, or calcific uremic arteriolopathy, is a rare but highly morbid disorder of vascular calcification and skin necrosis, affecting 1%–4% of the population with end-stage renal disease (ESRD). It results from mural calcium deposits in small- and/or medium-sized vessels located in the dermis and subcutaneous fat, leading to vascular occlusion and tissue ischemia and is usually seen in uremic patients with secondary hyperparathyroidism.[57] Calciphylaxis in children is extremely rare and clinically different compared with adults as it involved the distal and acral parts of the skin, with acral calciphylaxis indicating a worse prognosis. Among the few cases reported in the literature, two had digital gangrene of the toes that, in one case, led to amputation.[57,58]

Endocrine Disorders

Diabetes

Capillaroscopy of the proximal nail fold may be used to detect microangiopathy in diabetic patients and could be a useful tool to detect the early changes of microangiopathy in children with diabetes type 1, being seen in about 30% of the cases.[59] The typical capillaroscopy features of diabetic children are an increase in the number of capillaries, with abnormal capillaries in irregular distribution, related to the prolonged time course of diabetes, megacapillaries, and deformed loops, which increase in relation to mean values of HbA1c, and intense red background.[60] The presence of an increased number of irregularly shaped capillary is considered a consequence of decreased baseline perfusion. Avascular areas are more common in patients with type 1 diabetes complications and indicate microvascular disease (retinopathy or microalbuminuria), while microhemorrhages are common in children with recently elevated HbA1c.[61]

Prevention of skin ulceration in adulthood may be done by appropriate education of children with diabetes to proper foot care and by treating biomechanical foot abnormalities. A large study evaluating foot care and frequency of foot problems in more than 500 children and adolescents with type I and II diabetes revealed poor toenail care as the most common feature, with long toenails and bitten/picked toenails.[62] Ingrown toenail was another common finding, seen in 2.8% of the cases, and was related to the body mass index (BMI) *z*-score.

Parathyroid Disease

Pseudohypoparathyroidism is a heterogeneous group of disorders characterized by hypocalcemia, hyperphosphatemia, increased serum concentration of parathyroid hormone (PTH), and insensitivity to the biologic activity of PTH. Typical clinical features include short stature, rounded face, shortened fourth metacarpals and other bones of the hands and feet, obesity, dental hypoplasia, and soft-tissue calcifications/ossifications. Brachydactyly, broad thumb, and nail pitting were reported in a child with pseudohypoparathyroidism and visual disturbances.[63]

Pituitary Disease

Sotos syndrome (SS, MIM#117550), also known as cerebral gigantism, is a prenatal and postnatal over-growth syndrome characterized by excessive growth resulting in tall stature and macrocephaly, distinctive craniofacial features, and developmental delay. Three of twenty-two adolescent patients with SS were found to have thin and brittle nails.[64]

Thyroid Disease

Brittle nails are a typical finding of hypothyroidism. The nails are dry, brittle, may have longitudinal and transverse striations (Figure 11.11), and are dull in appearance. Slow nail growth rate and oncholysis are other possible symptoms.[65,66] Brittle nails and slow nail growth are also present in congenital hypothyroidism.[67]

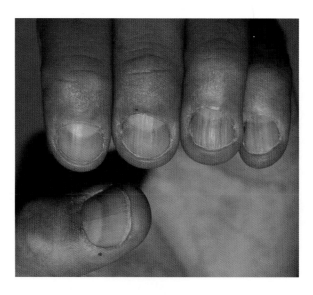

FIGURE 11.11 A 13-year-old child with hypothyroidism: the nails are thin, brittle with longitudinal striations.

Plummer's nails are considered a typical sign of hyperthyroidisms: the nails are onycholytic with an upward distal edge. They are reported in 5% of adult patients with hyperthyroidism, but in children the reports are very scarce.[68] In the same way, there are few data on the prevalence of thyroid acropachy in children with hyperthyroidism. Thyroid acropachy is a triad consisting of digital clubbing, soft-tissue swelling of the hands and feet, and periosteal new bone formation.[69]

Hematological and Lymphatic Disorders

Anemia

Iron deficiency with decreased red blood cells (RBC) production is the most common cause of anemia in children and adolescents (see section "Iron Deficiency").

Dyskeratosis Congenita

Dyskeratosis congenita (DC) is a multisystem inherited syndrome characterized by mucocutaneous abnormalities, bone marrow failure, and a predisposition to cancer. Mode of inheritance includes autosomal dominant, autosomal recessive, and X-linked recessive. Reticular hyperpigmentation of the skin and nail changes usually appear first, often below the age of 10 and then bone marrow failure develops frequently below the age of 20, with up to 80% of patients showing signs of bone marrow failure by the age of 30. Mucosal leukoplakia is a pathognomonic feature and occurs in approximately 80% of patients. Nail abnormalities include longitudinal splitting and ridging, nail thinning, and nail atrophy (Figure 11.12).[70,71] These lichenoid changes may resemble the nail signs seen in graft versus host disease (GVHD).[72]

Langerhans Cell Histiocytosis

Langerhans cell histiocytosis (LCH) is a dendritic cell histiocytosis and the most common of the histiocytic disorders. Most often children are affected, with a peak incidence of 0.2–1.0/100,000

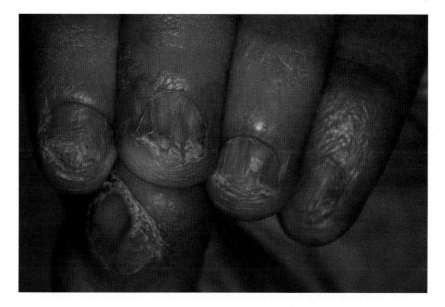

FIGURE 11.12 Dyskeratosis congenita in a 9-year-old boy: the nails are thinned, with multiple longitudinal striations and fissures, resembling lichen planus and graft-versus-host disease. Note multiple viral warts of the digits due to immunodepression.

children per year from 1 to 4 years of age.[73] LCH encompasses a number of diseases, including the acute, fulminant, disseminated Letterer–Siwe disease, the solitary or few, indolent and chronic lesions of bone or other organs called eosinophilia granulomas (EG), and the intermediate clinical form called Hand–Schuller–Christian disease, characterized by multifocal, chronic involvement with the triad of exophthalmos, diabetes insipidus, and calvarial lytic lesions. More than 60% of patients have single-system disease, which mostly involves bone, skin, or lymph nodes. Fingernails and toenails are rarely affected.

Nail changes involve all/several nails and include onycholysis with redness of the nail plate, subungual hyperkeratosis with hemorrhages, and pustule formation or cheesy discharge.[74] Other possible symptoms include periungual inflammation with paronychia, helkonyxis,[75] purpuric striae,[76] and onycholysis.[77] Severe pulmonary involvement maybe associated with clubbing.[78] Nail lesions may precede the onset of other symptoms of LCH.[79–81] Histologically, nail lesions have the same characteristics of skin lesions and not always regress with therapy.[82] In other cases, nail changes regress with treatment but recur when the disease progresses.[83] For these reasons, nail involvement is considered a bad prognostic sign, also because nail changes occur in patients with multisystem disease and involvement of high-risk organs.[80] However, there is little evidence about the use of nail involvement as an independent prognostic marker.

Connective Tissue Disorders

Nail fold capillaroscopy visualizes the capillary network and is a noninvasive painless technique. Capillaroscopy examinations of healthy persons, including children and adolescents, show a homogeneous, ordered distribution of capillaries, which are located in parallel, at regular distances, displaying narrow distances between ascending and descending arms. The shape of regular capillaries resembles the letter "U" upside down or a hairpin, with a narrower arterial arm, an upper part, and a venous arm, the latter larger than the arterial one. The median linear capillary density in healthy children is 6.7 capillaries/mm (range 5.3–9.3), with younger children having fewer capillaries.[84,85] Young control children of preschool age have evenly distributed, wide capillaries with many tortuous, bizarre shapes, compared with adults.

The most common capillary abnormalities include (1) alteration of density, with loss of capillaries and/or avascular areas, (2) alteration of capillary length (normal values 200–500 microns), (3) alteration of shape, with tortuous or branched capillary loops, giant or bushy capillaries, (4) alteration of arrangement, where capillaries are not in parallel rows but disarranged, and (5) presence of microhemorrhages. Capillary abnormalities can be seen in several diseases of different etiology, but they are typical of autoimmune rheumatic diseases, where capillary changes are similar to those seen in adults. The so-called scleroderma (SD) pattern, characterized by the presence of avascular areas and enlarged or giant loops, is diagnostic of several connective tissue diseases and is seen in about 50% of children with mixed connective tissue disease (MCTD) and in 90% of children with systemic SD.[85,86] A follow-up study on nail fold capillaroscopy in 150 children and adolescents with primary Raynaud phenomenon showed that the presence of sclerodermatous type of capillary changes has a high prognostic value of development SD spectrum disorders.[87] In childhood systemic lupus erythematosus (SLE), capillaroscopy shows major capillary abnormalities in 35% of the patients, without a specific pattern (Figure 11.13a and b).[88]

Gottron's papules, corresponding to symmetric, pink to violaceous, raised or macular areas on the dorsal aspect of metacarpophalangeal and interphalangeal joints, elbows, patellae, and medial malleoli are seen in 60%–80% of children and are pathognomonic of dermatomyositis (DM). Among the highly characteristic skin lesions of DM there is also the grossly visible periungual telangiectasia with or without dystrophic cuticles[89] (Figure 14a). Capillaroscopy of children with juvenile dermatomyositis shows the SD pattern in approximately 60% of the patients (Figure 14b), and the intensity of the morphological changes correlates with the clinical course.[85,86,90,91]

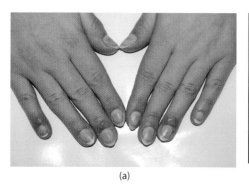
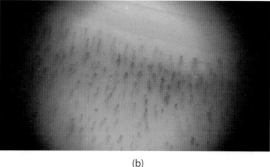

FIGURE 11.13 Systemic lupus erythematosus in a 13-year-old girl showing periungual inflammation (a) that at capillaroscopy (b) reveals edema and dilated tortuous capillary vessels.

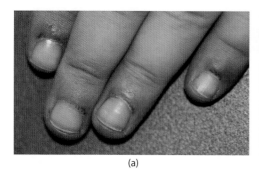
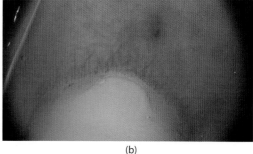

FIGURE 11.14 Juvenile dermatomyositis in a 7-year-old girl: periungual telangiectasia of the fingernails (a), associated with SD pattern capillary changes at capillaroscopy (b).

Immunological Disorders

Primary Immunodeficiency Disorders

Primary immunodeficiency disorders (PID) refer to a large heterogeneous group of rare disorders characterized by poor or absent function in one or more components of the immune system. Most PIDs result from inherited defects in immune system development and/or function; however, acquired forms have also been described. PIDs can be divided into disorders of adaptive immunity, which include T-cell and B-cell immunodeficiencies and combined (B- and T-cell) immunodeficiency disorders and disorders of innate immunity, which include phagocyte defects and complement defects. Most disorders involve at least an increased susceptibility to infections. Nail changes often are due to fungal infections, due to *Candida*, and due to dermatophytes.[92,93] In chronic mucocutaneous candidiasis, persistent and/or recurrent candidiasis of the skin, nails, and mucous membranes is typical (Figure 11.15), and the nails are the initial target of the infection.[94] Other nail abnormalities can be due to associated autoimmune phenomena, as in the case of trachyonychia reported in a child with selective IgA deficiency.[95]

Graft versus Host Disease

GVHD is an immune-mediated disease that often develops after allogeneic hematopoietic-cell transplantation and results from the interaction between donor and recipient adaptive immunity. Chronic GVHD in children is associated with 41% mortality and usually develops after the third month posttransplant, with the skin as the most commonly affected organ. Nail changes occur in half of the children, and are more

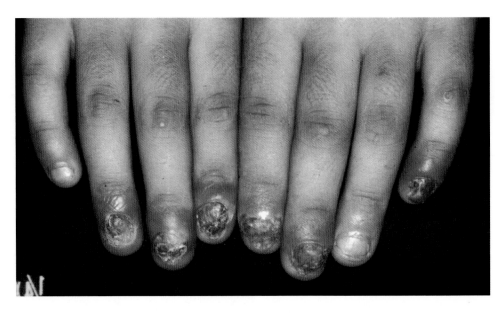

FIGURE 11.15 Candida onychomycosis in a 9-year-old child with chronic mucocutaneous candidiasis: nail invasion with nail plate damage and subungual hyperkeratosis is associated with periungual inflammation.

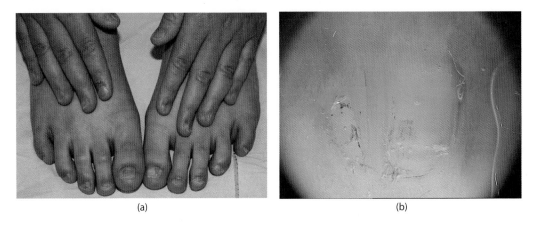

(a)   (b)

FIGURE 11.16 GVHD in an 8-year-old boy: the nails are thinned with multiple longitudinal striations and some show dorsal pterygium (a). Dermoscopy of dorsal pterygium (b) shows the scarring that produces a V-shaped extension of the proximal nail fold that divides the nail plate in two parts.

common in the sclerotic variant of GVHD, where they are detected in two-thirds of the patients.[96] Nail abnormalities may appear before the development of GVHD. Dorsal pterygium, longitudinal ridging, and distal splitting of the fingernails are the typical features (Figure 11.16a and b). Nail involvement, together with persistent peripheral edema and persistent peripheral eosinophilia, is considered a bad prognostic sign, as patients with nail dystrophy are more likely to have steroid-resistant disease and lung GVHD.

Orthopedic and Rheumatologic Disorders

Chronic Recurrent Multifocal Osteomyelitis

Chronic recurrent multifocal osteomyelitis (CRMO) is an autoinflammatory bone disease occurring primarily in children and adolescents, characterized by the insidious onset of pain with swelling and tenderness over the affected bones. The clavicle and the metaphyses and epiphyses of long bones are the

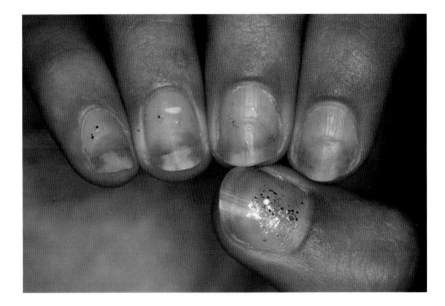

FIGURE 11.17 Chronic recurrent multifocal osteomyelitis in an 8-year-old girl: the nail shows onycholysis with erythematous border and Beau's lines. (Courtesy of Blume-Peytavi U).

most frequently affected. Some authors believe that CRMO is the pediatric presentation of synovitis, acne, pustulosis, hyperostosis, osteitis (SAPHO).[97] Skin changes are uncommon and include psoriasis and palmoplantar pustulosis[98] (Figure 11.17). A case of a 9-year-old girl with psoriasiform lesions of the soles and nails, consisting of periungual inflammation, onycholysis, and subungual hyperkeratosis with salmon patches of the NB and pitting has recently been described. Nail lesions improved with oral methotrexate therapy (15 mg/week).[99]

Adult-Onset Still Disease

Splinter hemorrhages of the nails were present in two adolescents with a febrile illness associated with an urticarial rash with linear dermatographism that flared during fever spikes and severe malaise, myalgia, arthralgia, and leukocytosis. These patients were difficult to diagnose as the clinical and laboratory findings were consistent for an adult-onset Still disease or systemic juvenile idiopathic arthritis sine arthritis.[100]

Infective Disorders

Human Immunodeficiency Virus Infection

Skin and mucosal conditions are extremely common in human immunodeficiency virus (HIV)-infected children, especially in those with CD4 count below 200 cells/mm³. Nail changes may be due to opportunistic fungal infections, especially due to *Candida*, with total onychomycosis often associated with periungual inflammation. Extensive *Trichophyton rubrum* infection of the skin with onychomycosis of the fingernails and toenails is also reported.[101] Other infective conditions that involve the nails and that are more common and more severe in HIV-infected than in healthy children include severe herpetic whitlow, periungual warts (Figure 11.18),[102] and Norwegian scabies. Nail symptoms may also be due to the drugs used to cure HIV infection (see Chapter 6 on drug-induced nail diseases). Other nail signs described in children with acquired immunodeficiency syndrome (AIDS) include transitory transverse leukonychia[103] and finger clubbing, which is reported in 9% of the cases[104] and is related to cardiac and pulmonary complications associated with HIV infection.

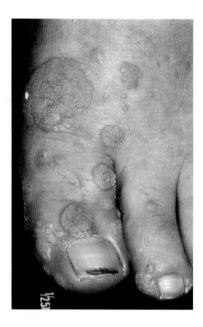

FIGURE 11.18   Multiple human papilloma virus (HPV)–induced periungual warts in an HIV-infected 15-year-old boy.

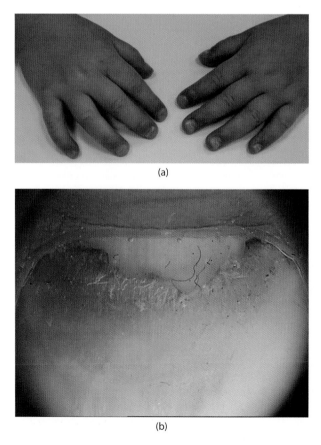

FIGURE 11.19   Onychomadesis of several nails after HFMD (a). Dermoscopy shows the detachment of the proximal nail plate that follows a transient arrest of nail growth (b).

Hand, Foot, and Mouth Disease

Hand, foot, and mouth disease (HFMD) is a viral illness caused by various strains of enterovirus type A, most commonly coxsackie virus A16 and enterovirus 71 (EV71), which typically occur in children less than 10 years of age. Beau's lines and, more commonly, onychomadesis of several/all nails (Figure 11.19a and b) are a common sequela, being reported in several epidemics and in single-case reports.[105] Onychomadesis appears 30–50 days from the onset of HFMD and is followed by nail shedding and complete regrowth of the nail as normal. The reason for the high frequency of onychomadesis after HFMD is not explained: Onychomadesis is not rare in children after viral illnesses[106] and is considered to be due to the systemic sufferance related to the disease. In 2009, a coxsackie virus was isolated both from the vesicle fluids and also in a fragment of shedded nail, suggesting the theory that virus replication may directly damage the nail matrix resulting in temporary arrest of nail growth.[107]

Deficiencies

Deficiency disorders are uncommon in modern industrialized societies where nutritional supplementation of foodstuff is common. However, they may still manifest in vulnerable population, such as infants.

Nail fragility is the most common sign of nutritional deficiencies, especially those due to low protein intake, such as protein energy malnutrition (PEM) (marasmus and kwashiorkor), where the nails are soft, thin, brittle, slow glowing, and often show Beau's lines and onychomadesis,[108] and anorexia nervosa, where nail fragility may be associated with other symptoms.[109,110]

Iron Deficiency

Iron deficiency is not unusual in children, with the highest prevalence in toddlers and adolescents because the increment in hemoglobin per unit body weight is greatest at these ages. The most common nail sign of iron deficiency anemia is koilonychia, reported in about 2% of anemic children.[111] Mild-to-moderate nail pallor is another common finding that, however, is considered less sensitive than conjunctival pallor for screening purposes.[112] NB pallor is 85% sensitive and 41% specific in identifying parasitemic children with acute anemia who need antimalarial treatment.[113]

Selenium

Leukonychia can be a sign of selenium deficiency, which may affect patients who are maintained for long periods through parenteral nutrition and/or enteral nutrition with either reduced or no dose of selenium. Nail discoloration resolves when selenium levels return to normal.[114] In a case series on 95 children, nail whitening associated with hair browning, macrocytemia, and cardiac dysfunction was seen in three of five patients with serum levels of selenium below 2 μm/dL.[115]

Zinc Deficiency

Zinc deficiency can be genetic, as in acrodermatitis enteropathica, or acquired. Acrodermatitis entheropathica (AE) is a rare autosomal recessive disorder due to mutation of the gene *SLC39A4* (solute carrier family 39 [zinc transporter], member 4) on chromosome 8q24.3, which encodes for the Zip4 intestinal zinc transporter. The mutation induces the inability to absorb sufficient zinc. The clinical features are growth retardation, immune system dysfunction, alopecia, severe dermatitis, diarrhea, and occasionally mental disorders. Symptoms typically manifest when the child is weaned from breast milk and are characterized by the typical triad of diarrhea, acral, and periorificial dermatitis and alopecia. When the fingers and toes are involved, there is marked erythema and swelling of the periungual tissues, Beau's

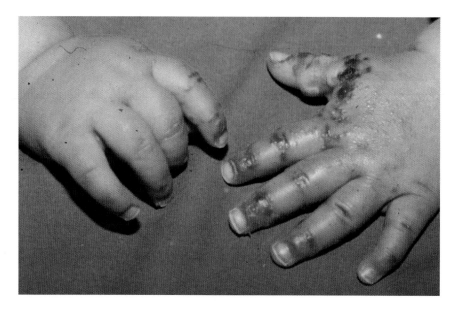

FIGURE 11.20 Acrodermatitis entheropathica in a young child: periungual inflammatory changes with bullae.

lines, and often onycholysis and subungual hyperkeratosis. Periungual formation of bullae is also possible (Figure 11.20).

In children and adolescents, acquired zinc deficiency can result from decreased dietary intake, due to low breast milk zinc levels, anorexia nervosa, total parenteral nutrition, or diet high in cereal grains and low in meats. Low breast milk zinc results from zinc deficiency in the mother or from an inherited mutation in the *SLC30A2* gene, which encodes the transporter responsible for secreting zinc into human breast milk (MIM609617).[116] Premature infants are at risk of zinc deficiency because of high metabolic demand from rapid growth, inadequate stores, poor absorption, and increased urinary and fecal losses. Zinc deficiency can also be one of the presenting signs of cystic fibrosis.

Nail signs of zinc deficiency include paronychia and slow nail growth.[117] Muehrcke's lines, onychorrhexis, leukonychia, and Beau's lines have also been described in these children.[118]

Neurological Disorders

Carpal Tunnel Syndrome

Carpal tunnel syndrome (CTS) during childhood is very rare and often has an unusual presentation. Causes of CTS in infancy may be hereditary, as in primary familial CTS, or genetic, especially lysosomal storage diseases such as mucopolysaccaridosis.[119] Individuals with Down's syndrome are at a greater risk of developing CTS. Other less common causes of CTS in children include intensive sports practice (golf, weight lifting, and basketball), traumas, and local tumors.[119] Idiopathic CTS has also been reported.[120]

Diagnosis of CTS in children is often delayed, as they have modest complaints such as clumsiness and/or weakness, wrist or hand pain, thenar atrophy, and thenar weakness. Moreover, children often are too young to communicate their problem. Cutaneous manifestations secondary to the sensory and autonomic damage of the median nerve fibers are rare, unilateral, and associated with long-standing severe cases. They typically involve the index, middle, or ring fingers and present as nonhealing ulcers

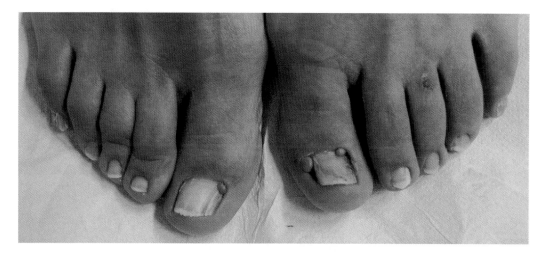

FIGURE 11.21 Tuberous sclerosis in a 14-year-old girl: Koenen's tumors (fibrokeratomas) of the proximal nail fold of several digits appearing as pink nodules associated with longitudinal furrows of the nail plate due to nail matrix compression.

and various types of nail dystrophies, including Beau's lines, nail thickening, and striate leukonychia. Shortening of the distal phalanges due to acroosteolysis is extremely rare.[121]

Congenital Insensitivity to Pain

Congenital insensitivity to pain with anhidrosis, or hereditary sensory and autonomic neuropathy type IV (MIM 256800), is a rare autosomal recessive disorder characterized by a decrease in the number of myelinated and nonmyelinated nerve fibers of peripheral nerves, which causes diminished or absent pain sensation leading to increase in self-mutilative habits. The most important characteristic of the disease is the self-mutilating behavior that leads the child to oral ulcerations on lips, tongue, and cheeks, self-extraction of teeth, and also finger and hand biting. Severe biting injuries of the fingertips appear at the time of tooth eruption and include nail and pulp injuries with skin scarring and finger mutilations.[122]

Tuberous Sclerosis

Tuberous sclerosis (TS) complex is an autosomal dominant, neurocutaneous, multisystem disorder characterized by cellular hyperplasia and tissue dysplasia. Skin changes include hypomelanotic macules, facial angiofibromas, shagreen patches, fibrous facial plaques, and ungual fibromas. The major diagnostic criteria are nontraumatic ungual or periungual fibromas (Koenen tumors). Koenen tumors develop in up to 50% of cases of TS, with the onset occurring around puberty. They are more common in the toenails and usually arise from the proximal nail fold, appearing as pink filiform or nodular skin-colored masses. Compression of the underlying nail matrix produces a longitudinal groove in the nail plate (Figure 11.21).

Psychiatric Disorders

Anorexia Nervosa and Other Eating Disorders

Anorexia and bulimia nervosa are common in female adolescents and young adults between 15 and 24 years and are typically associated with skin changes.[109,110,123] Cutaneous signs resulting from malnutrition include xerosis, diffuse hypertricosis, acrocianosis, perniosis, telogen effluvium, and brittle nails

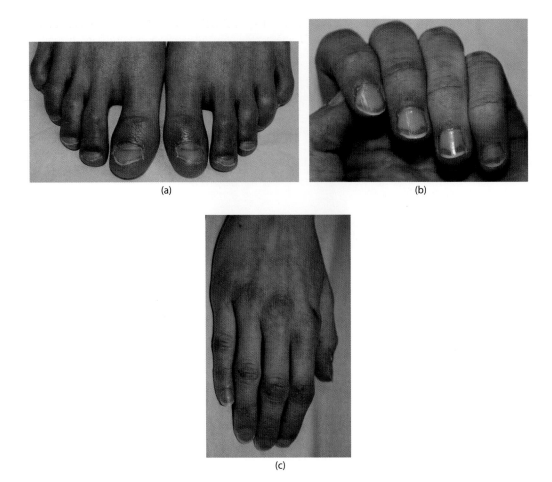

FIGURE 11.22 Anorexia nervosa in a 16-year-old girl: (a) nail fragility and acrocianosis of the toes, (b) half and half nails, and (c) excoriations of the dorsum of the hand (Russell's sign).

(Figure 11.22a), reported in about 30% of the cases. Other reported nail signs include longitudinal striae, onychocryptosis, and periungual erythema (Figure 11.22b). Skin signs caused by self-induced vomit include erosions, scars, and calluses on the dorsal surface of the dominant hand (Figure 11.22c), mainly located at the base of the third digit (Russell's sign, knuckle calluses). Other skin changes may be related to concomitant drug consumption or self-aggressing behaviors, which are seen very often in young patients with eating disorders. Among the latter, severe onychophagia is common.

Drug-Induced Nail Changes

Reports of drug-induced nail changes in children are uncommon and mainly related to the same classes of drugs reported to cause nail signs in adults. Drug-induced nail changes usually involve several or all 20 nails and appear in temporal correlation with drug intake. Nail abnormalities may result from toxicity to the matrix, the NB, or the periungual tissues or acute damages to the nail blood vessels. Some drugs may also deposit in the NB. Drug-induced nail abnormalities are usually transitory and disappear with drug withdrawal, but sometimes persist over time. Some nail changes are asymptomatic and only cause cosmetic problems, while others cause pain and discomfort.

Cancer chemotherapeutic agents are reported to induce nail changes in about 10% of the children.[124] Nail signs caused by chemotherapy in children include Beau's lines, trachyonychia, and different types of leukonychia, i.e., Mees' line Muehrcke's lines and half and half nails.[124–126] Transverse, longitudinal, or total melanonychia may also occur.[127,128] Chemotherapy with Adriamycin (doxorubicin), bleomycin, vinblastine, and dacarbazine (ABVD) for Hodgkin's lymphoma may induce hemorrhagic painful onycholysis with NB erosions (Figure 11.23).

Longitudinal or total melanonychia, sometimes associated with skin hyperpigmentation, is a common side effect of hydroxyurea in children, being reported in up to 10% of thalassemic children receiving the drug (Figure 11.24).[129] Other nail signs due to hydroxyurea in children include leukonychia and nail ridging.[130]

Longitudinal melanonychia is also reported in up to 5% of HIV children treated with zidovudine.[131,132]

Another common nail sign associated with drug intake in children is onychomadesis: single-case reports describe its occurrence after the intake of carbamazepine,[133] trimethoprim–sulfamethoxazole,[134] and valproic acid.[135] Onychomadesis has also been reported following an allergic reaction to penicillin in a 23-month-old child.[136]

Other nail signs due to drugs reported in children include periungual pyogenic granulomas due to isotretinoin (Figure 11.25),[137] brown NB discoloration due to doxycycline dermal deposition,[138] and doxycycline-induced photo-onycholysis.[139]

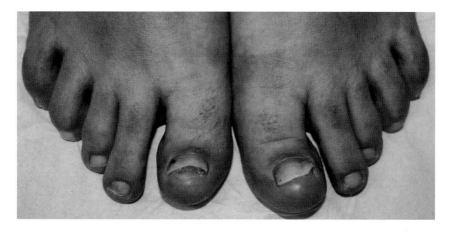

FIGURE 11.23 Painful onycholysis due to Adriamycin (doxorubicin), bleomycin, vinblastine, and dacarbazine (ABVD) chemotherapy in a 17-year-old girl.

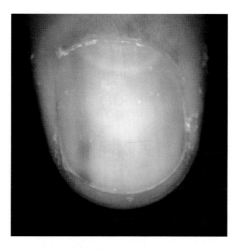

FIGURE 11.24 Longitudinal melanonychia after therapy with hydroxyurea in an 8-year-old boy with sickle cell anemia.

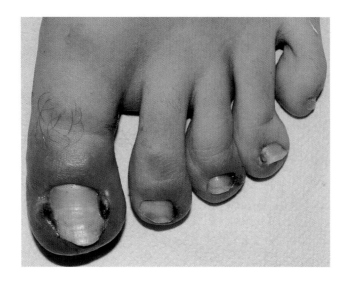

FIGURE 11.25   Multiple periungual pyogenic granulomas in a 15-year-old boy treated with isotretinoin for acne.

REFERENCES

1. Shah KN and Rubin AI. Nail disorders as signs of pediatric systemic disease. *Curr Probl Pediatr Adolesc Health Care*. 2012; 42: 204–211.
2. Zaiac MN and Walker A. Nail abnormalities associated with systemic pathologies. *Clinics Dermatol*. 2013; 31: 627–649.
3. Fawcett RS, Linford S, Stulberg DS. Nail abnormalities: Clues to systemic disease. *Am Fam Physician*. 2004; 69: 1417–1424.
4. Iglesias A, Tamayo L, Sosa-de-Martìnez C et al. Prevalence and nature of nail alterations in pediatric patients. *Ped Dermatol*. 2001; 18: 107–109.
5. Sarifakioglu E, Yilmaz AE, Gorpelioglu C. Nail alterations in 250 infant patients: A clinical study. *J Eur Acad Dermatol Venereol*. 2008; 22: 741–744.
6. Spicknall KE, Zirwas MJ, English JC 3rd. Clubbing: An update on diagnosis, differential diagnosis, pathophysiology, and clinical relevance. *J Am Acad Dermatol*. 2005; 52: 1020–1028.
7. Waring WW, Wilkinson RW, Wiebe RA et al. Quantitation of digital clubbing in children. Measurements of casts of the index finger. *Am Rev Respir Dis*. 1971; 104: 166–174.
8. Paton JY, Bautista DB, Stabile MW et al. Digital clubbing and pulmonary function abnormalities in children with lung disease. *Pediatr Pulmonol*. 1991; 10: 25–29.
9. Lemen RJ, Gates AJ, Mathé AA et al. Relationships among digital clubbing, disease severity, and serum prostaglandins F2alpha and E concentrations in cystic fibrosis patients. *Am Rev Respir Dis*. 1978; 117: 639–646.
10. Nakamura CT, Ng GY, Paton JY et al. Correlation between digital clubbing and pulmonary function in cystic fibrosis. *Pediatr Pulmonol*. 2002; 33: 332–338.
11. Augarten A, Goldman R, Laufer J et al. Reversal of digital clubbing after lung transplantation in cystic fibrosis patients: A clue to the pathogenesis of clubbing. *Pediatr Pulmonol*. 2002; 34: 378–380.
12. Borkar VV, Poddar U, Kapoor A et al. Hepatopulmonary syndrome in children: A comparative study of non-cirrhotic vs. cirrhotic portal hypertension. *Liver Int*. 2015; 35: 1665–1672.
13. Richet H, Casalta JP, Thuny F et al. Development and assessment of a new early scoring system using non-specific clinical signs and biological results to identify children and adult patients with a high probability of infective endocarditis on admission. *J Antimicrob Chemother*. 2008; 62: 1434–1440.
14. Staalman CR and Umans U. Hypertrophic osteoarthropathy in childhood malignancy. *Med Pediatr Oncol*. 1993; 21: 676–679.
15. Drakonaki EE, Bradley KM, Khan ZA et al. Hypertrophic osteoarthropathy in a child due to thoracic Hodgkin's disease. *Skeletal Radiol*. 2012; 41: 1027–1028.

16. Goodyer MJ, Cronin MC, Ketsitlile DG et al. Hodgkin's lymphoma with digital clubbing. *J Clin Oncol.* 2009; 27: e95–e96.

17. Narváez-Moreno B, Bernabeu-Wittel J, Fernández-Pineda I. Unilateral clubbing as a clinical manifestation of lower limb venous malformation. *Int J Dermatol.* 2014; 53: e382–e383.

18. Garganese MC, De Sio L, Serra A et al. Rhabdomyosarcoma associated hypertrophic osteoarthropathy in a child: Detection by bone scintigraphy. *Clin Nucl Med.* 2009; 34: 155–157.

19. Mohindra S, Yachha SK, Srivastava A et al. Coeliac disease in Indian children: Assessment of clinical, nutritional and pathologic characteristics. *J Health Popul Nutr.* 2001; 19: 204–208.

20. Grosfeld JL and West KW. Generalized juvenile polyposis coli. *Arch Surg.* 1986; 121: 530–534.

21. Bowie MD, Morison A, Ireland JD, Duys PJ. Clubbing and whipworm infestation. *Arch Dis Child.* 1978; 53: 411–413.

22. Rubinstein A, Morecki R, Silverman B et al. Pulmonary disease in children with acquired immune deficiency syndrome and AIDS-related complex. *J Pediatr.* 1986; 108: 498–503.

23. Martínez-Lavín M, Bobadilla M, Casanova J et al. Hypertrophic osteoarthropathy in cyanotic congenital heart disease: Its prevalence and relationship to bypass of the lung. *Arthritis Rheum.* 1982; 25: 1186–1193.

24. Pal P and Giri PP. Orange-brown chromonychia, a novel finding in Kawasaki disease. *Rheumatol Int.* 2013; 33: 1207–1209.

25. Thapa R and Pal P. Transverse orange-brown chromonychia in Kawasaki disease. *Int J Dermatol.* 2009; 49: 227–235.

26. Tessarotto L, Rubin G, Bonadies L et al. Orange-brown chromonychia and Kawasaki disease: A possible novel association? *Pediatr Dermatol.* 2015; 32: e104–e105.

27. Huang MY, Huang JJ, Huang TY et al. Deterioration of cutaneous microcirculatory status of Kawasaki disease. *Clin Rheumatol.* 2012; 31: 847–852.

28. Lindsley CB. Nail bed lines in Kawasaki disease. *Am J Dis Child.* 1992; 146: 659–660.

29. Baran R and Perrin C. Nail degloving: Polyetiologic condition with three main patterns: A new syndrome. *J Am Acad Dermatol.* 2008; 58: 232–237.

30. Vanderhooft SL and Vanderhooft JE. Pincer nail deformity after Kawasaki disease. *J Am Acad Dermatol.* 1999; 41: 341–342.

31. Ames EL, Jones JS, Van Dommelen B, Posch JL. Bilateral hand necrosis in Kawasaki syndrome. *J Hand Surg Am.* 1985; 10: 391–395.

32. Martino F, Agolini D, Tsalikova E et al. Nailfold capillaroscopy in Henoch-Schönlein purpura: A follow-up study of 31 cases. *J Pediatr.* 2002; 141: 145.

33. Zampetti A, Rigante D, Bersani G et al. Longitudinal study of microvascular involvement by nailfold capillaroscopy in children with Henoch-Schönlein purpura. *Clin Rheumatol.* 2009; 28: 1101–1105.

34. Mazzone L and Schiestl C. Management of septic skin necroses. *Eur J Pediatr Surg.* 2013; 23: 349–358.

35. Nanda A, Al-Essa FH, El-Shafei WM, Alsaleh QA. Congenital yellow nail syndrome: A case report and its relationship to non immune fetal hydrops. *Pediatr Dermatol.* 2010; 27: 533–534.

36. Semiz S, Dagdeviren E, Ergin H et al. Congenital lymphoedema, bronchiectasis and seizure: Case report. *East Afr Med J.* 2008; 85: 145–149.

37. Dessart P, Deries X, Guérin-Moreau M et al. Yellow nail syndrome: Two pediatric case reports. *Ann Dermatol Venereol.* 2014; 141: 611–619.

38. Cecchini M, Doumit J, Kanigsberg N. Atypical presentation of congenital yellow nail syndrome in a 2-year-old female. *J Cutan Med Surg.* 2013; 17: 66–68.

39. Kamatani M, Rai A, Hen H et al. Yellow nail syndrome associated with mental retardation in two siblings. *Br J Dermatol.* 1978; 99: 329–333.

40. Lambert EM, Dziura J, Kauls L et al. Yellow nail syndrome in three siblings: A randomized double-blind trial of topical vitamin E. *Pediatr Dermatol.* 2006; 23: 390–395.

41. Baran R and Thomas L. Combination of fluconazole and alpha-tocopherol in the treatment of yellow nail syndrome. *J Drugs Dermatol.* 2009; 8: 276–278.

42. Seyhan M, Erdem T, Ertekin V, Selimoğlu MA. The mucocutaneous manifestations associated with celiac disease in childhood and adolescence. *Pediatr Dermatol.* 2007; 24: 28–33.

43. Kitis G, Thompson H, Allan RN. Finger clubbing in inflammatory bowel disease: Its prevalence and pathogenesis. *BMJ.* 1979; 2: 825–828.

44. Munck A, Murciano D, Pariente R et al. Latent pulmonary function abnormalities in children with Crohn's disease. *Eur Respir J.* 1995; 8: 377–380.

45. Max JE and Shawayder TA. Pyogenic granulomas of the nail beds in a patients with ulcerative colitis. Poster presented at the American Academy of Dermatology 57th Annual Meeting, March 1999.

46. Lazzerini M, Bramuzzo M, Maschio M et al. Thromboembolism in pediatric inflammatory bowel disease: Systematic review. *Inflamm Bowel Dis.* 2011; 17: 2174–2183.

47. Talbot RW, Heppell J, Dozois RR, Beart RW Jr. Vascular complications of inflammatory bowel disease. *Mayo Clin Proc.* 1986; 61: 140–145.

48. Shah KR, Boland CR, Patel M et al. Cutaneous manifestations of gastrointestinal disease: Part I. *J Am Acad Dermatol* 2013; 68: 189.e1–21.

49. Gandhi V, Nagral A, Philip S et al. Reversal of nail changes after liver transplantation in a child. *Indian J Gastroenterol.* 2009; 28: 154–156.

50. Wheeler DA, Edmondson HA, Reynolds TB. Spontaneous liver cell adenoma in children. *Am J Clin Pathol.* 1986; 85: 6–12.

51. Seyhan M, Erdem T, Selimoğlu MA, Ertekin V. Dermatological signs in Wilson's disease. *Pediatr Int.* 2009; 51: 395–398.

52. Masmoudi A, Hajjaji Darouiche M, Ben Salah H et al. Cutaneous abnormalities in patients with end stage renal failure on chronic hemodialysis. A study of 458 patients. *J Dermatol Case Rep.* 2014; 8: 86–94.

53. Udayakumar P, Balasubramanian S, Ramalingam KS et al. Cutaneous manifestations in patients with chronic renal failure on hemodialysis. *Indian J Dermatol Venereol Leprol.* 2006; 72: 119–125.

54. Attia EA, Hassan SI, Youssef NM. Cutaneous disorders in uremic patients on hemodialysis: An Egyptian case-controlled study. *Int J Dermatol.* 2010; 49: 1024–1030.

55. Abdelaziz AM, Mahmoud KM, Elsawy EM, Bakr MA. Nail changes in kidney transplant recipients. *Nephrol Dial Transplant.* 2010; 25: 274–277.

56. Menni S, Beretta D, Piccinno R, Ghio L. Cutaneous and oral lesions in 32 children after renal transplantation. *Pediatr Dermatol.* 1991; 8: 194–198.

57. Feng J, Gohara M, Lazova R, Antaya RJ. Fatal childhood calciphylaxis in a 10-year-old and literature review. *Pediatr Dermatol.* 2006; 23: 266–272.

58. Bakkaloglu SA, Dursun I, Kaya A et al. Digital calciphylaxis progressing to amputation in a child on continuous ambulatory peritoneal dialysis. *Ann Trop Paediatr.* 2007; 27: 149–152.

59. Karahanyan E, Boikinov B, Pechilkova M et al. Degenerative vascular changes in children with diabetes mellitus. *Folia Med (Plovdiv).* 1994; 36: 19–25.

60. Kaminska-Winciorek G, Deja G, Polańska J, Jarosz-Chobot P. Diabetic microangiopathy in capillaroscopic examination of juveniles with diabetes type 1. *Postepy Hig Med Dosw.* 2012; 30: 51–59.

61. Hosking SP, Bhatia R, Crock PA et al. Non-invasive detection of microvascular changes in a paediatric and adolescent population with type 1 diabetes: A pilot cross-sectional study. *BMC Endocr Disord.* 2013; 5: 41.

62. Rasli MH and Zacharin MR. Foot problems and effectiveness of foot care education in children and adolescents with diabetes mellitus. *Pediatr Diabetes.* 2008; 9: 602–608.

63. Maheshwari R, Rani RP, Prasad RN et al. Visual disturbances as a presenting feature of pseudohypoparathyroidism. *Indian J Endocrinol Metab.* 2013; 17: S219–S220.

64. Wit JM, Beemer FA, Barth PG et al. Cerebral gigantism (Sotos syndrome). Compiled data of 22 cases. Analysis of clinical features, growth and plasma somatomedin. *Eur J Pediatr.* 1985; 144: 131–140.

65. Keen MA, Hassan I, Bhat MH. A clinical study of the cutaneous manifestations of hypothyroidism in Kashmir valley. *Indian J Dermatol.* 2013; 58: 326.

66. Doshi DN, Blyumin ML, Kimball AB. Cutaneous manifestations of thyroid disease. *Clin Dermatol.* 2008; 26: 283–287.

67. Leonhardt JM and Heymann WR. Thyroid disease and the skin. *Dermatol Clin.* 2002; 20: 473–481, vii.

68. Onyiriuka AN, Atamah CA, Onyiriuka LC. Plummer's nails (onycholysis) in an adolescent Nigerian girl with hyperthyroidism due to Graves' disease. *Aristotle Univ Med J.* 2012; 39: 13–16.

69. Thomas J, Collipp PJ, Sharma RK. Thyroid acropachy. *Am J Dis Child.* 1973; 125: 745–746.

70. Keeling B, Antia C, Steadmon M et al. Dyskeratosis congenita. *Dermatol Online J.* 2014; 16.

71. Ibrahim A and Halima K. Dyskeratosis congenita in a Nigerian boy. *Niger Med J.* 2014; 55: 173–175.

72. Ling NS, Fenske NA, Julius RL et al. Dyskeratosis congenita in a girl simulating chronic graft-vs-host disease. *Arch Dermatol.* 1985; 121: 1424–1428.

73. Salotti JA, Nanduri V, Pearce MS et al. Incidence and clinical features of Langerhans cell histiocytosis in the UK and Ireland. *Arch Dis Child.* 2009; 94: 376–380.

74. Sabui TK and Purkait R. Nail changes in Langerhans cell histiocytosis. *Indian Pediatr.* 2009; 46: 728–729.

75. de Berker D, Lever LR, Windebank K. Nail features in Langerhans cell histiocytosis. *Br J Dermatol.* 1994; 130: 523–527.

76. Ottink M, Feijen S, Rosias P et al. Langerhans cell histiocytosis presenting with complicated pneumonia, a case report. *Respir Med Case Rep.* 2013; 17: 28–31.

77. Chander R, Jaykar K, Varghese B et al. Pulmonary disease with striking nail involvement in a child. *Pediatr Dermatol.* 2008; 25: 633–634.

78. Schulze J, Kitz R, Grüttner HP et al. Severe isolated pulmonary Langerhans cell histiocytosis in a 6-year-old girl. *Eur J Pediatr.* 2004; 163: 320–322.

79. Ashena Z, Alavi S, Arzanian MT, Eshghi P. Nail involvement in Langerhans cell histiocytosis. *Pediatr Hematol Oncol.* 2007; 24: 45–51.

80. Mataix J, Betlloch I, Lucas-Costa A et al. Nail changes in Langerhans cell histiocytosis: A possible marker of multisystem disease. *Pediatr Dermatol.* 2008; 25: 247–251.

81. Yazc N, Yalçn B, Ciftci AO et al. Langerhans cell histiocytosis with involvement of nails and lungs in an adolescent. *J Pediatr Hematol Oncol.* 2008; 30: 77–80.

82. Holzberg M, Wade TR, Buchanan ID. Nail pathology in histiocytosis X. *J Am Acad Dermatol.* 1985; 13: 522–524.

83. Timpatanapong P, Hathirat P, Isarankura A. Nail involvement in Histiocytosis X. A 12 year retrospective study. *Arch Dermatol.* 1984; 120: 1052–1056.

84. Dolezalova P, Young SP, Bacon PA, Southwood TR. Nailfold capillary microscopy in healthy children and in childhood rheumatic diseases: A prospective single blind observational study. *Ann Rheum Dis.* 2003; 62: 444–449.

85. Ingegnoli F, Zeni S, Gerloni V, Fantini F. Capillaroscopic observations in childhood rheumatic diseases and healthy controls. *Clin Exp Rheumatol.* 2005; 23: 905–911.

86. Piotto DG, Len CA, Hilário MO, Terreri MT. Nailfold capillaroscopy in children and adolescents with rheumatic diseases. *Rev Bras Rheumatol.* 2012; 52: 722–732.

87. Pavlov-Dolijanović S, Damjanov N, Ostojić P et al. The prognostic value of nailfold capillary changes for the development of connective tissue disease in children and adolescents with primary Raynaud phenomenon: A follow-up study of 250 patients. *Pediatr Dermatol.* 23 (2006): 437–442.

88. Ingegnoli F, Zeni S, Meani L et al. Evaluation of nailfold video capillaroscopic abnormalities in patients with systemic lupus erythematosus. *J Clin Rheumatol.* 2005; 11: 295–298.

89. Euwer RL and Sontheimer RD. Dermatologic aspects of myositis. *Curr Opin Rheumatol.* 1994; 6: 583–589.

90. Christen-Zaech S, Seshadri R, Sundberg J et al. Persistent association of nailfold capillaroscopy changes and skin involvement over thirty-six months with duration of untreated disease in patients with juvenile dermatomyositis. *Arthritis Rheum.* 2008; 58: 571–576.

91. Schmeling H, Stephens S, Goia C et al. Nailfold capillary density is importantly associated over time with muscle and skin disease activity in juvenile dermatomyositis. *Rheumatology.* 2011; 50: 885–893.

92. Cobos G, Rubin AI, Gober LM, Treat JR. A case of exuberant candidal onychomycosis in a child with hyper IgE syndrome. *J Allergy Clin Immunol Pract.* 2014; 2: 99–100.

93. Olaiwan A, Chandesris MO, Fraitag S et al. Cutaneous findings in sporadic and familial autosomal dominant hyper-IgE syndrome: A retrospective, single-center study of 21 patients diagnosed using molecular analysis. *J Am Acad Dermatol.* 2011; 65: 1167–1172.

94. Tosti A, Piraccini BM, Vincenzi C, Cameli N. Itraconazole in the treatment of two young brothers with chronic mucocutaneous candidiasis. *Pediatr Dermatol.* 1997; 14: 146–148.

95. Leong AB, Gange RW, O'Connor RD. Twenty-nail dystrophy (trachyonychia) associated with selective IgA deficiency. *J Pediatr.* 1982; 100: 418–420.

96. Huang JT, Duncan CN, Boyer D et al. Nail dystrophy, edema, and eosinophilia: Harbingers of severe chronic GVHD of the skin in children. *Bone Marrow Transplant.* 2014; 49: 1521–1527.

97. Tlougan BE, Podjasek JO, O'Haver J et al. Chronic recurrent multifocal osteomyelitis (CRMO) and synovitis, acne, pustulosis, hyperostosis, and osteitis (SAPHO) syndrome with associated neutrophilic dermatoses: A report of seven cases and review of the literature. *Pediatr Dermatol.* 2009; 26: 497–505.

98. Job-Deslandre C, Krebs S, Kahan A. Chronic recurrent multifocal osteomyelitis: Five-year outcomes in 14 pediatric cases. *Joint Bone Spine.* 2001; 68: 245–251.

99. Bachmann F, Stieler K, Garcia Bartels N et al. Skin manifestations associated with chronic recurrent multifocal osteomyelitis in a 9-year-old girl. *J Am Acad Dermatol.* 014; 71: 218–219.

100. Prendiville JS, Tucker LB, Cabral DA, Crawford RI. A pruritic linear urticarial rash, fever, and systemic inflammatory disease in five adolescents: Adult-onset still disease or systemic juvenile idiopathic arthritis sine arthritis? *Pediatr Dermatol.* 2004; 21: 580–588.

101. Prose NS. Cutaneous manifestations of pediatric HIV infection. *Pediatr Dermatol.* 1992; 9: 326–328.

102. Doni SN, Mitchell AL, Bogale Y, Walker SL. Skin disorders affecting human immunodeficiency virus-infected children living in an orphanage in Ethiopia. *Clin Exp Dermatol.* 2012; 37: 15–19.

103. de Carvalho VO, da Cruz CR, Marinoni LP, Lima JH. Transverse leukonychia and AIDS. *Arch Dis Child.* 2006; 91: 326.

104. Sehgal R, Baveja UK, Chattopadhya D et al. Pediatric HIV infection. *Indian J Pediatr.* 2005; 72: 925–930.

105. Apalla Z, Sotiriou E, Pikou O et al. Onychomadesis after hand-foot-and-mouth disease outbreak in northern Greece: Case series and brief review of the literature. *Int J Dermatol.* 2015; 54(9): 1039–1044.

106. Kocak AY and Koçak O. Onychomadesis in two sisters induced by varicella infection. *Pediatr Dermatol.* 2013; 30: e108–e109.

107. Osterback R, Vuorinen T, Linna M et al. Coxsackievirus A6 and hand, foot, and mouth disease, Finland. *Emerg Infect Dis.* 2009; 15: 1485–1488.

108. Yan AC and Jen MV. Skin signs of pediatric nutritional disorders. *Curr Probl Pediatr Adolesc Health Care.* 2012; 42: 212–217.

109. Gupta MA, Gupta AK, Haberman HF. Dermatologic signs in anorexia nervosa and bulimia nervosa. *Arch Dermatol.* 1987; 123: 1386–1390.

110. Strumia R. Eating disorders and the skin. *Clin Dermatol.* 2013; 31(1): 80–85.

111. Ayogu RN, Okafor AM, Ene-Obong HN. Iron status of schoolchildren (6–15 years) and associated factors in rural Nigeria. *Food Nutr Res.* 2015; 59: 26223.

112. Thaver IH and Baig L. Anaemia in children: Part I. Can simple observations by primary care provider help in diagnosis? *J Pak Med Assoc.* 1994; 44: 282–284.

113. Redd SC, Kazembe PN, Luby SP et al. Clinical algorithm for treatment of Plasmodium falciparum malaria in children. *Lancet.* 1996; 347: 223–227.

114. Kien CL and Ganther HE. Manifestations of chronic selenium deficiency in a child receiving total parenteral nutrition. *Am J Clin Nutr.* 1983; 37: 319–328.

115. Etani Y, Nishimoto Y, Kawamoto K et al. Selenium deficiency in children and adolescents nourished by parenteral nutrition and/or selenium-deficient enteral formula. *J Trace Elem Med Biol.* 2014; 28: 409–413.

116. Chowanadisai W, Lonnerdal B, Kelleher SL. Identification of a mutation in SLC30A2 (ZnT-2) in women with low milk zinc concentration that results in transient neonatal zinc deficiency. *J Biol Chem.* 2006; 281: 39699–39707.

117. Corbo MD, Lam J. Zinc deficiency and its management in the pediatric population: A literature review and proposed etiologic classification. *J Am Acad Dermatol.* 2013; 69: 616–624.e1.

118. Cashman MW and Sloan SB. Nutrition and nail disease. *Clin Dermatol.* 2010; 28: 420–425.

119. Van Meir N and De Smet L. Carpal tunnel syndrome in children. *Acta Orthop Belg.* 2003; 69: 387–395.

120. Batdorf NJ, Cantwell SR, Moran SL. Idiopathic carpal tunnel syndrome in children and adolescents. *J Hand Surg Am.* 2015; 40: 773–777.

121. Maldonado García C, Valente Duarte de Sousa IC, López Cepeda L. Necrotic carpal tunnel syndrome in a child. *Pediatr Dermatol.* 2014; 31: 500–503.

122. Ravichandra KS, Kandregula CR, Koya S, Lakhotia D. Congenital insensitivity to pain and anhydrosis: Diagnostic and therapeutic dilemmas revisited. *Int J Clin Pediatr Dent.* 2015; 8: 75–81.

123. Schulze UM, Pettke-Rank CV, Kreienkamp M et al. Dermatologic findings in anorexia and bulimia nervosa of childhood and adolescence. *Pediatr Dermatol.* 1999; 16: 90–94.
124. Chen W, Yu YS, Liu YH et al. Nail changes associated with chemotherapy in children. *J Eur Acad Dermatol Venereol.* 2007; 21: 186–190.
125. Afsar FS, Ozek G, Vergin C. Half-and-half nails in a pediatric patient after chemotherapy. *Cutan Ocul Toxicol.* 2015; 19: 1–2.
126. Yoruk A and Yukselgungor H. Chemotherapy induced transverse leukonychia in children. *Int J Dermatol.* 2003; 42: 468–469.
127. Issaivanan, M and Khairkar PH. Doxorubicin induced melanonychia. *Indian Pediatr.* 2003; 40: 1094–1095.
128. Naithani R, Kumar R, Mahapatra M, Seth T. Melanonychia after allogenic hematopoietic stem cell transplantation. *Indian J Pediatr.* 2009; 76: 1179–1180.
129. Strouse JJ, Lanzkron S, Beach MC et al. Hydroxyurea for sickle cell disease: A systematic review for efficacy and toxicity in children. *Pediatrics.* 2008; 122: 1332–1342.
130. Zargari O, Kimyai-Asadi A, Jafroodi M. Cutaneous adverse reactions to hydroxyurea in patients with intermediate thalassemia. *Pediatr Dermatol.* 2004; 21: 633–635.
131. Doni SN, Mitchell AL, Bogale Y, Walker SL. Skin disorders affecting human immunodeficiency virus-infected children living in an orphanage in Ethiopia. *Clin Exp Dermatol.* 2012; 37: 15–19.
132. Tukei VJ, Asiimwe A, Maganda A et al. Safety and tolerability of antiretroviral therapy among HIV-infected children and adolescents in Uganda. *J Acquir Immune Defic Syndr.* 2012; 59: 274–280.
133. Baheti NN, Kabra D, Chandak NH et al. Reversible onychomadesis following exposure to carbamazepine. *Neurol India.* 2015; 63: 120–122.
134. Slaughenhoupt BL, Adeagbo S, Van Savage JG. A suspected case of trimethoprim-sulfamethoxazole-induced loss of fingernails and toenails. *Pediatr Infect Dis J.* 1999; 18: 76–77.
135. Poretti A, Lips U, Belvedere M, Schmitt B. Onychomadesis: A rare side-effect of valproic acid medication? *Pediatr Dermatol.* 2009; 26: 749–750.
136. Shah RK, Uddin M, Fatunde OJ. Onychomadesis secondary to penicillin allergy in a child. *J Pediatr.* 2012; 161: 166.
137. Armstrong K and Weinstein M. Pyogenic granulomas during isotretinoin therapy. *J Dermatol Case Rep.* 2011; 26: 5–7.
138. Akcam M, Artan R, Akcam FZ, Yilmaz A. Nail discoloration induced by doxycycline. *Pediatr Infect Dis J.* 2005; 24: 845–846.
139. Atiq N and van Meurs T. A boy with nail abnormalities. *Ned Tijdschr Geneeskd.* 2013; 157: A6429.

12

Nail Alterations in Cutaneous Porphyrias

Jose M. Mascaró Sr. and Paula Aguilera

The porphyrias are a group of diseases characterized by genetic or acquired enzyme deficiencies in the metabolic pathway of heme, resulting in the accumulation of heme precursors: 5-deltaaminolevulinic acid (ALA), porphobilinogen (PBG), and/or porphyrins (Tables 12.1 through 12.3).

Based on clinical manifestations, it is possible to divide the porphyrias into three categories:

1. *Cutaneous porphyrias* with acute phototoxic responses (acute cutaneous syndrome) or skin fragility (subacute cutaneous syndrome).
2. *Acute porphyrias* characterized by acute abdominal and neurological attacks without cutaneous manifestation.
3. *Mixed porphyrias* with the possibility of both acute attacks and cutaneous lesions.

Pathogenesis

Reactive oxygen species, inflammatory mediators, and inflammatory cells have been shown to contribute to the development of cutaneous lesions in porphyrias.[1] Porphyrias with only elevated levels of ALA and PBG have no cutaneous manifestations.

Upon exposure to the Soret band (400–410 nm) from the sun or artificial light, "excited state" porphyrins are generated, which can interact with the oxygen molecules to form singlet oxygen. Reactive oxygen species and peroxides damage cell membranes, resulting in the release of mediator from the mast cells and also damage hepatic and epidermal microsomal cytochrome P450, as well as lysosomal and mitochondrial membranes.[1] Mast cells, neutrophils, and the complement system also participate in the porphyrin-induced phototoxicity.

Protoporphyrin, but not uroporphyrin, is able to induce mast cell mediator release under the Soret band radiation action.[2] This appears to be because protoporphyrin is lipophilic, while uroporphyrin is hydrophilic. This effect may account for the sunburn-like manifestations of porphyrias presenting with acute syndrome (congenital erythropoietic porphyria [CEP], hepatoerythropoietic porphyria [HEP], and erythropoietic protoporphyria [EPP]). All of them are associated with a raised protoporphyrin level (see Tables 12.1 through 12.3).

Cutaneous Porphyrias

Dermatological manifestations of cutaneous porphyrias appear in two different forms.

1. An acute syndrome of photosensitivity with cutaneous manifestations resembling sunburn, due to sunlight exposure or, less commonly, to artificial light sources: This is very characteristic of EPP in which there is an overproduction of protoporphyrin. However, the acute photosensitivity may also develop in homozygous porphyrias when there is an overproduction of hydrophilic porphyrins as it occurs in CEP and HEP.

TABLE 12.1

Classification of Porphyrias

Hepatic porphyrias

1. Acute intermittent porphyria
2. Porphyria variegata
3. Hereditary coproporphyria
4. Porphyria cutanea tarda

Erythropoietic porphyrias

1. Erythropoietic protoporphyria
2. Congenital erythropoietic porphyria

Note: Based on the site of abnormal porphyrin overproduction (traditional since Schmid R, Schwartz S, Watson CJ. *Acta Haematol,* 1953; 10(3): 150–64.).

TABLE 12.2

Porphyria Algorithm

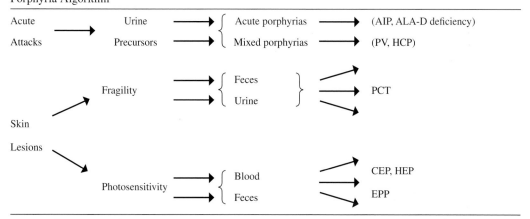

Notes: AIP, acute intermittent porphyria; ALA-D, 5-deltaaminolevulinic acid dehydratase; PV, porphyria variegate; HCP, hereditary coproporphyria; PCT, porphyria cutanea tarda; CEP, congenital erythropoietic porphyria; HEP, hepato-erythropoietic porphyria; EPP, erythropoietic protoporphyria.

TABLE 12.3

Excretion Patterns of Porphyrias

Disease	Enzyme Deficiency	Urine	Feces	RBC
AIP	PBG-D	ALA, PBG		
ALA-D deficiency	ALA-D	ALA	CP, PP	ZnPP
PV	PPO	CP	PP, CP	
		Acute attack: ALA, PBG		
HCP	CO	CP	CP	
		Acute attack: ALA, PBG		
PCT	UP-D	UP, 7-COOH	Iso-CP	
HEP	UP-D	UP, 7-COOH	Iso-CP	ZnPP
EPP	FeCh	PP	PP	
CEP	UPIII-S	UP, CP (isomers I)	CP (isomers I)	UP, CP (isomers I) PP

Notes: RBC, red blood cells; ALA, 5-deltaaminolevulinic acid; PBG-D, porphobilinogen deaminase; CP, coproporphyrin; PP, protoporphyrin; PPO, protoporphyrinogen oxidase; CO, coproporphyrinogen oxidase; UP-D, uroporphyrinogen decarboxylase; UP, uroporphyrin; 7-COOH, hepta-carboxylic porphyrin; Iso-CP, iso-coproporphyrin; FeCh, ferrochelatase; UPIII-S, uro III synthase; ZnPP, zinc protoporphyrin.

2. A subacute syndrome of cutaneous hyperfragility with vesiculobullous and erosive lesions developing after minimal trauma: This symptom is characteristic of the porphyrias with the overproduction of hydrophilic porphyrins: porphyria cutanea tarda (PCT), CEP, HEP, and the mixed porphyrias (porphyria variegata [PV], hereditary coproporphyria [HCP]).

a. *Porphyria cutanea tarda (PCT)*: PCT caused by uroporphyrinogen decarboxylase (UPD) deficiency is divided into four distinct clinical types. PCT I is a sporadic variant that develops in adults with no familial or inherited background. PCT types II and III are familial and may appear in children; UPD deficiency may be expressed in all tissues (type II) or may be absent in erythrocytes (type III). Despite these differences, clinical manifestations are identical in all three forms. PCT type IV is toxic porphyria and the best-known responsible toxic agent is hexochlorobenzene. In PCT I, it has been found that patients are often homozygous, heterozygous, or compound heterozygous carriers of familial hemochromatosis genes, particularly of the *C282Y* gene[3,4] and it is why sideremia and ferritin are elevated.

The onset of manifestations of familial PCT usually occurs in childhood. In some cases, a toxic agent may induce the disease. In other patients, particularly in PCT I, an infection, especially viral hepatitis or in some cases human immunodeficiency virus (HIV), may trigger it.[5]

Skin hyperfragility is usually the first clinical manifestation. Small serous or hemorrhagic vesicles or blisters, in general, without any erythematous halo, develop after minimal trauma; less frequently, lesions may be sunlight induced.

The lesions appear most commonly on the dorsum of the hands, but may also occur on other areas, such as the face or limbs. The rupture of the blisters results in superficial erosions. Finally, superficial scars develop and are sometimes covered by milia cysts. Simultaneous occurrences of vesiculobullous lesions, erosions, scars, and milia produce a characteristic polymorphous appearance.[6]

Tangential pressure on the patient's sun-exposed skin may provoke a blister similar to the Nikolsky sign in pemphigus. Erosions by hyperfragility without previous blisters may also develop.

Nail alterations: Minimal trauma may cause the formation of vesiculobullous lesions under the nail plates. Yellow, bluish, or violaceous (hemorrhagic) discoloration of the nail

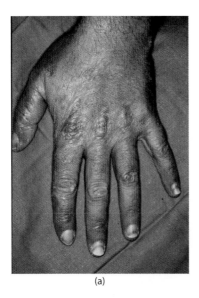

(a)

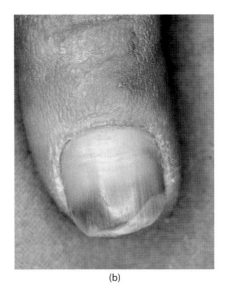

(b)

FIGURE 12.1   (a and b) Porphyria cutanea tarda (PCT). Light and minimal trauma-induced onycholysis. Reiterate vesiculo-bullous lesions produce an atrophic appearance of dorsal hands' skin.

plate may be visible with or without moderate pain. Disappearance of the lunula, onycholysis, and onychodystrophy may also occur (Figure 12.1).

Hypertrichosis of the facial area is also a common feature of PCT. In children with PCT II and III, this may also develop in the extremities.

A diffuse or reticulate tanned discoloration of sun-exposed areas can occur. Premature aging of the skin of the face and neck is a characteristic of chronic PCT. Scleroderma-like lesions could develop mainly in adulthood after a long evolution of the disease, particularly on the head, neck, and scalp.

Rarely, patients may present increased ocular photosensitivity, conjunctivitis, photophobia, and excessive tearing.

Liver involvement is found in most cases of PCT I; however, cirrhosis is uncommon. Hepatitis C antibodies, present in 89% of sporadic PCT patients,[7] are usually absent in familial PCT.

In all PCT types, the urine is dark brown and shows red fluorescence under Wood's light due to its porphyrin content. The most abundant porphyrin in urine is uroporphyrin (UP) followed by 7-carboxylic porphyrin (7-COOH). In feces, it is the very characteristic of the presence of a 5-carboxylic porphyrin named iso-coproporphyrin (iso-CP).

Phlebotomy is an old but still a valuable treatment for PCT. However, it is not utilized for the children. Chloroquine, at a weekly dosage of 3 mg/kg divided in 2 nonconsecutive days, is usually effective and well tolerated by the children. In addition, as in all cutaneous forms of porphyria, photo and trauma protection must be recommended.

b. *Erythropoietic protoporphyria (EPP):* After PCT, EPP due to ferrochelatase (FeCh) deficiency is the most common variety of porphyria. The inheritance of EPP has not been clearly established. Autosomal dominant inheritance with variable expressivity and incomplete penetrance has been considered.[8] In fact, heredity is complex and to develop EPP it appears that the patient must have inherited the deficiency from a biochemically abnormal asymptomatic relative (parent) and also a variant of FeCh (that 10% of population carries) with the reduced expression of the gene.[9,10]

The onset of the disease usually occurs before the age of 6 years.[11] Often, the family is not aware of their child's photosensitivity and is concerned by the tendency of these children to cry without apparent cause; for that reason, in some cases, they have been referred to a pediatric psychiatrist.

The primary cutaneous manifestation is increased photosensitivity. Usually, visible manifestations are preceded by itch, a burning sensation, or pain. Fever, malaise, and insomnia may also occur. Subjective manifestations may be mild or severe and cause crying.[11] Erythema, edema, and even purpura (similar to severe sunburn) may appear on sun-exposed areas. Symptoms may also develop following exposure to artificial light. Shaded facial areas are usually spared. Acute light-induced manifestation may also develop in the dorsal periungueal area of fingers.

Nail alterations are not very common; however, mild-to-moderate nail plate dystrophies and photo-onycholysis may appear if sun exposure is not avoided.

Progressively, by repetition of acute outbreaks, the skin of the exposed areas becomes thickened and yellowish. The presence of deep wrinkles in the nasolabial folds, below the lower eyelids, transversely over the nose and around the mouth, is characteristic. Multiple varioliform scars are often visible on the cheeks, nose, and forehead. On the dorsa of the hands, the skin of the knuckle is characteristically thickened with deep folds (Figure 12.2).

Defective FeCh is responsible for the PP overproduction. However, as PP is lipophilic but nonhydrophilic, urinary porphyrin levels are normal but raised in plasma, erythroblasts, and erythrocytes with a transient fluorescence under Wood's light due to the rapid transformation of PP in nonfluorescent oxyporphyrin.

The biopsy of chronic cutaneous lesions, particularly of the skin of dorsa of hands, fingers, and facial lesions, shows the presence of dense eosinophilic homogeneous hyaline deposits, initially perivascular, and very characteristic.

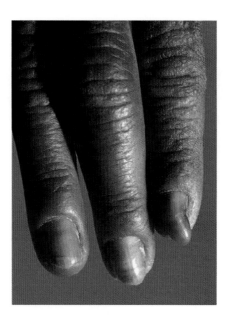

FIGURE 12.2 Erythropoietic protoporphyria (EPP). Recurrent acute light-induced episodes progressively produce thickening of dorsal hands' skin and variable degree of nail dystrophies.

Severe liver disease progressing to cirrhosis appears in 5%–10% of adult patients. The autosomal recessive variant of EPP has been proved to be associated with severe liver disease.[12] Some clinical and analytical signs predict liver failure: aggravation of photosensitivity, unexpected increase of plasma protoporphyrin, presence of porphyrins in urine (not PP because it is not hydrosoluble), and disappearance of porphyrins in the feces. These severe complications appear in adults.

There are also other very uncommon forms of EPP as a recessive type (less than 4% of cases) in double heterozygous or due to a X-linked increased activity of delta-aminolevulinate synthase 2 with also a raised risk of liver disease.[13]

Finally, there is also an uncommon form of EPP associated to a seasonal palmoplantar keratoderma and with no liver disease.[14,15]

Photoprotection is really important in EPP. However, the common sunscreen is not useful because it protects the skin from the sunburn band (290–320 nm) but not from longer wavelengths that are particularly harmful in these patients (400–410 nm or even longer). Physical sunscreens are more useful. In adults and children's nails, a colored nail lacquer is useful to protect the nail plate and prevent photo-onycholysis. Systemic betacarotene (15–90 mg daily for a child) provides a relative outdoor light tolerance. Antihistaminic drugs are able to reduce the symptom intensity. Psoralen and ultraviolet A radiation (PUVA), useful for adults, is not recommended for children. The recent development of a synthetic analog of alpha-melanocyte-stimulating hormone (MSH) subcutaneously implanted appears to be a significant advance in EPP treatment by increasing ultraviolet (UV) and visible light tolerance.[16] Liver transplantation has been successfully performed in adults with severe liver disease.[17]

Homozygous Porphyrias

The homozygous expression of an enzymatic deficiency in the heme pathway produces severe disease. This may occur where clinical manifestations appear exclusively in the homozygous state (the autosomal recessive porphyrias). Homozygous forms of autosomal dominant porphyrias may occur rarely. Two forms of homozygous porphyrias are of special interest.

1. *Congenital erythropoietic porphyria (CEP):* Günther disease due to uroporphyrinogen III synthase (UPIII-S) deficiency is a rare recessive disease. The onset of the disease occurs in infancy and is characterized by cutaneous hyperfragility and photosensitivity. Children develop post-traumatic or light-induced vesiculobullous lesions that evolve into erosions and scars on uncovered areas, especially the face and hands. The urine is dark and fluorescent under Wood's light, staining baby diapers.

   Clinical manifestations of CEP are initially similar to those of infantile PCT. However, in CEP, the deciduous teeth are dark red in color (erythrodontia) and fluoresces red due to the porphyrin deposition (Figure 12.3).

   Hypertrichosis is also a prominent and a constant feature on the light-exposed skin, such as the face and limbs.

   The disease gradually progresses toward soft tissue and bone destruction. Successive blistering episodes produce scars and fibrosis. Progressively, the skin of exposed regions (face and hands) becomes hard and pigmented. These alterations produce severe mutilations of the centrofacial area, especially the mouth and nose, as well as of the hands.

   Nail alterations: Sclerodactyly and nail dystrophy develop on the hands, with an eventual progressive loss of the terminal phalanges and finger nails (Figures 12.4 and 12.5). Toe nails are almost always preserved by socks and shoes. There is also the possibility of the preservation of fingers and nails, if they are continuously protected by gloves.

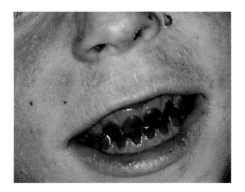

FIGURE 12.3 Congenital erythropoietic porphyria (CEP). Deciduous teeth are red (erythrodontia) and fluorescent under Wood's light due to porphyrin deposition.

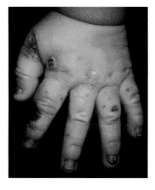

FIGURE 12.4 CEP. Light and repeated trauma initially produce vesiculo-bullous lesions and nail dystrophies.

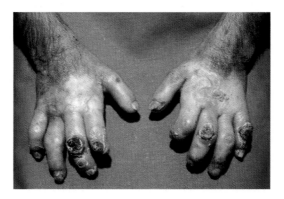

FIGURE 12.5 CEP. Progressive severe finger mutilations due to long term action of light and repeated trauma.

All these manifestations progress slowly but may also be severe from childhood. However, the gravity of evolution and mutilations is variable, depending on individual genotype and phenotype characteristics.

In CEP, the erythrocytes and bone marrow erythroblasts show strong red fluorescence upon exposure to Wood's light as they contain large amounts of isomer I porphyrins. Mild-to-severe hemolytic anemia and progressive splenomegaly are common.

Other noncutaneous manifestations may include ocular alterations such as photophobia, excessive tearing, keratoconjunctivitis, loss of eyelashes, ectropion, and a scleroconjunctival nonpainful ulcer (*scleromalacia perforans*).

Bone alterations are also frequent and severe. A distinctive osteodystrophy, with osteolysis of light-exposed extremities and high turnover osteoporosis, may develop. Light avoidance and the resultant vitamin D deficiency may contribute to the problem.

Rare cases of late-onset mild CEP (without erythrodontia or hemolytic anemia) have been reported. They may mimic PCT or EPP, lacking the typical mutilating tendency of Günther disease. Diagnosis is only made by biochemical or/and enzyme studies. An explanation for these mild forms of CEP has recently been found. In one clinical series, the "classic" patients with severe disease were noted to be homozygous for a single mutation (C73R, a cystine-to-arginine substitution at position 73). Mild or moderate disease appeared in compound heterozygotes of two different mutations, only one being C73R.[18,19] This was the first report of a genotype–phenotype correlation; observations of this sort may provide insight into the variability of clinical expression of the porphyrias.

The disease is due to a deficiency of UPgen-III-cosynthase and feedback activation of ALAS2 to overproduce isomer I porphyrins. The molecular defects observed in CEP are heterogeneous and have been found with variable frequencies. Missense mutation C73R represents 38.5% of the disease alleles. ALAS2 acts as a modifier gene; mutations that activate it are responsible for a more severe disease phenotype.[20]

There are also CEP cases with normal UPIII-S activity due to erythroid transcription factor gene mutations[21] as well as extremely rare cases with a late onset in adulthood associated to a myelodysplasic syndrome.[22]

Gene studies represent a promising field to evaluate the patient and also permit the prenatal diagnosis[23] and guess a possible gene therapy.[24]

2. *Hepatoerythropoietic porphyria (HEP):* It is a rare autosomal recessive disease that presents in infancy, with manifestations identical to those of CEP. However, erythrodontia, hemolytic anemia, and splenomegaly do not occur.

Patients present with photo-induced and post-traumatic vesiculobullous lesions. The urine is dark and progressive hypertrichosis, scleroderma, and ocular lesions are noted. The clinical evolution, including the development of severe mutilation of the centrofacial area and hands, is identical to CEP (Figures 12.6 and 12.7).

Nail alterations: Nails present with identical modifications similar to those of CEP. These range from mild dystrophy to complete disappearance of the distal phalanx. In general, because patients wear socks and shoes, the toe nails are preserved.

On the other hand, the biochemical pattern is identical to that of PCT. Uroporphyrin and 7-COOH porphyrin in the urine and iso-CP in the feces are markedly elevated. Different mutations or large deletions that account for an extremely severe UP-D deficiency (less than 10% of normal controls) have been found, thus proving the genetic heterogenicity of the disease; in fact, HEP is the homozygous or double heterozygous form of familial PCT (PCT II–III).[25]

In all homozygous porphyrias (CEP and HEP), it is crucial to protect patients, particularly children, from trauma. This is principally important for hands as feet are protected by socks and shoes. Photoprotection is also mandatory but, as in EPP, common sunscreen protects the skin from the

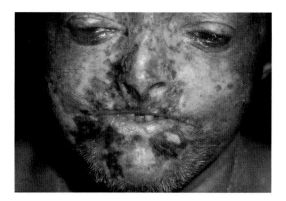

FIGURE 12.6 Hepatoerythropoietic porphyria (HEP). Clinically HEP looks like CEP, with severe sun exposed area mutilations.

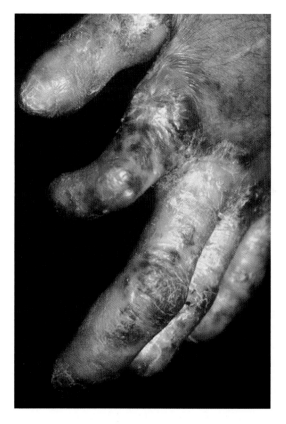

FIGURE 12.7 Hepatoerythropoietic porphyria (HEP). Light and repeated trauma produce severe finger mutilation as in CEP.

sunburn band but not from the longer wavelengths; physical sunscreens are more useful. Trauma and light protection may prevent severe facial and finger alterations. To wear gloves is indeed advisable when possible.

REFERENCES

1. Lim HW. Pathophysiology of cutaneous lesions in porphyrias. *Semin Hematol.* 1989; 26: 114–119.
2. Lim HW, Wasserman SI, Gigli I. Differential effects of protoporphyrin and uroporphyrin on murine mast cells. *J Invest Dermatol.* 1987; 88: 281–286.
3. de Villiers JN, Hillermann R, Loubser L, Kotze MJ. Spectrum of mutations in the HFE gene implicated in haemochromatosis and porphyria. *Hum Mol Genet.* 1999; 8: 1517–1522.
4. Bulaj ZJ, Phillips JD, Ajioka RS et al. Hemochromatosis genes and other factors contributing to the pathogenesis of porphyria cutanea tarda. *Blood.* 2000; 95: 1565–1571.
5. Aguilera P, Laguno M, To-Figueras J. Treatment of chronic hepatitis with boceprevir leads to remission of porphyria cutanea tarda. *Br J Dermatol.* 2014: 171: 1595–1596.
6. Mascaro JM, Herrero C, Lecha M, Muniesa AM. Uroporphyrinogen-decarboxylase deficiencies: Porphyria cutanea tarda and related conditions. *Semin Dermatol.* 1986; 5: 115–124.
7. Herrero C, Vicente A, Bruguera M et al. Is hepatitis C infection a trigger of porphyria cutanea tarda? *Lancet.* 1993; 341: 788–789.
8. Reed WB, Wuepper KD, Epstein JH et al. Erythropoietic protoporphyria. A clinical and genetic study. *J Am Med Assoc.* 1970; 214: 1060–1068.
9. Went L, Klassen EC. Genetic aspects of erythropoietic protoporphyria. *Ann Hum Genet.* 1984; 48: 105–117.
10. Gouya L, Puy H, Lamoril J et al. Inheritance in erythropoietic protoporphyria: A common wild-type ferrochelatase allelic variant with low expression accounts for clinical manifestation. *Blood.* 1999; 6: 2105–2110.
11. Todd DJ. Erythropoietic protoporphyria. *Br J Dermatol.* 1994; 131: 751–766.
12. Sarkany RP, Alexander GJ, Cox TM. Recessive inheritance of erythropoietic protoporphyria with liver failure. *Lancet.* 1994; 343: 1394–1396.
13. Whatley SD, Mason NG, Holme SA et al. Molecular epidemiology of erythropoietic protoporphyria in the U.K. *Br J Dermatol.* 2010; 162: 642–646.
14. Holme SA, Whatley SD, Roberts AG et al. Seasonal palmar keratoderma in erythropoietic protoporphyria indicates autosomal recessive inheritance. *J Invest Dermatol.* 2009; 129: 599–605.
15. Minder EI, Schneider-Yin X, Mamet R et al. A homoallelic FECH mutation in a patient with both erythropoietic protoporphyria and palmar keratoderma. *J Eur Acad Dermatol Venereol.* 2010; 24: 1349–1353.
16. Luger TA, Böhm M. An α-MSH analog in erythropoietic protoporphyria. *J Invest Dermatol.* 2015; 135(4): 929–931.
17. Polson RJ, Lim CK, Rolles K et al. Liver transplantation in a 13-year-old boy with erythropoietic protoporphyria. *Transplantation.* 1988; 46: 386–389.
18. Warner CA, Yoo HW, Roberts AG, Desnik RJ. Congenital erythropoietic porphyria: Identification and expression of exonic mutations in the uroporphyrinogen III synthase gene. *J Clin Invest.* 1992; 89: 693–700.
19. Deybach JC, de Verneuiilh H, Phung N et al. Congenital erythropoietic porphyria (Günther's disease). Enzymatic studies of two cases of late onset. *J Lab Clin Med.* 1981; 97: 551–558.
20. To-Figueras J, Badenas C, Mascaró JM et al. Study of the genotype–phenotype relationship in four cases of congenital erythropoietic porphyria. *Blood Cells Mol Dis.* 2007; 38: 242–246.
21. Phillips JD, Steensma DP, Pulsipher MA et al. Congenital erythropoietic porphyria due to a mutation in GATA1: The first trans-acting mutation causative for a human porphyria. *Blood.* 2007; 109: 2618–2621.
22. Sarkany RP, Ibbotson SH, Whatley SD et al. Erythropoietic uroporphyria associated with myeloid malignancy is likely distinct from autosomal recessive congenital erythropoietic porphyria. *J Invest Dermatol.* 2011; 131: 1172–1175.
23. Ged C, Moreau-Gaudry F, Taine L et al. Prenatal diagnosis in congenital erythropoietic porphyria by metabolic measurement and DNA mutation analysis. *Prenat Diag.* 1996; 16: 83–86.
24. Fontanellas A, Mazurier F, Moreau-Gaudry F et al. Correction of uroporphyrinogen decarboxylase deficiency (hepatoerythropoietic porphyria) in Epstein–Barr virus-transformed B-cell lines by retrovirus-mediated gene transfer: Fluorescence-based selection of transduced cells. *Blood.* 1999; 94: 465–474.
25. Elder GH, Smith SG, Herrero C et al. Hepatoerythropoietic porphyria: A new uroporphyrinogen decarboxylase defect or homozygous porphyria cutanea tarda? *Lancet.* 1981; I: 916–919.

13

Melanonychia

Eckart Haneke

Definition

The term *melanonychia* is derived from the Greek words *melas,* for black (brown), and *onyx,* for nail, and simply means a (brown to) black nail. Although the term is neutral concerning the nature of the pigment causing this discoloration, most clinicians mean melanin pigmentation when speaking of melanonychia.

Frequency

Melanonychia is rare in fair-skinned children but is a relatively common condition in individuals with dark complexion. Melanonychia is caused by melanocyte activation, lentigo, nevus, or melanoma. However, the exact percentages of melanonychia in general and particularly in children are not known. A systematic examination of 1000 consecutive patients with dark nail pigmentation showed eight subungual hematomas but no melanocytic lesion.[1]

Acquired melanocytic nevi of the lateral and proximal nail folds are surprisingly rare; they do not cause a brown streak in the nail.

Gender and Age

There is no clear-cut gender predominance. Melanonychias may be inborn, but this is rare. Most brown nail streaks develop between the age of 6 months and 5 years, but later appearance is not uncommon.

Etiology

Melanocytes are present in the nail, but more in the matrix than in the nail bed.[2] They are functionally inactive in fair-skinned people, but a great variety of stimuli may induce the melanin production and it is physiologic in individuals with dark complexions.

Functional hypermelanosis, lentigines, and nevi are the most frequent causes of melanonychia, with ungual melanoma being exceedingly rare in children. The exact numbers for melanocyte activation, lentigo, and nevus-derived melanonychias do not exist. Functional melanonychia is probably more frequent than matrix lentigo, and this is, again, more frequent than nevus. Acquired subungual lentigines and nevi occur both in Caucasians and, probably even more frequently, in Asians[3] and are often a matter of concern for patients and/or their parents. They are rare in blacks.[4] Congenital nevi causing melanonychia are also very rare. Blue nevi are rare[5–8] and do not produce a brown streak. Congenital blue nevi of the nail are exceptional.[9] It is not known whether lentigines and nevi exist in the nail bed; however, as the nail bed does not produce nail substance, it does not give rise

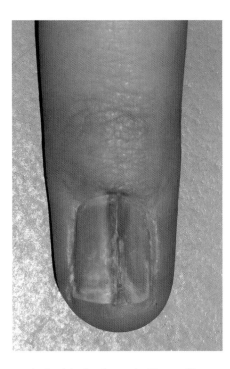

FIGURE 13.1   Recurrent matrix nevus in the right ring finger of a 25-year-old woman. The nevus had been known since the age of 4 years. A subtotal excision had been performed roughly 2 years prior to consultation at our department. A homogeneous brown streak is visible in addition to the postbiopsy nail dystrophy. Re-excision by the tangential biopsy method remained without a recurrence after 3 years.

to a brown streak and is visible as a brown spot under the nail. However, there are some examples of subungual nevi localized both in the matrix and in the nail bed and they give rise to longitudinal melanonychia.

Melanonychia develops when the matrix keratinocytes are unable to disintegrate the excess melanin in the matrix. The melanin is transferred into matrix keratinocytes that migrate obliquely upward and distally during nail plate genesis.

Nevi represent a manifestation of a punctual mosaicism as they develop from a postzygotic mutation.[10,11] This means that the size of a nevus is genetically predetermined, which may be the cause of recurrence in seemingly completely excised matrix nevi (Figure 13.1). Since a lentigo is probably the first stage of nevus development, this can be estimated to be true also for matrix lentigines.

Clinical Features

A brown band running from the matrix, usually emerging from under the proximal nail fold, to the free end of the nail is called a longitudinal melanonychia. It may be light to dark brown. Sometimes the streak is so light that it is barely visible, sometimes it is virtually black.

The so-called functional melanonychias are usually light brown with a grayish background. Dermatoscopically, they appear as regular brown bands with evenly distributed narrow streaks. The grayish background may be more obvious using a dermatoscope. The darker pigmentation of the proximal nail fold skin is a common feature in dark-skinned individuals and should not be confused with Hutchinson's sign.

Longitudinal melanonychia due to a lentigo is usually more brown, and the longitudinal streaks within it are regular on a brown-to-grayish background. This pattern is again more clearly seen with the dermatoscope (Figure 13.2).

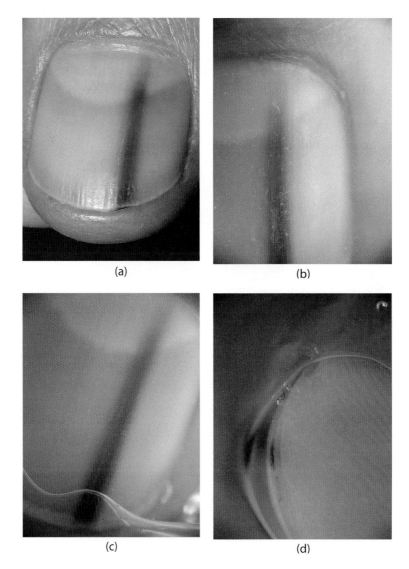

(a)

(b)

(c)

(d)

FIGURE 13.2 Lentigo of the nail matrix in the thumb nail of a 12-year-old girl, causing a regular brown streak in the nail. (a) Clinical photo. (b) Macrophoto without an optical medium. (c) Macrophoto with a laser contact gel as an optical medium. (d) End-on dermatoscopy shows pigment in the lower half of the nail plate, evidencing its origin from the distal matrix.

Nevi give rise to brown bands, with their color being more pronounced. Particularly in young children, they often display brown spots that are visible to the naked eye and represent intraungual collections of nevus cells. Periungual pigmentation is frequent in children (Figure 13.3). Dermatoscopy makes this pattern more clearly visible. This phenomenon is not seen in melanocyte activation and lentigines.

Acquired melanonychias are usually not wider than 5 mm, although they may widen insidiously or even abruptly to occupy almost the whole nail width. On the other hand, subungual melanomas of 2 mm diameter have been described in adults.[12]

Although the presence of periungual micropigmentation is highly indicative of a malignant melanoma in adults, this is not uncommonly seen in children (Figure 13.4).

Longitudinal melanonychias always run from the matrix into the free margin of the nail as the melanin is incorporated in the nail substance. The melanin cannot be scraped off like superficial and exogenous pigmentations caused by certain bacteria and stains. Dermatoscopy of the free end of the nail plate usually allows the melanin within the nail plate to be localized. Pigment in the upper layers is seen when the

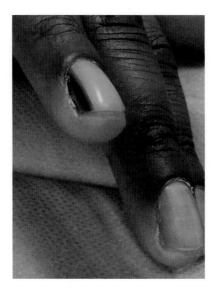

FIGURE 13.3   Nevus of the matrix of the right little fingernail of a 31-year-old dark-skinned nurse who had been present as long as she could remember. The brown band is regular, the central portion is darker than the margins.

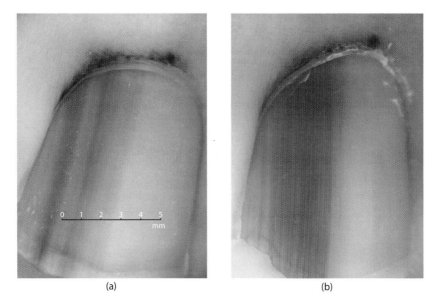

FIGURE 13.4   Longitudinal melanonychia in a 5-year-old child showing rapid change in width and periungual pigmentation. (a) Clinical presentation at first consultation. (b) Presentation 12 weeks later shows a more homogeneous pigmentation with regularly spaced brown lines in the band.

responsible lentigo or nevus is in the proximal matrix, in the middle nail layers when it is located in the middle matrix, and in the deep layers when the melanocyte nidus is present in the distal matrix. Pigment in the entire nail thickness indicates active melanocytes in the entire length of the matrix. Nail clippings stained with Fontana–Masson's argentaffin reaction permit a more precise estimate of the melanin localization under the microscope. New sophisticated and expensive techniques like optical coherence microscopy and reflectance confocal laser scanning microscopy permit the melanin to be precisely localized in the nail plate. Confocal laser microscopy enables the examiner also to discern single melanocytes and nevus cell nests in the nail. Nevus nests can also be demonstrated with a high-frequency ultrasound.

Histopathology

Depending on the material available for histopathological examination, different alterations are seen. In the nail clippings, particularly when the streak is only light brown, hematoxylin and eosin (H&E)-stained sections often do not exhibit a clear-cut melanin pigmentation. However, Fontana–Masson stain usually shows melanin granules in the nail plate, which is not seen in normal nails. Melanin is commonly seen in H&E sections of melanonychias due to lentigines and nevi, and occasionally, the latter may also show an intraungual nevus cell nest.

Nail biopsies must be taken from the matrix. Depending on the width of the brown band, a punch with a maximal diameter of 3 mm, a transversely oriented fusiform, or a slightly crescentic matrix biopsy, and in the case of lateral localization a lateral longitudinal nail biopsy or, particularly for wider melanonychias, a tangential excisional biopsy is preferred. In most cases, it is recommended to gently separate the nail plate from the matrix before taking the biopsy. This nail may be laid back after the biopsy and fixed with a suture strip or one or two stitches, which facilitates wound healing. The specimen should be marked to allow it to be oriented in the histopathology laboratory.[13,14] Formalin fixation is sufficient. In addition to H&E stain, Fontana–Masson and immunohistochemical demonstration of one or several melanocyte markers are generally recommended; MelanA and HMB45 are safe to demonstrate intraepithelial melanocytes, whereas protein S100 more reliably stains intradermal melanocytes. Sox10 and microphthalmia associated transcription factor (MITF) are not generally used; however, they have the advantage of not being melanosome stains but demonstrate the nuclei of melanocytes. It has to be stressed that the staining of serial sections of the same specimen very often yields different staining intensity and patterns with the various melanocyte markers and is thus useful in doubtful cases.

Functional melanonychia exhibits just an increase of melanin granules with a normal melanocyte count, which is about 6.5 melanocytes/mm stretch of the basal layer.[15] Although often performed, the immunohistochemical demonstration of matrix melanocytes is not really helpful; to visualize the increased pigmentation, a Fontana–Masson stain is necessary and usually confirms the hyperpigmentation. The discrepancy between a normal H&E stain and normal immunohistochemistry on one side and the increased pigmentation seen in the argentaffin reaction of Fontana–Masson allows the diagnosis of functional melanonychia to be made.

A matrix lentigo is characterized by a numerical increase of melanocytes with marked pigmentation (Figure 13.5). To make this visible, melanocyte markers are needed. A nevus has in addition at least one nest of melanocytes. In contrast to normal matrix melanocytes that are frequently localized above the basal row of matrix keratinocytes, melanocytes in lentigines often mainly occupy the basal layer. Immunohistochemically and with special melanin stains, long but slender dendrites can be identified (Figure 13.6).

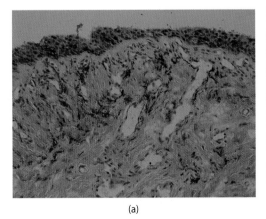
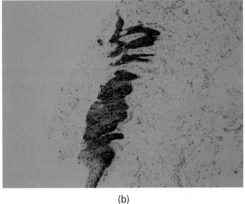

(a)   (b)

FIGURE 13.5 Histology of a matrix lentigo with many melanocytes and huge masses of melanophages. (a) Hematoxylin and eosin (H&E)-stained section of a tangential excision specimen showing an increased number of melanocytes in the matrix epithelium and melanophages in the dermis. (b) MelanA staining demonstrates a tremendous increase in the number of active melanocytes, but the melanophages are not stained (Pap method).

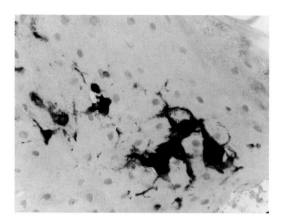

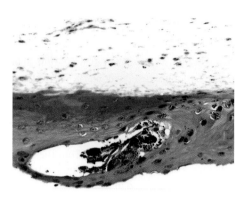

FIGURE 13.7   Nevus cell nest in the matrix epithelium with dark pigmentation seen to ascend obliquely distally. There are also pigmented nail cells in the nail plate. H&E, original magnification, ×200.

FIGURE 13.6   Melanocytes with long dendrites in a case of infantile matrix lentigo. Original magnification, ×400.

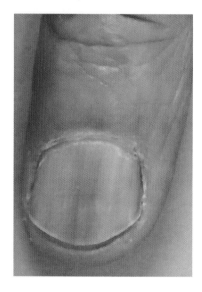

FIGURE 13.8   Laugier–Hunziker–Baran syndrome in a 53-year-old female patient, starting in infancy.

The melanocyte nests of a nevus are usually oval and may sometimes be taken up with the maturing cells of the keratogenous zone to finally be included in the nail plate (Figure 13.7). The degree of pigmentation varies from light brown to almost black; the color intensity does not reflect the dignity of the lesion.

The number of matrix melanocytes is either normal or increased in the Laugier–Hunziker–Baran syndrome,[16–18] which is characterized by lenticular brown spots of the oral mucosa, sometimes also the genito-anal mucosa and brown streaks in some nails (Figure 13.8). Peutz–Jeghers syndrome, defined by multiple colon polyps and periorificial lentigines, was also observed to cause nail involvement with longitudinal melanonychia.[19]

Congenital nevi sometimes affect the nail unit. They are usually much larger and darker than acquired ones and the entire nail plus periungual tissue may be involved, occasionally leading to nail deformation.[20–22] Malignant degeneration or development of an ungual melanoma from a congenital nevus has not (yet) been reported.

Blue nevi of the nail are very rare. They do not cause longitudinal melanonychia. However, a very large congenital blue nevus involving the entire big toenail and periungual tissue was observed with the so-called benign lymph node metastasis.

In adults, the Hutchinson's sign is commonly seen as a reliable marker of ungual melanoma. However, particularly in Japanese subjects, periungual pigmentation has also been observed in benign longitudinal melanonychia[23,24] and it is not uncommon in congenital melanocytic nevi of the nail.[25]

The diagnosis of a subungual melanoma is extremely delicate in children.[26-30] Melanocyte atypia is occasionally seen in pediatric melanonychia, but severe, widespread atypia must be interpreted as melanoma.[31] The melanocyte count as proposed recently for adults[32] is not applicable for childhood melanonychia.

Significance and Risk of Malignant Degeneration

Melanonychias in children are almost always benign,[33-36] but they are a matter of concern when they arise in adults. A particular cut-off age, up to which a brown band can be considered to be benign, is yet to be established. Since the underlying cause of melanonychia—simple hypermelanosis, lentigo, nevus, or melanoma—cannot be diagnosed with certainty on clinical grounds and nail plate histopathology alone, one has to be particularly prudent in light-skinned individuals. Dermatoscopy gives little more accuracy, although criteria like background color, evenness of striation, regular distance of striae within the band, and micro-Hutchinson sign are more easily evaluated.[37] A brown band in the nail of a child that has been present for many years without alteration but all of a sudden widens or becomes darker must raise concern and requires excisional biopsy with histopathologic examination. On the other hand, long-standing melanonychias in children have been observed to gradually lighten and finally disappear.

More than 35 years ago, it was stated that an acquired longitudinal melanonychia in a fair-skinned adult should rather be seen as malignant than benign,[38] which contrasts with melanonychia in children. Congenital nevi may give rise to very dark and wide bands, often associated with nevus spread to a part of the surrounding periungual skin; this periungual pigmentation is not suspicious of melanoma.

Since approximately two-thirds to three-quarters of all nail melanomas start as a longitudinal melanonychia,[39] they theoretically offer an excellent chance for early diagnosis.

Diagnosis

For the clinical differential diagnosis of benign from malignant melanonychia, the ABCDEF rule was designed.[40] However, although this is useful for adults, its value for children is limited.

Dermatoscopy is a useful adjunct to the clinical diagnosis.[41] A gray background and thin gray lines were associated with melanocyte activation, ethnic, and drug-induced pigmentation. A brown background and regular brown lines were linked with nevus, whereas melanoma shows a brown background and irregular brown lines.[42] However, both in children and in congenital nevi irregularities may be seen that are commonly observed in adults with subungual melanoma.[43] Direct matrix inspection and matrix dermatoscopy reliably differentiate lentigines and nevi from melanoma.[44-46]

In a study of 137 cases of longitudinal melanonychia, 72 were considered type I due to functional melanocyte activation, lentigo, and nevus; they did not show enlargement during a follow-up of a mean 5 years. Fifty-two were classified as type II melanonychia and five of them demonstrated enlargement during follow-up; they were biopsied and three showed lentigo or nevus, whereas two were in situ melanomas. The remaining 13 brown bands were classified as type III melanonychias and histologically diagnosed as melanoma in situ.[47]

The diagnostic gold standard is the histopathologic examination of an adequate biopsy specimen, ideally an excisional biopsy. Depending on the width of the melanonychia, different techniques such as punch, fusiform, crescentic, or lateral longitudinal biopsies are available. The superficial tangential biopsy allows large areas of the matrix to be biopsied virtually without the risk of postbiopsy nail dystrophy.[48] A quantitative study of the density of melanocytes yielded a mean melanocyte count of 15.3 and a median of 14 and a range of 5–31 per millimeter stretch of basal layer for lentigines in contrast to mean and median counts of 7.7 and 7.5, range 4–9 for controls, and a much higher number for invasive (102 and 92.5, range 52–212) and in situ melanoma (58.9 and 51, range 39–156), respectively.[32] However, we have seen higher numbers of melanocytes per millimeter stretch of the basal layer of the matrix epithelium in many cases of lentigines (Figure 13.7a and b).

DNA ploidy investigations were used to differentiate subungual nevi from melanoma.[49] Multiple gene amplifications are found in subungual melanomas early in their progression, about one half of them in the cyclin D1 locus.[50] Comparative genomic hybridization also allowed the diagnosis of a subungual melanoma to be made in a 13-year-old girl.[51]

Differential Diagnosis

The clinical differential diagnosis of lentigines and nevi comprises virtually all melanocytic processes such as functional melanonychia and melanoma; inflammatory nail diseases in darker-pigmented individuals; hormonal diseases such as Addison and Nelson syndrome[52]; nail pigmentation in malnutrition and vitamin B_{12} deficiency as well as from many drugs; epithelial tumors with melanocyte population such as pigmented Bowen disease, onychopapilloma, and onychomatricoma (Figure 13.9) but also nonmelanocyte causes such as subungual hematoma; infections with chromogenic bacteria such as pigmentation due to *Proteus* spp., *Klebsiella* spp., and *Pseudomonas aeruginosa*; fungal melanonychia from *Trichophyton rubrum* var. *nigricans* (Figure 13.10) and a variety of molds; exogenous nail pigmentation due to silver nitrate, dirt, tar, ornamental stains (Figure 13.11), and heavy smoking; and many more. Fumagoid bodies (Medlar bodies) were once seen to cause longitudinal melanonychia.[53] Except for the melanocytic processes, the other pigmentations are not fine granular and argentaffin. Staining from enterobacteria is usually on the nail surface and can be scraped off as can many other exogenous discolorations. Nail clippings may contain nests of nevus cells but intraungual single melanocytes are considered to be melanoma cells. Hematomas are not included in the free margin of the nail plate and their entire appearance is different; it is easy to differentiate them from melanin pigmentation. Furthermore, the material is scraped out and it can be differentiated using the benzidine reaction: the clotted blood is collected in a tiny test tube, a drop of water is added, and a test stripe for the diagnosis of blood in urine or feces is dipped into the test tube after a few minutes; in the case of blood, the test stripe turns positive. This is a very safe test for blood, but it has to be kept in mind that a bleeding melanoma will also be positive.[54]

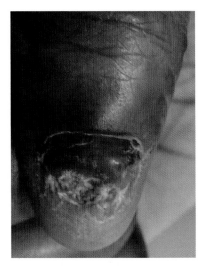

FIGURE 13.10 Post-traumatic single-digit black onychomycosis due to *Trichophyton rubrum* in a 34-year-old black cook. Note the increased pigmentation of the proximal nail fold (false Hutchinson sign), which was not associated with his onychomycosis. He had dark fingernails since adolescence.

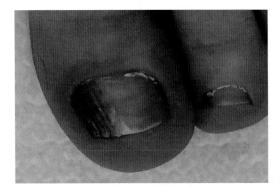

FIGURE 13.9 Pigmented onychomatricoma of the big toe in a 51-year-old woman starting in late adolescence. Histopathology showed a slight increase in the number of melanocytes.

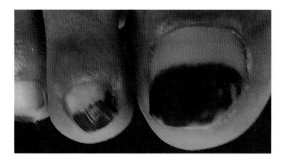

FIGURE 13.11 Toenails of a 34-year-old black woman with a dark stain due to *p*-phenylene diamine adulterated henna applied for ornamental reasons. The staining grows out with its proximal margin being parallel to the free margin of the nail fold, which is proof of the exogenous nature of the dark nail stain. She had painted her nails since preschool age.

Natural Course

The natural course of longitudinal melanonychias has not been systematically studied. Parents presenting their child with a brown streak in the nail are either worried about the prognosis or embarrassed because of the unusual cosmetic appearance. A few large studies have observed the children over a period of 10 years and more. It is said that a certain percentage will fade after the age of 14 years, but this does not give any information for a single case allowing the patients and parents to be reassured on a scientific ground.

Sun exposure was claimed to alter the intensity of the pigmentation of longitudinal melanonychia[55]; however, this is highly unlikely as the origin of the melanonychia is under the proximal nail fold and nail plate: The nail plate is a very effective ultraviolet (UV) shield[56] and the proximal nail fold is too thick to be penetrated by the UV light.

Treatment of Nail Lentigines and Nevi

Whereas it is our policy to remove acquired lentigines and nevi of the nail whenever the patient or his or her parents are concerned, many patients try to avoid surgery and instead rely on conservative diagnostic measures such as dermatoscopy or laser scanning microscopy. This may be correct for many cases, particularly in children; however, over a period of more than 30 years the number of invasive thick ungual melanomas that we have seen has dramatically decreased, and we believe that the early excision of suspicious lesions is the right way to avoid thick melanomas.[57] For lentigines and acquired nevi, which are almost invariably junctional and very rarely compound nevi, the diagnostic tangential excision is usually sufficient and therapeutic (Figures 13.2 and 13.5). Even when a light brown streak reoccurs, the histopathologic diagnosis has been made with certainty.

Outlook—Future Developments

Although quite common, particularly in more deeply pigmented individuals, melanonychias are still often overlooked or incorrectly diagnosed. It is not rare that a patient presents to his family physician for years or decades with a brown nail streak that gradually increases in color intensity and widens—unmistakable signs of proliferation and in most cases of malignancy. It is not the lack of examination tools but the lack of awareness of potential malignant development that delays the diagnosis of ungual melanomas. Certainly, more precise criteria for the diagnosis of matrix lentigines and nevi will be developed and the refinement of confocal laser scanning microscopy criteria will enable us to differentiate, at least in many cases, lentigines from nevi and above all from subungual melanoma.

REFERENCES

1. Shukla VK, Hughes LE. How common are benign subungual naevi? *Eur J Surg Oncol.* 1992; 18: 249–250.
2. Perrin CH, Michiels JF, Pisani A, Ortonne JP. Anatomic distribution of melanocytes in normal nail unit. An immunohistochemcial investigation. *Am J Dermatopathol.* 1997; 19: 462–467.
3. Leung AK, Woo TY. A subungual nevus in a Filipino child. *Pediatr Dermatol.* 2004; 21: 462–465.
4. Libow LF, Casey TJ, Varela CD. Congenital subungual nevus in a black infant. *Cutis.* 1995; 56: 154–156.
5. Vidal S, Sanz A, Hernández B et al. Subungual blue naevus. *Br J Dermatol.* 1997; 137: 1023–1025.
6. Causeret AS, Skowron F, Viallard AM et al. Subungual blue nevus. *J Am Acad Dermatol.* 2003; 49: 310–312.
7. Dalle S, Ronger-Savle S, Cicale L et al. A blue-gray subungual discoloration. *Arch Dermatol.* 2007; 143: 937–942.
8. Lee EJ, Shin MK, Lee MH. A subungual blue naevus showing expansile growth. *Acta Derm Venereol.* 2012; 92: 162–163.
9. Gershtenson PC, Krunic A, Chen H et al. Subungual and periungual congenital blue naevus. *Australas J Dermatol.* 2009; 50: 144–147.
10. Happle R. Wie häufig sind genetische Mosaike in der Haut? *Hautarzt.* 2014; 65: 536–541.
11. Happle R. *Mosaicism in Human Skin: Understanding Nevi, Nevoid Skin Disorders, and Cutaneous Neoplasia.* Berlin, Germany: Springer; 2014.
12. Rosendahl C, Cameron A, Wilkinson D et al. Nail matrix melanoma: Consecutive cases in a general practice. *Dermatol Pract Concept.* 2012; 2(2): 202–213.
13. Richert B, Theunis A, Norrenberg S et al. Tangential excision of pigmented nail matrix lesions responsible for longitudinal melanonychia: Evaluation of the technique on a series of 30 patients. *J Am Acad Dermatol.* 2013; 69: 96–104.
14. Reinig E, Rich P, Thompson CT. How to submit a nail specimen. *Dermatol Clin.* 2015; 33: 303–307.
15. Tosti A, Piraccini BM, Baran R. The melanocyte system of the nails and its disorders. In Nordlund JJ, Boissy RE, Hearing VJ et al. (eds.), *The Pigmentary System.* New York, NY: Oxford University Press; 1998. pp. 937–942.
16. Haneke E. Laugier–Hunziker–Baran Syndrom. *Hautarzt.* 1991; 42: 512–515.
17. Makhoul EN, Ayoub NM, Helou JF, Abadjian GA. Familial Laugier–Hunziker syndrome. *J Am Acad Dermatol.* 2003; 49: S143–S145.
18. Moore RT, Chae KA, Rhodes AR. Laugier and Hunziker pigmentation: A lentiginous proliferation of melanocytes. *J Am Acad Dermatol.* 2004; 50: S70–S74.
19. Valero A, Sherf K. Pigmented nails in Peutz–Jeghers syndrome. *Am J Gastroenterol.* 1965; 43: 56–59.
20. Ohtsuka H, Hori Y, Ando M. Nevus of the little finger with a remarkable nail deformity. *Plast Reconstr Surg.* 1978; 61: 108–111.
21. Coskey RJ, Magnel TD, Bernacki EG. Congenital subungual nevus. *J Am Acad Dermatol.* 1983; 9: 747–751.
22. Pomerance J, Kopf AW, Ramos L et al. A large, pigmented nail bed lesion in a child. *Ann Plast Surg.* 1994; 33: 80–82.
23. Asahina A, Matsuyama T, Tsuchida T et al. Two cases of infantile subungual pigmented nevi with Hutchinson's sign. *Nihon Hifuka Gakkai Zasshi.* 1989; 99: 899–906.
24. Kawabata Y, Ohara K, Hino H, Tamaki K. Two kinds of Hutchinson's sign, benign and malignant. *J Am Acad Dermatol.* 2001; 44: 305–307.
25. Agusti-Mejias A, Messeguer F, Febrer I, Alegre V. Congenital subungual and periungual melanocytic nevus. *Acta Dermosifiliograf.* 2013; 104: 446–448.
26. Kato T, Usuba Y, Takematsu H et al. A rapidly growing pigmented nail streak resulting in diffuse melanosis of the nail. A possible sign of subungual melanoma in situ. *Cancer.* 1989; 64: 2191–2197.

27. Molina D, Sanchez JL. Pigmented longitudinal bands of the nail. A clinicopathologic study. *Am J Dermatopathol.* 1995; 17: 539–541.

28. Kiryu H. Malignant melanoma in situ arising in the nail unit of a child. *J Dermatol.* 1998; 25: 41–44.

29. Motta A, López C, Acosta A, Peñaranda C. Subungual melanoma in situ in a Hispanic girl treated with functional resection and reconstruction with onychocutaneous toe free flap. *Arch Dermatol.* 2007: 143: 1600–1602.

30. Iorizzo M, Tosti A, Di Chiacchio N et al. Nail melanoma in children: Differential diagnosis and management. *Dermatol Surg.* 2008: 34: 974–978.

31. Tosti A, Piraccini BM, Cagalli A, Haneke E. In situ melanoma of the nail unit in children: Report of two cases in fair-skinned Caucasian children. *Pediatr Dermatol.* 2012; 29: 79–83.

32. Amin B, Nehal KS, Jungbluth AA et al. Histologic distinction between subungual lentigo and melanoma. *Am J Surg Pathol.* 2008; 32: 835–843.

33. Léauté-Labrèze C, Biouliac-Sage P, Taïeb A. Longitudinal melanonychia in children. *Arch Dermatol.* 1996; 132: 167–169.

34. Tosti A, Baran R, Piraccini BM et al. Nail matrix nevi: A clinical and histopathologic study of twenty-two patients. *J Am Acad Dermatol.* 1996; 34: 765–771.

35. Goettmann-Bonvallot S, André J, Bélaich S. Longitudinal melanonychia in children: A clinical and histopathologic study of 40 cases. *J Am Acad Dermatol.* 1999; 41: 17–22.

36. Theunis A, Richert B, Sass U et al. Immunohistochemical study of 40 cases of longitudinal melanonychia. *Am J Dermatopathol.* 2011: 33: 27–34.

37. Di Chiacchio N, Cadore De Farias D, Piraccini BM et al. Consenso sobre dermatoscopia da placa ungueal em melanoníquias [Consensus on melanonychia nail plate dermoscopy]. *An Bras Dermatol.* 2013; 88: 313–317.

38. Kopf AW, Waldo E. Melanonychia striata. *Australas J Dermatol.* 1980; 21: 59–70.

39. Tomizawa K. Early malignant melanoma manifested as longitudinal melanonychia: Subungual melanoma may arise from suprabasal melanocytes. *Br J Dermatol.* 2000; 143: 431–434.

40. Levit EK, Kagen MH, Scher RK et al. The ABC rule for clinical detection of subungual melanoma. *J Am Acad Dermatol.* 2000; 42: 269–274.

41. Braun RP, Baran R, Le Gal FA et al. Diagnosis and management of nail pigmentations. *J Am Acad Dermatol.* 2007; 56: 835–847.

42. Ronger S, Touzet S, Ligeron C et al. Dermoscopic examination of nail pigmentation. *Arch Dermatol.* 2002; 138: 1327–1333.

43. Goldminz AM, Wolpowitz D, Gottlieb AB, Krathen MS. Congenital subungual melanocytic nevus with a pseudo-Hutchinson sign. *Dermatol Online J.* 2013; 19(4): 8.

44. Hirata SH, Yamada S, Almeida FA et al. Dermoscopy of the nail bed and matrix to assess melanonychia striata. *J Am Acad Dermatol.* 2005; 53: 884–886.

45. Hirata SH, Yamada S, Almeida FA et al. Dermoscopic examination of the nail bed and matrix. *Int J Dermatol.* 2006; 45: 28–30.

46. Hirata SH, Yamada S, Enokihara MY et al. Patterns of nail matrix and bed of longitudinal melanonychia by intraoperative dermatoscopy. *J Am Acad Dermatol.* 2011; 65: 297–303.

47. Sawada M, Yokota K, Matsumoto T et al. Proposed classification of longitudinal melanonychia based on clinical and dermoscopic criteria. *Int J Dermatol.* 2014; 53: 581–585.

48. Haneke E. Operative Therapie akraler und subungualer Melanome. In Rompel R, Petres J (Hrsg.) (eds.), *Operative und Onkologische Dermatologie. Fortschritte der Operativen und Onkologischen Dermatologie*, Vol. 15. Berlin, Germany: Springer; 1999. pp. 210–214.

49. Asahina A, Chi HI, Otsuka F. Subungual pigmented nevus: Evaluation of DNA ploidy in six cases. *J Dermatol.* 1993; 20: 466–472.

50. Bastian BC. Understanding the progression of melanocytic neoplasia using genomic analysis: From fields to cancer. *Oncogene.* 2003; 22: 3081–3086.

51. Takata M, Maruo K, Kageshita T et al. Two cases of unusual acral melanocytic tumors: Illustration of molecular cytogenetics as a diagnostic tool. *Hum Pathol.* 2003; 34: 89–92.

52. Chang P, Román V, Monterroso MA et al. Síndrome de Nelson. *Dermatol Cosm Med Quir.* 2013; 11: 199–202.

53. Ko CJ, Sarantopoulos GP, Pai G, Binder SW. Longitudinal melanonychia of the toenails with presence of Medlar bodies on biopsy. *J Cutan Pathol.* 2005; 32: 63–65.
54. Haneke E, Baran R. Subunguale Tumoren. *Z Hautkr.* 1982; 57: 355–362.
55. Haenssle HA, Blum A, Hoffmann-Wellenhof R et al. When all you have is a dermatoscope—Start looking at the nails. *Dermatopathol Pract Concept.* 2014; 4(4): 2, 11–20.
56. Stern DK, Creasey AA, Quijije J, Lebwohl MG. UV-A and UV-B penetration of normal human cadaveric fingernail plate. *Arch Dermatol.* 2011; 147: 439–441.
57. Haneke E. Ungual melanoma—Controversies in diagnosis and treatment. *Dermatol Ther.* 2012; 25: 510–524.

14

Dermoscopy in Pediatric Longitudinal Nail Pigmentation

Luc Thomas

Nowadays, dermoscopy is considered as a mandatory step in the clinical evaluation of skin pigmented lesions. Several concordant meta-analysis proved that dermoscopy, performed by sufficiently trained observers, enhances the diagnostic performances of cutaneous nevi, melanomas, pigmented basal cell carcinomas, dermatofibromas, thrombotized angiomas, and seborrheic keratosis.[1–5]

In adults, after the publication by Ronger et al.,[6] several reports have further analyzed pigmented longitudinal bands of the nail plate. Even though some doubts have been initially expressed on the real value of dermoscopy of the nail,[7] many reports conclude that there is an increased accuracy of the diagnosis of nail tumors with dermoscopy compared with the naked eye and a consensus has been reached among the community of the nail melanoma specialists that dermoscopy gives interesting information in order to better determine if a nail matrix or nail-unit biopsy is needed in the case of longitudinal nail pigmentation.[8–16]

In children, however, nail tumors are quite rare and maybe excepted in the very peculiar setting of some genetic disorders like Gorlin–Goltz syndrome, xeroderma pigmentosum, and tuberous sclerosis. This is the reason why dermoscopy is mainly used in children in cases of *melanonychia striata longitudinalis* (MSL).

This chapter will focus only on the dermoscopical evaluation of MSL in prepubertal children. At this age, the main diagnostic dilemma is to diagnose nevi and exceptional (and, in several published cases, diagnostically debatable) cases of melanoma and to offer a reinsuring management of the longitudinal pigmented band to worried parents, once it is diagnosed in their child's nail.

Unfortunately, neither clinical nor dermoscopical criteria for benign and malignant MSL described in adolescents and adults apply to prepubertal patients leading to difficult choices in terms of diagnostic and/or therapeutic management. This is why our group proposed, 8 years ago, the creation of an international register of congenital or nearly congenital cases of nail pigmentation under the auspices of the International Dermoscopy Society (http://www.dermoscopy-ids.org/index.php/studies). More than 140 cases of MSL were discovered before the age of 5, and these have been gathered in this register. To date, no single case of undebatable histopathology-proven melanoma has been observed in this cohort recruited from more than 40 different countries. Indeed, continued follow-up of this cohort is necessary in order to better understand the evolution of these cases; however, our original and exclusive experience allows us to recommend (1) follow-up as the best management option and (2) continuous inclusion of new cases in our register in order to increase our knowledge and better support our conclusions.

Prepubertal Diagnostic Dilemma of MSL: Melanoma of Congenital Nevus?

Exceptional cases of prepubertal nail-unit melanoma have been published in the literature.[17–22] Even though some cases could be true malignant cases, many are debatable and one published case, reviewed by us both clinically and histopathologically after 7 years of evolution after partial (noncarcinologic) excision and locally recurrent pigmentation, corresponded to a congenital nevus of the nail unit.

In contrast, congenital (present at birth) and congenital type (not visible yet probably present at birth and then diagnosed before the age of 5) are rare but are not uncommon conditions.[23–28] It is noteworthy to say here that the concept of congenital-type nevus is nowadays widely acknowledged in skin; it corresponds to a malformation process rather than to a tumor process.[29–36] On skin, these nevi, also known as hamartomatous type of nevus, are raised, include terminal hair, and have brown globules as the dermoscopical signature feature. These lesions are observed early in life (at birth or shortly then after) and could involute through an inflammatory process (Sutton's halo nevus). Yet, in most cases, they stay in place through all ages and constitute the major part of nevi observed in elderly patients. Recent studies have shown that the major part of nevus-associated melanomas could be associated with this peculiar type of nevi.[37,38] On the opposite, acquired nevus will show reticulate pattern of their dermoscopical pigmentation and absence of terminal hair. This later type of nevi is mainly acquired after puberty and progressively involutes by progressively fading off during adulthood, and then being rarely observed in the elderly. Moreover, genotypical studies have shown that the *BRAF* mutation is more often observed in the acquired type of nevi (and acquired melanomas), whereas the *NRAS* mutation is more common in congenital-type ones (and nevus-associated melanomas).[39–43]

It is, in our view, a reasonable speculation to imagine that the figures could be similar in the nail unit. The discovery of a malformation-type mode of development of early-diagnosed nail-unit pigmented lesion, i.e., involving not only the melanocytes but also the epithelial and connective structures of the nail unit, further supports this hypothesis. Extrapolation of the natural history of the congenital-type nevi of the skin to their nail-unit counterparts indeed raises the question of possible malignant evolution of a proportion of the nail located ones. However, if the majority of nevus-associated melanomas on skin is found in combination with a congenital type of nevus, it is also widely accepted that in comparison with the very common prevalence of small-sized congenital nevi, the individual risk for each single one is very little.[44,45] However, a long-term follow-up of the cases included in the Lyons international congenital or nearly congenital nail pigmentation will be required in order to better evaluate this possible, yet probably individually rare, possibility.

Misleading Clinical Features of Congenital (or Congenital-Type) Nevus of the Nail Unit

In adults, MSL is considered suspicious[6] if (1) acquired during adulthood, (2) monodactylic, (3) triangular shaped, (4) multicolored, (5) associated with nail plate erosion, and (6) associated with periungual involvement (also known as Hutchinson's sign). Unfortunately, all but one of these criteria are commonly observed in congenital nevi of the nail unit.[22–26] Indeed, the lesion is diagnosed in childhood (we have set the threshold at age 5 for inclusion in the Lyons international register of congenital or congenital-type nail pigmentation); however, in early observations, the lesion if very often triangular shaped (Figure 14.1) is often multicolored with different shades of brown and gray-to-black (Figure 14.2) and is accompanied by longitudinal nail plate grooves (Figure 14.3). Periungual pigmentation is commonly observed (Figure 14.4) and the lesion is, in the vast majority of cases, monodactylic. We have observed only one case of involvement of two adjacent fingers in a case of medium-sized congenital nevus involving the hand of a 2-year-old patient.

Clinical features of adult's criteria for a malignant pigmentation are therefore frequently observed and constitute a major diagnostic pitfall. It augments the negative gestalt of the lesion in pediatric and unspecialized dermatologic clinics. The doctor's anxiety is then immediately transferred to the parents, unfortunately sometimes leading to precipitated surgical procedures. Surgery is often the source of complicated evolution: not only definitive functionally and significantly scarring but also recurrent pigmentation which is then extremely difficult to manage since anatomical changes led to difficult-to-diagnose pigmentation changes. Needless to say also that the histopathological evaluation of early biopsied congenital nevus is extremely difficult, especially in acral sites, with a high risk of overdiagnosis of melanoma.[24,27,28]

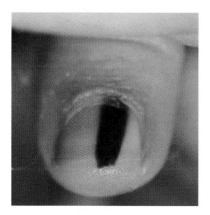

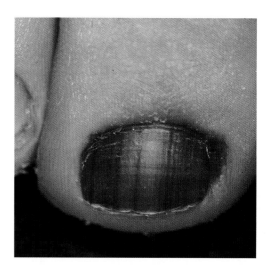

FIGURE 14.1 Triangular-shaped melanonychia striata longitudinalis (MSL) in a 3-day-old newborn male patient included in the Lyons international register of congenital or nearly congenital nail longitudinal pigmentation. This triangular-shaped pigmented band indicates that the causal lesion enlarges more rapidly than the speed of the growth of the nail. In adults, it is considered as highly indicative of malignancy. In contrast, this finding is not uncommon in the congenital nevus of the nail unit.

FIGURE 14.2 Multiple shades of brown within an MSL in a 1-year-old female patient included in the Lyons international register of congenital or nearly congenital nail longitudinal pigmentation.

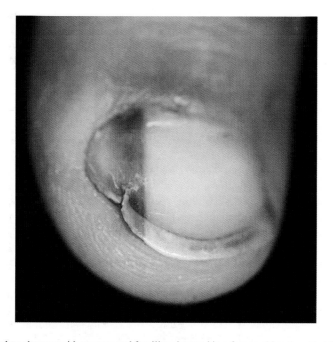

FIGURE 14.3 Nail plate changes with grooves and fragility observed in a 2-year-old male patient included in the Lyons international register of congenital or nearly congenital nail longitudinal pigmentation.

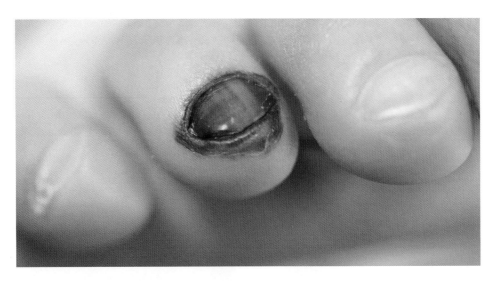

FIGURE 14.4 Periungual pigmentation in a 2-year-old female patient included in the Lyons international register of congenital or nearly congenital nail longitudinal pigmentation.

Misleading Dermoscopical Features of Congenital (or Congenital-Type) Nevus of the Nail Unit

In adults, the benign type of melanocytic pigmentation of the nail unit is typically quite easily opposed to the malignant one.[6,8–15] Both have a brown coloration of the background sign of the presence of a significant melanocytic hyperplasia in the nail matrix (on the opposite dermoscopical gray-yellowish pigmentation of longitudinal pigmented band of the nail is associated with conditions in which melanin content of the matric is increased in the absence of significant melanocytic hyperplasia: lentigo and lentiginosis, ethnic-type, drug-induced, repetitive trauma-induced pigmentations). After puberty, a nevus will typically show, on dermoscopy, a regular pattern of the longitudinal lines overlying the brown background and will be opposed to a melanoma showing irregular longitudinal lines with irregular coloration, irregular thickness, and irregular spacing of the bands; however, staying parallel along the nail plate at least during the early stages. Disruption of longitudinal parallelism of the longitudinal band is a feature dermoscopically observed in only advanced cases of nail-unit melanoma. Periungual pigmentation (Hutchinson's sign) is a clinical sign in favor of melanoma as described above. Yet this pigmentation might not be seen with the naked eye and only disclosed with the dermoscope. In this case, we have described this feature as a "micro-Hutchinson's sign."[6]

Unfortunately, congenital nevi of the nail unit, during early observations, share much more dermoscopical features with adult's melanoma than with postpuberty nevi.[26] After several years of follow-up, these initially very atypical, by adult's criteria evaluation, show a marked tendency to evolve toward a more benign appearance. At first or early evaluation, congenital nevi often show a markedly irregular pattern of the longitudinal bands with different shades of brown or gray and black with uneven width and spacing of the lines (Figure 14.5). Weakness of the nail plate is also often observed and responsible on nail plate erosions and grooves. Moreover periungual pigmentation, in most cases visible to a naked eye, is better visualized through the dermoscope (Figure 14.6). Interestingly enough, this periungual pigmentation is not only proximal, as seen in most cases of Hutchinson's sign in adult's melanoma, but often distal (Figure 14.7). We speculate that this distal location of the pigmentation is due to the very early development of the nevus during embryogenesis, before the formation of the nail folding process around the eighth week of gestation, resulting in the presence of nevus material on both proximal and

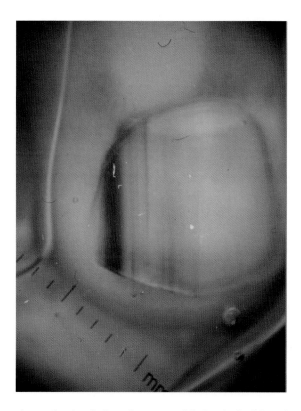

FIGURE 14.5 Dermoscopy image showing the irregular pattern of the longitudinal lines (irregular in color, width, and spacing of the longitudinal dermoscopical microlines) in 1-year-old male patient included in the Lyons international register of congenital or nearly congenital nail longitudinal pigmentation.

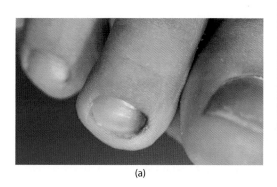

(a)

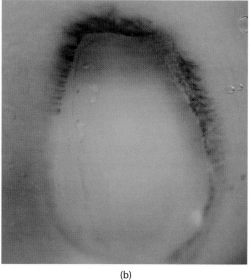

(b)

FIGURE 14.6 Periungual pigmentation is more visible on dermoscopy (b) than with naked-eye examination (a) in a 0.5-year-old male patient included in the Lyons international register of congenital or nearly congenital nail longitudinal pigmentation.

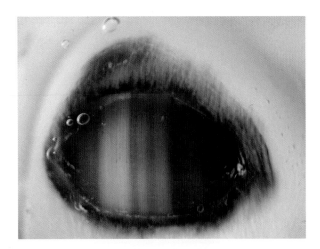

FIGURE 14.7   Dermoscopy image of proximal lateral and distal periungual pigmentation present since birth in a 1-year-old female patient included in the Lyons international register of congenital or nearly congenital nail longitudinal pigmentation. Note that periungual pigmentation in glabrous (plantar) skin shows a mix of parallel furrow pattern and fibrillar pattern, two well-known benign patterns of acral skin pigmentation.

distal part of the perionychium just like that observed in both eyelids in the case of congenital nevus of the periocular region.

A "Signature Dermoscopic Feature" of Congenital Nevi of the Nail Unit

As seen above, periungual pigmentation is very common in congenital nevi of the nail unit. However, our published work in adults has shown that the dermoscopical features observed in melanoma-associated periungual pigmentation show one or another or both classical features of acral melanoma that are the parallel ridge pattern of the pigmentation and irregular diffuse pattern of the acral pigmentation. In contrast, in nevi, even in newborn or prepubertal children, the perinungual pigmentation reproduces the benign features described on acral skin that are parallel furrow pattern (Figure 14.7) and, yet less commonly, lattice-like pattern and fibrillar pattern.

In our experience, the fibrillar distal pigmentation is composed of thin longitudinal parallel lines in the periungual area in distality of the hyponychium (Figures 14.8 and 14.9) and can be considered as the "signature feature" of the congenital nevi of the nail unit. It is not consistently found associated with this condition, but, when present, the diagnosis can be considered as almost certain.

Reinsuring Evolutive Behavior of Congenital Nevi of the Nail Unit

As seen previously, with the remarkable exception of the highly significant presence of a distal fibrillar pattern, neither the clinical features nor the dermoscopical observations of congenital nevi are specific. Moreover, the observed features at early stages are mimicking adult's melanoma. Therefore, it is often impossible to rely only on one single observation to establish the diagnosis. Repeated spaced observations of the case will therefore be of crucial importance in order to establish the final diagnosis, especially if, as we believe, it constitutes the best management; the lesion has not been biopsied.

Over time, the lesion will initially enlarge (Figure 14.10), then stabilize with a more homogeneous pattern of pigmentation (Figure 14.11), and, in a large number of cases, show a marked tendency to progressively fade away over time (Figure 14.12). However, the clinically unapparent lesion cannot probably be considered as the complete resolution of the entire lesion. As well-known in other cutaneous congenital

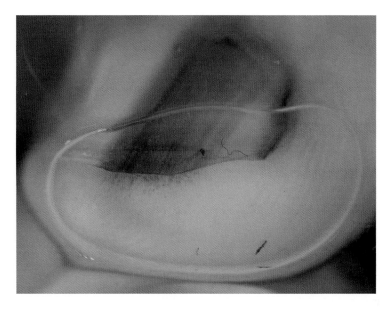

FIGURE 14.8 The "signature dermoscopy feature" of the congenital nevus of the nail unit: distal fibrillar pattern in the area corresponding to the nail pigmented band in a 1-year-old male patient included in the Lyons international register of congenital or nearly congenital nail longitudinal pigmentation.

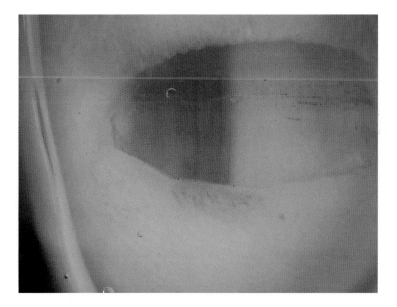

FIGURE 14.9 Less pigment is a clearly identifiable "signature dermoscopy feature" of the congenital nevus of the nail unit: distal fibrillar pattern in the area corresponding to the nail pigmented band in a 1-year-old female patient included in the Lyons international register of congenital or nearly congenital nail longitudinal pigmentation.

lesions and hamartomas, constituting elements may remain in the original site of the lesion and could hypothetically explain the latter onset of recurrences or, maybe, and malignant transformation.

We suggest that unexcised prepubertal MSL, especially if diagnosed under the age of 5, the chosen threshold age for our study, should be followed clinically and by digital dermoscopy after 4 months, then 12 months, and then every 6 months until stabilization, and then a yearly follow-up could be

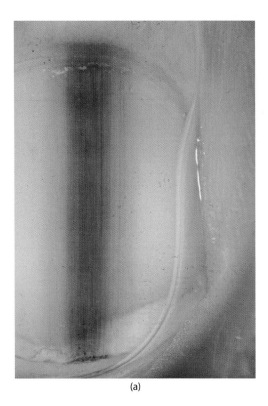
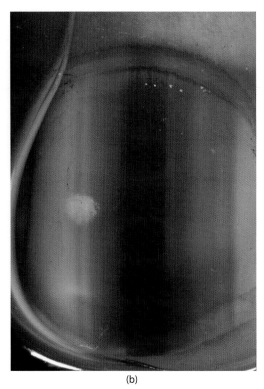

(a)   (b)

FIGURE 14.10   Dermoscopy image of the initial increase in the width of a congenital MSL in a (a) 3-month-old and then (b) 1-year-old male patient included in the Lyons international register of congenital or nearly congenital nail longitudinal pigmentation.

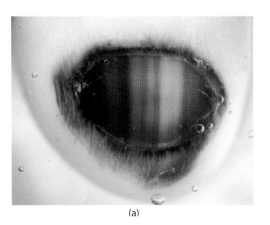
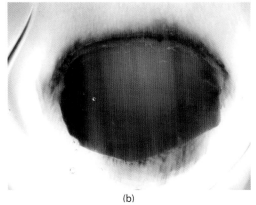

(a)   (b)

FIGURE 14.11   More homogeneous pattern of the pigmentation at age 5 (b) was initially recorded in a 1-year-old (a, also seen on Figure 14.7) female patient included in the Lyons international register of congenital or nearly congenital nail longitudinal pigmentation.

instituted. If fading off of the lesion is observed, follow-up should be continued until the complete disappearance of the pigmentation both clinically and dermoscopically. Then, continued follow-up of the patient might be of scientific interest yet difficult to justify in the parents' and patient's eyes.

Indeed, inclusion of the case in the Lyons international register of nail-unit congenital nevus is welcome and recommended (http://www.dermoscopy-ids.org/index.php/studies).

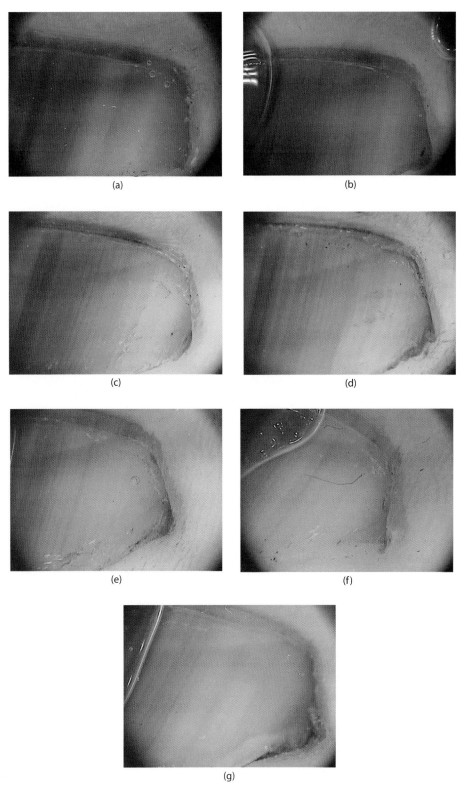

FIGURE 14.12. (a–g) Digital dermoscopy follow-up images taken in an initially 2-year-old male patient included in the Lyons international register of congenital or nearly congenital nail longitudinal pigmentation for congenital lesions and then observed at ages 3, 4, 5, 6, 7, and 8 years old.

REFERENCES

1. Kittler H, Pehamberger H, Wolff K, Binder M. Diagnostic accuracy of dermoscopy. *Lancet Oncol.* 2002; 3(3): 159–165.
2. Salerni G, Terán T, Puig S et al. Meta-analysis of digital dermoscopy follow-up of melanocytic skin lesions: A study on behalf of the International Dermoscopy Society. *J Eur Acad Dermatol Venereol.* 2013; 27(7): 805–814.
3. Vestergaard ME, Macaskill P, Holt PE, Menzies SW. Dermoscopy compared with naked eye examination for the diagnosis of primary melanoma: A meta-analysis of studies performed in a clinical setting. *Br J Dermatol.* 2008; 159(3): 669–676.
4. Bafounta ML, Beauchet A, Aegerter P, Saiag P. Is dermoscopy (epiluminescence microscopy) useful for the diagnosis of melanoma? Results of a meta-analysis using techniques adapted to the evaluation of diagnostic tests. *Arch Dermatol.* 2001; 137(10): 1343–1350.
5. Tromme I, Sacré L, Hammouch F et al. DEPIMELA study group. Availability of digital dermoscopy in daily practice dramatically reduces the number of excised melanocytic lesions: Results from an observational study. *Br J Dermatol.* 2012; 167(4): 778–786.
6. Ronger S, Touzet S, Ligeron C et al. Dermoscopic examination of nail pigmentation. *Arch Dermatol.* 2002; 138(10): 1327–1333.
7. Jellinek NJ. Dermoscopy between the lines. *Arch Dermatol.* 2010; 146(4): 431–433.
8. Koga H, Saida T, Uhara H. Key point in dermoscopic differentiation between early nail apparatus melanoma and benign longitudinal melanonychia. *J Dermatol.* 2011; 38(1): 45–52.
9. Di Chiacchio N, Hirata SH, Enokihara MY et al. Dermatologists' accuracy in early diagnosis of melanoma of the nail matrix. *Arch Dermatol.* 2010; 146(4): 382–387.
10. Phan A, Dalle S, Touzet S et al. Dermoscopic features of acral lentiginous melanoma in a large series of 110 cases in a white population. *Br J Dermatol.* 2010; 162(4): 765–771.
11. Bilemjian AP, Piñeiro-Maceira J, Barcaui CB, Pereira FB. Melanonychia: The importance of dermatoscopic examination and of nail matrix/bed observation. *An Bras Dermatol.* 2009; 84(2): 185–189.
12. Bristow IR, Bowling J. Dermoscopy as a technique for the early identification of foot melanoma. *J Foot Ankle Res.* 2009; 2: 14.
13. Tosti A, Piraccini BM, de Farias DC. Dealing with melanonychia. *Semin Cutan Med Surg.* 2009; 28(1): 49–54.
14. Thomas L, Dalle S. Dermoscopy provides useful information for the management of melanonychia striata. *Dermatol Ther.* 2007; 20(1): 3–10.
15. Braun RP, Baran R, Le Gal FA et al. Diagnosis and management of nail pigmentations. *J Am Acad Dermatol.* 2007; 56(5): 835–847.
16. Tosti A, Argenziano G. Dermoscopy allows better management of nail pigmentation. *Arch Dermatol.* 2002; 138(10): 1369–1370.
17. Bonamonte D, Arpaia N, Cimmino A, Vestita M. In situ melanoma of the nail unit presenting as a rapid growing longitudinal melanonychia in a 9-year-old white boy. *Dermatol Surg.* 2014; 40(10): 1154–1157.
18. Tosti A, Piraccini BM, Cagalli A, Haneke E. In situ melanoma of the nail unit in children: Report of two cases in fair-skinned Caucasian children. *Pediatr Dermatol.* 2012; 29(1): 79–83.
19. Iorizzo M, Tosti A, Di Chiacchio N et al. Nail melanoma in children: Differential diagnosis and management. *Dermatol Surg.* 2008; 34(7): 974–978.
20. Antonovich DD, Grin C, Grant-Kels JM. Childhood subungual melanoma in situ in diffuse nail melanosis beginning as expanding longitudinal melanonychia. *Pediatr Dermatol.* 2005; 22(3): 210–212.
21. Kiryu H. Malignant melanoma in situ arising in the nail unit of a child. *J Dermatol.* 1998; 25(1): 41–44.
22. Haneke E. Ungual melanoma—Controversies in diagnosis and treatment. *Dermatol Ther.* 2012; 25(6): 510–524.
23. Goettmann-Bonvallot S, André J, Belaich S. Longitudinal melanonychia in children: A clinical and histopathologic study of 40 cases. *J Am Acad Dermatol.* 1999; 41(1): 17–22.
24. Buka R, Friedman KA, Phelps RG et al. Childhood longitudinal melanonychia: Case reports and review of the literature. *Mt Sinai J Med.* 2001; 68(4–5): 331–335.
25. Yan AC, Smolinski KN. Melanocytic nevi: Challenging clinical situations in pediatric dermatology. *Adv Dermatol.* 2005; 21: 65–80.

26. Lazaridou E, Giannopoulou C, Fotiadou C et al. Congenital nevus of the nail apparatus—Diagnostic approach of a case through dermoscopy. *Pediatr Dermatol.* 2013; 30(6): e293–e294.

27. Theunis A, Richert B, Sass U et al. Immunohistochemical study of 40 cases of longitudinal melanonychia. *Am J Dermatopathol.* 2011; 33(1): 27–34.

28. Domínguez-Cherit J, Chanussot-Deprez C, Maria-Sarti H et al. Nail unit tumors: A study of 234 patients in the dermatology department of the "Dr Manuel Gea González" General Hospital in Mexico City. *Dermatol Surg.* 2008; 34(10): 1363–1371.

29. Pellacani G, Scope A, Farnetani F et al. Toward an in vivo morphologic classification of melanocytic nevi. *J Eur Acad Dermatol Venereol.* 2014; 28(7): 864–872.

30. Haliasos EC, Kerner M, Jaimes N et al. Dermoscopy for the pediatric dermatologist part III: Dermoscopy of melanocytic lesions. *Pediatr Dermatol.* 2013; 30(3): 281–293.

31. Moscarella E, Zalaudek I, Cerroni L et al. Excised melanocytic lesions in children and adolescents—A 10-year survey. *Br J Dermatol.* 2012; 167(2): 368–373.

32. Piliouras P, Gilmore S, Wurm EM et al. New insights in naevogenesis: Number, distribution and dermoscopic patterns of naevi in the elderly. *Australas J Dermatol.* 2011; 52(4): 254–258.

33. Zalaudek I, Schmid K, Marghoob AA et al. Frequency of dermoscopic nevus subtypes by age and body site: A cross-sectional study. *Arch Dermatol.* 2011; 147(6): 663–670.

34. Haliasos HC, Zalaudek I, Malvehy J et al. Dermoscopy of benign and malignant neoplasms in the pediatric population. *Semin Cutan Med Surg.* 2010; 29(4): 218–231.

35. Zalaudek I, Manzo M, Savarese I et al. The morphologic universe of melanocytic nevi. *Semin Cutan Med Surg.* 2009; 28(3): 149–156.

36. Zalaudek I, Hofmann-Wellenhof R, Kittler H et al. A dual concept of nevogenesis: Theoretical considerations based on dermoscopic features of melanocytic nevi. *J Dtsch Dermatol Ges.* 2007; 5(11): 985–992.

37. Shitara D, Nascimento M, Ishioka P et al. Dermoscopy of naevus-associated melanomas. *Acta Derm Venereol.* 2015; 95(6): 671–675.

38. Kolm I, French L, Braun RP. Dermoscopy patterns of nevi associated with melanoma. *G Ital Dermatol Venereol.* 2010; 145(1): 99–110.

39. Zalaudek I, Guelly C, Pellacani G et al. The dermoscopical and histopathological patterns of nevi correlate with the frequency of BRAF mutations. *J Invest Dermatol.* 2011; 131(2): 542–545.

40. Shitara D, Tell-Martí G, Badenas C et al. Mutational status of naevus-associated melanomas. *Br J Dermatol.* 2015; 173(3): 671–680.

41. Salgado CM, Basu D, Nikiforova M et al. BRAF mutations are also associated with neurocutaneous melanocytosis and large/giant congenital melanocytic nevi. *Pediatr Dev Pathol.* 2015; 18(1): 1–9.

42. Lu C, Zhang J, Nagahawatte P et al. The genomic landscape of childhood and adolescent melanoma. *J Invest Dermatol.* 2015; 135(3): 816–823.

43. Dubruc E, Balme B, Dijoud F et al. Mutated and amplified NRAS in a subset of cutaneous melanocytic lesions with dermal spitzoid morphology: Report of two pediatric cases located on the ear. *J Cutan Pathol.* 2014; 41(11): 866–872.

44. Price HN, O'Haver J, Marghoob A et al. Practical application of the new classification scheme for congenital melanocytic nevi. *Pediatr Dermatol.* 2015; 32(1): 23–27.

45. Krengel S, Scope A, Dusza SW et al. New recommendations for the categorization of cutaneous features of congenital melanocytic nevi. *J Am Acad Dermatol.* 2013; 68(3): 441–451.

15

Nail Tumors in Children

Marcel Pasch

Introduction

A nail tumor may be defined as a swelling of the nail, the nail bed, or the periungual tissues, generally without inflammation, caused by an abnormal growth of tissue, whether benign or malignant. Nail tumors in children occur infrequently and the vast majority of these tumors are benign. Malignant nail tumors, however, despite their rarity in children, cannot be completely disregarded or ignored.

Nail tumors may also be classified by location: nail plate, nail bed, nail fold, digital pulp, and distal phalanx. The distinct localization of tumors of the nail results in a particular clinical picture. The interpretation of the modes of clinical expression will be discussed briefly in this chapter. Not only skin tumors may present as a nail tumor but also tumors containing cells of a different origin may give the impression of a nail tumor if located around the nail unit.

The name of the tumor generally is based upon the parenchymal cell they arise from. In this chapter, a classification based upon cells and tissue of origin will be used (Table 15.1). Pyogenic granulomas, hamartomas, vascular and lymphatic tumors, pigmented lesions, and ingrown toenails are discussed as separate entities in Chapters 6, 9, 10, 13, and 17, respectively.

Presentation

A nail tumor may differ from tumors developing at other sites. These differences are sometimes caused by differences in biologic behavior compared with neoplasms that originate from the same cell type at other locations, but differences in clinical expression may also be explained by anatomical reasons: The location of the tumor will have consequences for the anatomical integrity of the nail plate. As a rule of thumb, a benign tumor does not destroy the surrounding tissues, while a malignant tumor will not accept the integrity of the surrounding tissues. The consequences for nail tumors will be that a benign tumor or an early (pre-) malignant tumor in the vicinity of the nail matrix will result in a change of the shape of the nail plate but not in the destruction of the nail plate. A benign tumor arising in the dorsal part of the proximal nail fold will cause compression on the nail matrix from above, which can be recognized as a longitudinal groove in the intact nail plate distal from the tumor (Figure 15.1), while a benign tumor arising in the ventral part of the proximal nail fold will cause an upward pressure on the nail matrix from the phalangeal side. Clinically, this results in ridging of the nail plate distal from the tumor or in an overcurvature of the entire nail (Figure 15.2). A malignant tumor, however, will, regardless whether it is located dorsal or ventral from the matrix, result in a partial destruction of the matrix causing a longitudinal defect or fissure of the nail plate (Figure 15.3), or result in the complete destruction of the matrix, causing anonychia if the destructive process has involved the entire nail matrix.

The nail plate is in direct contact with the underlying nail bed. Development of a tumor in the tiny anatomical niche between the distal phalanx and the nail plate may cause deformity of the nail, onycholysis,

TABLE 15.1

Tumors That May Occur in or around the Nail of Children (Modified WHO Classification)

Keratinocyte tumors

1. Warts
2. Bowen's disease and squamous cell carcinoma
3. Onychopapilloma
4. Knuckle pads
5. Onychomatricoma
6. Onychocytic matricoma
7. Acanthoma: acantholytic dyskeratotic acanthoma
8. Nail cysts

Melanocytic tumors

1. Nevus
2. Lentigo
3. Melanoma

Soft tissue tumors

1. Vascular tumors
   a. Hemangioma of infancy
   b. Epithelioid hemangioma of bone
   c. Angiomas
   d. Capillary malformations
   e. Venous malformations
   f. Digital arteriovenous malformations
   g. Angiokeratoma circumscriptum
   h. Pyogenic granuloma
   i. Malignant hemangioendothelioma
2. Lymphatic tumors: Lymphangioma circumscriptum
3. Fibrous, fibrohistiocytic and histiocytic tumors
   a. Digital fibrokeratoma
   b. Superficial acral fibromyxoma
   c. Keloid scar
4. Fibrogenic/fibroblastic/myofibroblastic tumors
   a. Congenital infantile fibrosarcoma
   b. Fibrosarcoma
   c. Infantile digital fibromatosis
5. Chondro-osseous tumors: Soft tissue chondroma
6. Smooth muscle tumors: Leiomyosarcoma
7. Pericytic (perivascular) tumors: Glomus tumor
8. Nerve sheath tumors
   a. Neurofibroma
   b. Schwannoma, plexiform schwannoma, and malignant schwannoma
9. Soft tissue tumor of uncertain differentiation: Epithelioid sarcoma

Cartilage and bone tumors

1. Osteochondroma and exostosis
2. Enchondroma
3. Chondrosarcoma
4. Chondromyxoid fibroma

(Continued)

TABLE 15.1 (*CONTINUED*)

Tumors That May Occur in or around the Nail of Children (Modified WHO Classification)

   5. Osteoid osteoma

   6. Ewing's sarcoma

   7. Aneurysmal bone cyst

   8. Giant cell tumor of the bone

Neural tumors

   1. Merkel cell carcinoma

   2. Granular cell tumor

Hematolymphoid tumors

   1. Langerhans cell histiocytosis

   2. Juvenile xanthogranuloma

   3. APACHE

Congenital nail tumors and nail tumors in inherited syndromes

   1. Epidermal nevi

   2. Hereditary multiple exostosis

   3. Ollier disease

   4. Neurofibromatosis type 1

   5. Tuberous sclerosis

   6. Incontinentia pigmenti

   7. Digitocutaneous dysplasia

   8. Juvenile hyaline fibromatosis

   9. Congenital hypertrophic lip of the hallux

Abbreviations: WHO, World Health Organization; APACHE, acral pseudolymphomatous angiokeratoma of children.

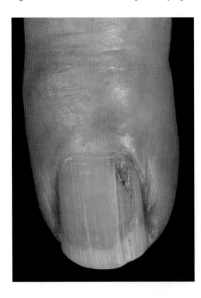

FIGURE 15.1   A tumor arising in the dorsal part of the proximal nail fold will cause compression on the nail matrix from above, resulting in a longitudinal groove in the intact nail plate distal from the tumor (digital fibrokeratoma).

and pain due to swelling and compression. Tumors that normally reside within the upper parts of the skin may deform or invade the bone of the distal phalanx if they arise in this tiny niche. A tumor originating from the bone of the distal phalanx, or subcutaneously located, may cause bulbous enlargement of the distal part of the finger (Figure 15.4) and nail clubbing due to widening of the bone associated with the pressure beneath the nail bed.

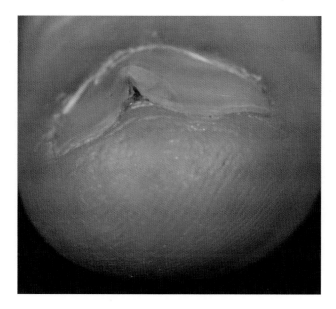

FIGURE 15.2 A tumor arising in the ventral part of the proximal nail fold will cause an upward pressure on the nail matrix from the phalangeal side, resulting in ridging of the nail plate distal from the tumor (glomus tumor).

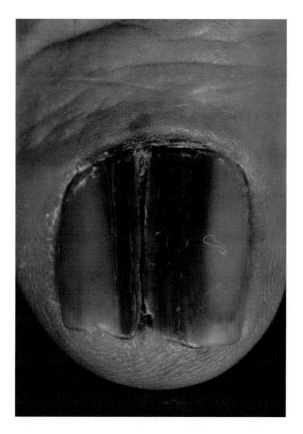

FIGURE 15.3 A malignant tumor destroys (part of) the matrix causing a longitudinal defect or fissure of the nail plate (melanoma).

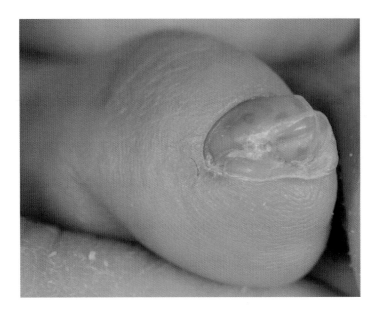

FIGURE 15.4   A tumor originating from under the nail plate may cause nail clubbing or bulbous enlargement of the distal part of the finger.

Evaluation of Nail Tumors

Many changes in the nail unit may be indicative of underlying tumor growth. In some cases, like uncomplicated periungual warts, clinical inspection will be sufficient for a certain diagnosis. Additional tests are required for the majority of nail tumors, since the clinical appearance of both benign and malignant nail tumors is nonspecific. Pathology is the cornerstone of the final classifying diagnosis. Tissue for histology can become available after the diagnostic excision of a tumor. In most cases, a (punch) biopsy will be sufficient to make the correct diagnosis. Radiology may be useful to rule out or to confirm certain clinical diagnoses. The most often used radiological techniques are X-ray, computed tomography (CT), magnetic resonance imaging (MRI), and ultrasound. Bone tumors or cartilaginous tumors will be detectable by conventional radiology, as well as bone invasion or deformation of other neoplasms. CT is able to assess tiny abnormalities of the cortex of the distal phalanx. Ultrasonography, in particular high-resolution ultrasonography with color Doppler studies, provides useful information regarding tumor size, location, shape, and internal characteristics (cystic, solid, or mixed) and may be helpful to visualize a vascular component of a tumor. MRI offers the advantage of imaging the soft parts of the nail unit or the underlying bone and may provide more accurate information about location and signal characteristics that reflect the underlying pathologic features of a tumor.[1,2] Radiological techniques are discussed in Chapters 20 and 21.

Keratinocyte Tumors

Warts

Warts are by far the most common tumor of the nail in children. Periungual and subungual warts are caused by many different genotypes of human papillomavirus (HPV). HPV 1, 2, 4, 27, and 57 are generally the cause of benign ungual warts.[3] HPV 16, 18, and 58 are rare causes but are associated with malignant transformation to squamous cell carcinoma.[3,4] Warts are caused by the infestation of the abraded or macerated skin with the HPV.[5] In particular, nail biting is a risk factor for ungual warts in children. Nail biting and picking may also result in the spreading of the condition to the face and lips.[6] HPV is very resistant to heat, desiccation, and detergents. Therefore, warts can also be acquired by indirect contact and not only by direct contact in a susceptible host.

Few weeks to more than 1 year after inoculation, clinical warts develop. Fingernails are involved more often than toenails, possibly because of more frequent exposure of the hands to the sources of HPV.

HPV may invade the skin from any epidermal side of the nail plate. This invasion induces hyperkeratotic growth of the epidermal compartment resulting in verrucous lesions, recognizable as warts. These warts are present as 1 mm–10 cm nodular or linear keratotic papules and plaques under or around the nail plate (Figure 15.5). Not infrequently warts of the proximal nail fold produce periungual hyperkeratosis simulating a hyperkeratotic cuticle. Epidermal ridges do not cross the wart and paring the wart surface produces characteristic pinpoint bleeding that can be observed in any common wart. Local nail bed destruction can result in significant deformities such as onycholysis or subungual hyperkeratosis without nail plate dystrophy. Although warts do not directly affect the nail matrix, they may produce slight matrix damage due to compression, resulting in nail plate ridging and grooving.[6] HPV-induced Bowen's disease or squamous cell carcinoma, which may clinically be indistinguishable from common ungual warts, has not been reported in children.

Periungual warts can be diagnosed clinically. Histology is useful in exceptional cases to exclude Bowen's disease or squamous cell carcinoma.

Treatment

Warts often disappear spontaneously, especially in healthy children. The duration of warts varies from a few months to many years but specific data on ungual warts are missing. Aggressive measures are not recommended because of this spontaneous resolution. Furthermore, aggressive measures do not offer a guarantee for definitive cure, recurrences are frequent in any treatment, and the warts may become larger and unmanageable after repetitive treatments. A stronger indication for treatment are warts in immunocompromised patients, which are often present for years and have an insidious growth.

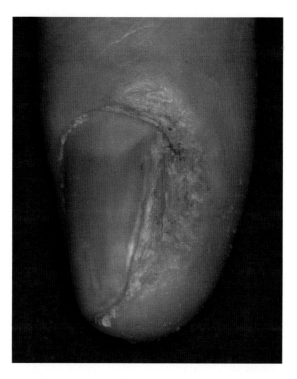

FIGURE 15.5 A typical wart of the proximal and lateral nail fold with extension under the nail plate with hyperkeratosis and characteristic pinpoint bleeding.

The decision to treat ungual warts in children is often pushed by parents who are afraid of stigmatizing. Other patient-dependent factors should also be taken in consideration to choose the optimal approach for an individual patient. Factors to consider are the number, size, location, and duration of the warts, age of the patient, and immunologic status.

Topical therapies may help to control the growth of the warts. Keratolytic agents are effective and mostly contain salicylic acid, sometimes lactic acid, bichloroacetic acid, or trichloroacetic acid. Virucidal agents contain glutaraldehyde or formaldehyde and are as effective as keratolytic agents. A more time-consuming and also an effective approach is topical immunotherapy with squaric acid dibutylether or diphenylcyclopropenone.[7] This topical immunotherapy is an interesting option for a painless mode of treatment in patients with multiple warts. Topical immunomodulatory therapy using imiquimod 5% cream may be considered in more recalcitrant cases.[8] Also, photodynamic therapy using 20% delta-aminolevulinic acid has been reported to be effective in ungual warts.[9] Topical 5% 5-fluorouracil cream has not been investigated in ungual warts, but it was found to be effective in plantar warts.[10] More aggressive topical therapy, such as intralesional injection of the antimitotic bleomycin, has shown good results,[11,12] but this treatment may occasionally result in permanent nail damage.[13] Systemic treatments with cimetidine have been advocated in the past[14] but its efficacy has never been definitively proven. Surgical treatment of warts includes cryotherapy, excision, and laser therapy. Cryotherapy with liquid nitrogen is often the first choice for small warts. In children, its use is limited by the pain that patients may experience. Cryotherapy in the vicinity of the matrix should be performed carefully to prevent permanent damage of this nail-forming organ. Excision is less favorable due to the high rate of recurrence and resultant deformity. More recently, several lasers have been used, including the CO_2, pulsed dye, and Yag laser,[15,16] but in daily practice their efficacy is not always convincing. Laser therapy is recommended as a second line for recalcitrant warts.

Conclusions

Periungual warts in healthy children mostly disappear spontaneously. A wait-and-see policy or use of mild topical keratolytics is justified in most of the cases. Aggressive treatments should be used with reluctance, because recurrences and permanent scarring of the nail unit are not uncommon.

HPV-associated Bowen's disease or squamous cell carcinoma are reported in persistent and recalcitrant verrucae[17] but have not been reported in children. However, suspicion is justified in those situations in which the nail plate is damaged, because a common wart does not invade the nail matrix.

Bowen's Disease and Squamous Cell Carcinoma

Malignant transformation of epithelial surfaces of the nail unit is rare in children and adolescents. Bowen's disease, the clinical term for in situ squamous cell carcinoma of the skin, and invasive squamous cell carcinoma have nevertheless been reported in a number of cases in children of 4 years old and up.[18–21] As discussed above, Bowen's disease and squamous cell carcinoma of the nail unit can often be attributed to HPV in adults[3,4] but no reported pediatric case can be related to warts or positive HPV test. Other risk factors for malignant transformation are radiation therapy, immunodeficiency, arsenic, pesticides, and subungual tumors of incontinentia pigmenti[22,23] (see also the section "Ollier Disease" and Chapters 1 and 9.

Bowen's disease of the nail unit is a special type of in situ squamous cell carcinoma, which seems to evolve relatively often toward an invasive form but squamous cell carcinoma of the nail unit metastasizes less often than other primary cutaneous squamous cell carcinoma. This relative benign behavior results in a very good prognosis.

Diagnosis of Bowen's disease and squamous cell carcinoma of the nail unit is often delayed or incorrect. Because of their benign appearance they are often misdiagnosed as a viral wart (Figure 15.6). Lesions mostly are present for several years before the correct diagnosis can be made. The fingers are more often involved than the toes.

Bowen's disease and squamous cell carcinoma of the nail unit may not only present as warty lesions but also as longitudinal melanonychia, onychopapilloma, fibrokeratoma, or onychomatricoma-like

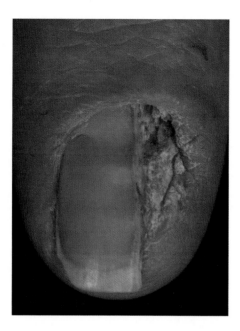

FIGURE 15.6 Diagnosis of Bowen's disease (and squamous cell carcinoma) of the nail unit is often delayed or incorrect; because of their benign appearance, they are often misdiagnosed as a viral wart.

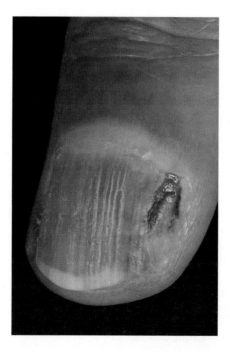

FIGURE 15.7 In particular, the nail plate destruction is a discriminating feature of Bowen's disease and squamous cell carcinoma with viral warts. The integrity of the nail is lost because this squamous cell carcinoma infiltrates the nail matrix.

lesions. The nail bed is most commonly involved. The commonest clinical signs are, in decreasing order, subungual hyperkeratosis, onycholysis, oozing, and nail plate destruction.[24] In particular the nail plate destruction is a discriminating feature with viral warts (Figure 15.7); the integrity of the nail is lost if the destructive malignant tumor infiltrates the nail matrix.

Generally, a punch biopsy from the lesion is sufficient to allow histological confirmation of the diagnosis of Bowen's disease or squamous cell carcinoma. It should be noted, however, that an incisional biopsy specimen may only reveal an in situ carcinoma but examination of the whole residual lesion may show overt invasive or microinvasive clusters. The preoperative evaluation should include radiography to exclude osseous involvement because bony invasion is reported regularly in invasive squamous cell carcinoma.[24]

Surgery is the preferred treatment for both Bowen's disease and squamous cell carcinoma of the nail unit. Nonsurgical treatments with CO_2 laser, photodynamic therapy, imiquimod cream, or 5% 5-fluorouracil cream, with or without prior curettage, have been used for the treatment of Bowen's disease of the nail unit. Considering the doubt one might have about the certainty a biopsy can offer in differentiating Bowen's disease from invasive squamous cell carcinoma, one might prefer a treatment that is also effective against invasive squamous cell carcinoma.[25] The recurrence rate of all treatments taken together was reported to be 30.6%.[24] The first-line surgical treatment of in situ or invasive squamous cell carcinoma of the nail unit can be a conventional surgical resection or Mohs micrographic surgery. The value of Mohs micrographic surgery in invasive squamous cell carcinoma of the nail unit is a matter of debate. Some authors prefer this treatment to prevent amputation,[19,24] while others find rather high recurrence rates, up to 56%.[26] Amputation of the distal phalanx is generally accepted to be the first choice when there is bone involvement. Another reason is because radiation therapy has been associated with bone necrosis.[13]

Onychopapilloma

Onychopapilloma was first reported in 1995 by Baran and Perrin.[27] It is a benign nail unit tumor that presents as a monodactylous linear streak under the nail plate. Linear erythronychia,[28] linear leukonychia,[29] or linear melanonychia[30] are all clinical signs seen in onychopapilloma. The streak mostly has interrupted splinter hemorrhages and distally, it ends in a visible hyperkeratotic papule that sticks out from under the nail plate (Figure 15.8). The nail plate usually shows distal splitting and a wedge-shaped notch. The hyperkeratotic plug at the distal end of the nail often is painful when pulled or clipped.

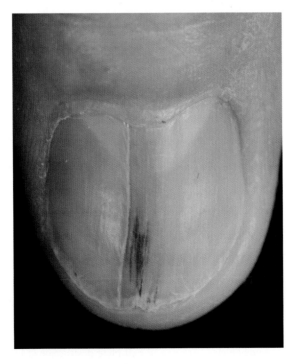

FIGURE 15.8 An onychopapilloma with an erythematous streak with interrupted splinter hemorrhages. The nail plate usually shows distal splitting and a wedge-shaped notch.

Mostly, the clinical expression mostly is very suggestive for onychopapilloma. However, the reliable diagnosis cannot be made solely on clinical characteristics because Baran and Perrin have shown presence of Bowen's disease in 2 out of 16 patients with the clinical picture of onychopapilloma.[31] The diagnosis onychopapilloma can be confirmed histologically. Onychopapilloma is usually seen in adults and also in adolescents.[28]

Management of monodactylous longitudinal streaks with subungual hyperkeratosis should be based on the patient's symptoms or changes in the lesion. Symptomatic lesions should be surgically excised. Sudden onset or changing streaks should be excised to rule out Bowen's disease and other causes of linear erythronychia.[32] Stable streaks can be re-evaluated in a few months. Punch biopsies can miss the diagnostic pathology or contribute to the recurrence of a lesion if only a portion of the tumor is sampled. Complete excision with a longitudinal nail unit biopsy from matrix to hyponychium that include the length of the lesion is recommended for these lesions. This is especially important in children to avoid trauma from two procedures.[28]

Knuckle Pads

Knuckle pads are discrete round, soft, and freely movable keratoderma, 0.5–1.5 cm in diameter, which may give a clue for another underlying or concomitant disorder. Mostly, they are skin-colored but hyperpigmentation or hypopigmentation has also been observed. The proximal interphalangeal joints are most frequently involved, but they have also been noted on the distal interphalangeal joints, metacarpophalangeal joints, and may occasionally occur on the thumbs and toes.

Primary knuckle pads appear as a spontaneous finding unassociated with other cutaneous disorders. Knuckle pads secondary to repeated trauma are called pseudo-knuckle pads,[33] or "chewing pads" in children. Knuckle pads may also be associated with fibrosing conditions, such as Dupuytren's contractures, Ledderhose disease, Peyronie's disease, and genetic disorders, such as epidermolytic palmoplantar keratoderma and Bart–Pumphrey syndrome. Severe knuckle pads in children have been attributed to G59A mutation in the GJB2 gene encoding connexin 26 in families with knuckle pads, palmoplantar keratoderma, and sensorineural hearing loss.[34]

Commonly, they appear between 15 and 30 years of age and persist through adulthood. The diagnosis of knuckle pads is primarily based on the clinical morphology of the skin lesions; biopsy of suspected lesions may be considered to exclude conditions with similar appearing morphology.[35] Knuckle pads are benign lesions that generally do not require treatment.

Onychomatricoma

Onychomatricoma is a rare benign tumor of the nail matrix presenting as a symptomless, slowly developing, focally or completely thickening of the nail plate.[36,37] The thickened area of the nail plate has prominent ridging, yellow discoloration along the length of the nail plate with multiple splinter hemorrhages involving the proximal nail plate, increased transverse curvature of the nail, and a funnel-shaped deformity (Figure 15.9). Very typical are filamentous extensions originating from the matrix, which become visible on nail avulsion and correspond with the funnel-shaped deformity of the nail plate. Onychomatricoma have some preference for fingernails above toenails but have no sex preference. The mean age of presentation is approximately 51 years[38] but a pediatric case has been reported.[39] Diagnosis can be confirmed with nail clipping and imaging methods including ultrasound and MRI. Histological examination reveals distinctive features that confirm the diagnosis. Surgery is the only option for treatment.

Onychocytic Matricoma

An onychocytic matricoma is a recently described rare tumor of the nail matrix. It is a benign acanthoma of the nail matrix producing onychocytes.[40] Clinically, the lesions were described as monodactylous longitudinal melanonychia. The main histological differential diagnosis is seborrheic keratosis. So far, five cases have been described but only one in a child, a 17-year-old adolescent.

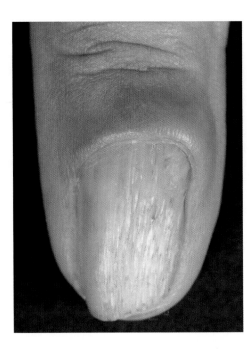

FIGURE 15.9 Onychomatricoma: The thickened area of the nail plate has prominent ridging, yellow discoloration along the length of the nail plate with some splinter hemorrhages involving the proximal nail plate and increased transverse curvature of the nail.

Acanthoma: Acantholytic Dyskeratotic Acanthoma

Acantholytic dyskeratosis is a histologic pattern defined by a hyperkeratotic and parakeratotic epidermis with intraepidermal clefts containing acantholytic and dyskeratotic keratinocytes. It usually is an accidental finding in histology and resembles Darier's disease or warty dyskeratoma but reflects a different tumorous process. Three cases involving the nail have been reported of which two were in children.[41] Both presented as median longitudinal hemorrhagic lesions in the thumbs, originating from the matrix and extending up to the distal part of the nail apparatus. This was accompanied by onycholysis and resembled onychopapilloma.

Nail Cysts

The nail cysts represent a broad group of lesions that differ in histogenesis and clinical picture. They may be small and subclinical, such as subungual epidermoid inclusions. Others are indistinguishable from epidermal inclusion cysts of the skin and are known as implantation epidermoid cysts. Finally, some cysts may contain epithelium that resembles that of the nail bed and are called onycholemmal cysts.[42] Of these, only subungual epidermoid inclusions[43] and implantation epidermoid cysts[44] have been reported in children.

Clinically, in subungual epidermoid inclusions the distal phalanx of the digit gradually increases in size with marked hyperplasia of the bed epithelium, resulting in subungual keratosis, onycholysis, or dystrophic nail plate.[45] Initially, this is painless but later pain appears due to bone compression or eventually fractures. Other clinical presentations include shooting pain or even an acquired pincer nail.[43] There is no pathognomonic clinical or radiologic sign. A nail bed biopsy is required for diagnosis because the reported inclusions are rather microscopic than macroscopic. Once the diagnosis on subungual epidermoid inclusions has been made, no clear treatment is curative, although simply making an accurate diagnosis may prevent inappropriate treatment.[45]

Implantation epidermoid cyst of the distal phalanx is a distinct and unrelated abnormality, although the clinical presentation may be identical.[45] It mostly is characterized by a solitary, painful, enlarged distal phalanx associated with recent trauma or surgery (Figure 15.10). Radiographic studies and

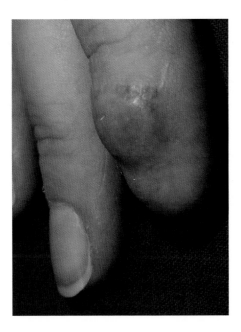

FIGURE 15.10 Implantation epidermoid cyst of the distal phalanx associated with recent surgery (skin graft after excision of the nail unit because of an in situ melanoma).

histology are both diagnostic, demonstrating that this cyst arises in the bone of the terminal phalanx. The occurrence of the cyst in children is very rare but an 8-year-old girl with two implantation epidermoid cysts of the distal phalanx following nail surgery has been reported by Baran and Bureau.[44] Implantation epidermoid cysts can be removed surgically.

Soft Tissue Tumors

Vascular Tumors

Hemangioma of Infancy

Hemangioma of infancy is the most common soft-tissue tumor in children, with an incidence of 1%–2% in the general population. They are discussed in Chapter 10.

Epithelioid Hemangioma of Bone

Epithelioid hemangioma, previously designated angiolymphoid hyperplasia with eosinophilia and histiocytoid hemangioma, is a vascular tumor mostly occurring in the skin and subcutis. Its presentation in the nail unit is discussed in Chapter 10.

Angioma

Subungual angioma often present as painful swellings with focal blue-red discoloration, mostly beneath the lunula. They are discussed in Chapter 10.

Capillary Malformations

Capillary malformations, port-wine stains, or nevus flammeus are the most common congenital vascular malformations, frequently occurring on the extremities. They are discussed in Chapter 10.

Venous Malformations

A common vascular malformation is the venous malformation. It is discussed in Chapter 10.

Digital Arteriovenous Malformations

Arteriovenous malformation is usually congenital but an acquired type is also known, of which most are due to an injury. It is discussed in Chapter 10.

Angiokeratoma Circumscriptum

Angiokeratoma circumscriptum presents as a hyperkeratotic plaque containing warty red–blue papules and nodules. These are present at birth and are discussed in Chapter 10.

Pyogenic Granuloma

Pyogenic granuloma mostly are reactive tumors occurring in the lateral nail folds. They are discussed in Chapter 6.

Malignant Hemangioendothelioma

Retiform hemangioendothelioma, epithelioid hemangioendothelioma, and congenital hemangioendo-thelioma are rare malignant tumors that may arise in the vicinity of the nail.

Retiform Hemangioendothelioma

Locally aggressive, low-grade angiosarcoma of unknown etiology that was first described in 1994. In 2011, Keiler reported of an 11-year-old girl with a rapidly enlarging and intermittently painful swelling of her left distal fourth finger.[46] Local recurrence is common, but no cases of distant metastasis, transformation to an aggressive vascular tumor, or tumor-related death have been observed.

Epithelioid Hemangioendothelioma

A borderline malignant vascular tumor that occurs mainly during the second and third decades of life. The most common symptoms are localized pain and swelling. Pediatric cases involving the phalanges have occasionally been reported.[47,48]

Congenital Hemangioendothelioma

Congenital hemangioendothelioma are extremely rare. Only one case describing an infant with a congenital lesion on the right index finger has been reported.[49]

Lymphatic Tumors: Lymphangioma Circumscriptum

Lymphangioma circumscriptum or superficial lymphatic malformation is the most common lymphangioma. It occurs in infancy or early childhood but the finger is an extremely unusual site. Clinically, the lesion generally presents as a cluster of small, cutaneous, translucent vesicles, which resemble frog spawn (Figure 15.11). One pediatric case has been reported in a 16-year-old girl.[50]

Fibrous, Fibrohistiocytic, and Histiocytic Tumors

Digital Fibrokeratoma

Digital fibrokeratomas (DF), also known as acquired ungual fibrokeratoma or garlic clove fibroma, are benign tumors of fibrous tissue. They present as solitary, smooth, dome-shaped or fingerlike, flesh-colored, asymptomatic papules with a hyperkeratotic tip and a narrow base mostly located in the periungual area (Figure 15.12). DF is a dermoepidermal tumor, covered by an orthokeratotic or hyperkeratotic,

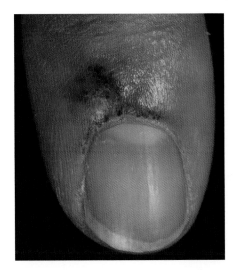

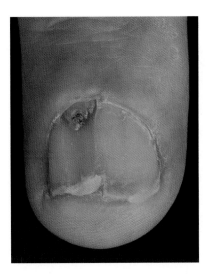

FIGURE 15.11 Lymphangioma circumscriptum presenting as a cluster of small, cutaneous, translucent, and hemorrhagic vesicles.

FIGURE 15.12 Digital fibrokeratoma: A solitary, smooth, dome-shaped, or fingerlike, flesh-colored, asymptomatic papules with a hyperkeratotic tip located in the periungual area.

papillomatous, acanthotic epidermis, with an underlying connective tissue proliferation. Trauma is thought to be a major causative factor, but the recollection of trauma is absent in many cases.

Mostly emerging from the dorsal side of the proximal nail fold, they induce pressure on the underlying matrix. As a consequence of this pressure an abnormal shaped nail plate is formed: a longitudinal groove runs the whole length of the plate. However, some DF origin from within the matrix, resulting in an intraungual DF which is like in an envelope, covered both ventrally and dorsally with nail plate (Figure 15.13). The latter are known as dissecting ungual fibrokeratomas. Occasionally DF find their origin in the nail bed and appear as a tumor at the hyponychium. Their sizes may vary from 1 to at least 10 mm.

Ungual or periungual fibroma are one of the major diagnostic criteria of tuberous sclerosis complex. These patients often present in puberty with multiple DF, which are called Koenen tumor. This is discussed in more detail in the section "Tuberous Sclerosis" and in Chapter 9.

While multiple DF appear early in life in tuberous sclerosis complex patients, isolated DF tend to occur later in life. However, diagnosis in young adolescents may occur.[51]

Verruca vulgaris, pyogenic granuloma, and neurofibromas are the common lesions that cause difficulty in the clinical differential diagnosis. The main diagnostic pitfall is Bowen's disease which may present as a DF. Therefore, histology, often as an excisional biopsy, is mandatory to exclude Bowen's disease. Removal from its very base is required to prevent recurrence.

Superficial Acral Fibromyxoma

Superficial acral fibromyxoma is a cutaneous neoplasm with a striking predilection for the subungual or periungual region of the hands and feet. It affects young adults, and a couple of cases have been reported in children and adolescents from the age of 4 years and above.[52–54]

It usually presents as a solitary erythematous elastic tumor under the nail plate or affecting the lateral nail fold (Figure 15.14). Ungual involvement may be present, induced by pressure on the nail or nail matrix. Patients may present with a painful mass, but almost as many are asymptomatic.

X-rays show bone alterations in about one-third of patients, commonly erosions.[54] An incisional biopsy is required to reveal the true nature of the tumor. However, it poses a diagnostic problem for pathologists, resulting in misclassification and overtreatment.[54] The distinction between digital fibromyxoma and malignant myxoid tumors is important since the latter often have a protracted clinical course characterized by multiple recurrences and metastasis.[54]

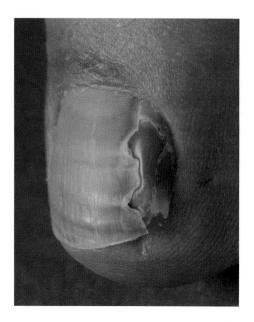

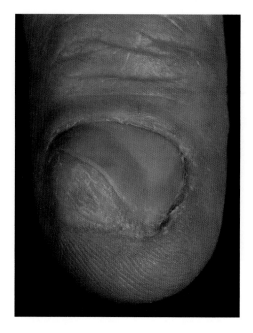

FIGURE 15.13 A digital fibrokeratoma originating from within the matrix, resulting in an intraungual or dissecting digital fibrokeratoma, which is covered both ventrally and dorsally with nail plate.

FIGURE 15.14 Superficial acral fibromyxoma presenting as a solitary erythematous elastic tumor under the nail plate or affecting the lateral nail fold.

Superficial acral fibromyxoma has a benign behavior and malignization has not been described. Complete excision is mandatory in order to prevent local recurrences.

Keloid Scar

Keloids are collagenous, cutaneous lesions acquired as a result of abnormal wound healing after trauma or after surgery of the skin. In contrast to hypertrophic scars, keloids exceed the boundaries of the initial injury, do not spontaneously regress and are difficult to revise surgically. Keloid formation of the fingers is in particular noticed after syndactyly release surgery.[55,56] Almost all of these patients were white in contrary to the usual keloid patients who are preferentially from African ancestry.

Treatment of keloid scars is problematic. Standard treatment (pressure, topical or intralesional corticosteroids, and re-excision) was unsuccessful in resolving the keloids. Adjunctive methotrexate treatment was successful in several patients.[55,56]

Fibrogenic/Fibroblastic/Myofibroblastic Tumors

Congenital Infantile Fibrosarcoma

Congenital infantile fibrosarcoma is a rare mesenchymal tumor that primarily develops in the soft tissue of distal extremities. It occurs mainly in children below the age of 5 years and is usually regarded as a tumor of borderline or low malignant potential.[57] One case involving the whole finger of a neonate was reported.[58] Clinically, congenital infantile fibrosarcoma presents with a rapidly expanding dusky firm swelling resembling hemangioma, lymphatic malformation, or a hemorrhagic vascular malformation. A biopsy will show histology that is identical to the classic fibrosarcoma of adults.[57]

Treatment modalities include resection, chemotherapy, or, rarely, radiotherapy. This tumor uncommonly metastasizes, but local recurrence may occur.

Fibrosarcoma

Fibrosarcoma is a malignant spindle cell tumor, which exhibits fibroblastic differentiation without synthesis of osseous or chondroid matrix. Fibrosarcoma may occur everywhere where fibrous connective tissue is found but is rare in hands and feet.[59] The diagnosis depends on histology. Adequate treatment requires at least wide surgical margins achieved either by en bloc resection or amputation.

Infantile Digital Fibromatosis

Infantile digital fibromatosis is an uncommon benign proliferation of fibroblastic and myofibroblastic cells that typically occur in the dermal tissue of the digits of young children. Several names exist for the same condition: Infantile digital fibromatosis, recurring digital fibrous tumors of childhood, benign juvenile digital fibromatosis, and inclusion body fibromatosis.

The appearance and consistency of infantile digital fibromatosis is similar to that of keloid: it presents as a firm, broad-based, nontender nodule, typically less than 2 cm in diameter, in the lateral side of the digits covered by smooth flesh-colored surface.[60,61] Single or multiple lesions can be observed. The lesions may result in deformity and functional impairment, and become clinically evident within the first year of age, and in up to one-third of cases immediately after the birth. There are also rare descriptions of this disease in older children, adolescents, and adults. The lesion has also been described after syndactyly release,[61] and in association with digitocutaneous dysplasia.[62]

Location and age are very suggestive for the diagnosis infantile digital fibromatosis, but histology is often required to confirm the diagnosis.[61]

Management of these lesions is controversial. Conservative, expectant observation is reasonable, given the benign nature of the lesions, potential for recurrence after surgery, and their tendency to spontaneously regress. However, lesions may cause functional impairment thereby warranting therapeutic intervention.[63] Options include amputation, excision, and skin grafting, Mohs micrographic resection, injection of chemotherapeutics, and observation. The recurrence rate can be as high as 60% following tumor excision, which is reflected in the name "recurring digital fibrous tumors of childhood."

Chondro-Osseous Tumors: Soft Tissue Chondroma

Soft tissue chondroma is a rare benign cartilaginous tumor that is not attached to the underlying bone. It mainly occurs on the hands or feet of individuals aged between 30 and 60 years[64] but pediatric cases have been reported in the literature.[65,66] Most cases of the soft tissue chondroma are characterized by a asymptomatic slowly growing mass. Over time, patients complain of symptoms such as local tenderness, and pain on action.

The clinical, radiological, and histological triad is important for the correct diagnosis of soft tissue chondroma. MRI is the method of choice in the evaluation of this entity. Histology often is required for the correct diagnosis, because cytology will show worrying cell atypia.[64] Treatment is recommended only for patients who have persistent pain or cosmetic concerns, such as nail deformity. Soft tissue chondroma shows a relatively high rate of local recurrence of 15%–25%.

Smooth Muscle Tumors: Leiomyosarcoma

Dermal or subcutaneous leiomyosarcoma is a rare smooth muscle cell neoplasm probably arising from the arrectores pilorum or vessel walls. They are usually asymptomatic, solitary, firm nodules measuring 0.5–3 cm in diameter, but pain and tenderness have been recorded. Two adolescent cases involving the distal phalanx have been reported.[67,68]

Histology has a central position in the diagnostic process. The treatment should be radical wide excision. Adjuvant radiotherapy or chemotherapy, or both, is of little, if any, benefit.[67]

Pericytic (Perivascular) Tumors: Glomus Tumor

Glomus tumor is a benign vascular hamartoma that contains all the neuromyoarterial cells of the normal glomus apparatus in the reticular dermis. Most likely, because of the high concentration of glomus bodies at this site, 75%–90% of glomus tumors are located in the subungual region. Reports on glomus tumors in children exist[69,70] and typical subungual glomus tumors are frequently reported in pediatric patients with neurofibromatosis type 1 (see the section "Neurofibromatosis Type 1" and Chapter 9). Clinically, often a red-purple macule is visible in the lunula (Figure 15.15). Splitting of the nail plate may occur later (Figure 15.16). Diagnosis is usually based on the presence of a characteristic classic triad of severe pain, pinpoint tenderness, and cold sensitivity. Radiography may reveal bone erosions and MRI with contrast may show a hot-spot. Also, ultrasound may be helpful to estimate the size of the lesion.

The treatment of choice for glomus tumors is total surgical excision. Malignant transformation has not been reported in children.

Nerve Sheath Tumors

Neurofibroma

Neurofibroma is a benign neoplasm containing fibroblasts, Schwann cells, and perineural cells. Neurofibromas may occur as a solitary tumor or as part of neurofibromatosis. Neurofibromas seldom occur in the nail region and less than 10 case reports of solitary subungual neurofibroma have been documented,[71] one of them in a 13-year-old girl.[72] These neurofibromas are difficult to diagnose, particularly as they are often small and without obvious symptoms. The symptoms described ranged from onychodystrophy, subungual hyperkeratosis, an increase in the size of the affected digit, and an increase in the curvature of the nail (Figure 15.17).[73]

Radiography may be part of the workup in order to evaluate bone involvement.[73] As the clinical features of this tumor are nonspecific, complete surgical excision should be considered as the curative treatment of choice for the correct diagnosis and treatment of the tumor.

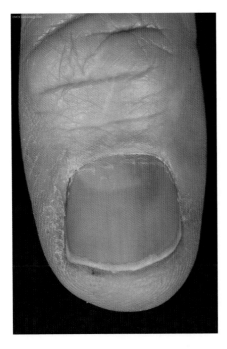

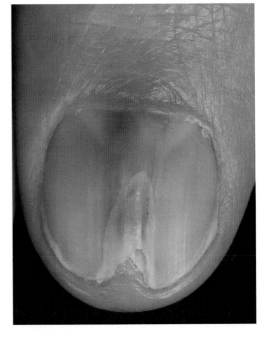

FIGURE 15.15 An "early" glomus tumor, presenting with a red-purple macule in the lunula.

FIGURE 15.16 An "older" glomus tumor with splitting of the nail plate distal from the red-purple macule.

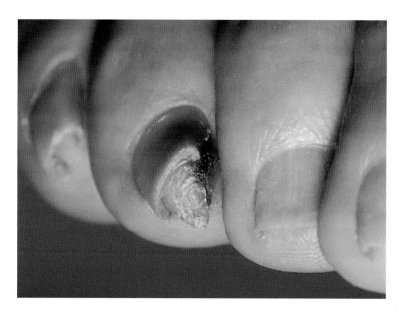

FIGURE 15.17 A subungual neurofibroma presenting as a partly hyperkeratotic and partly smooth subungual tumor.

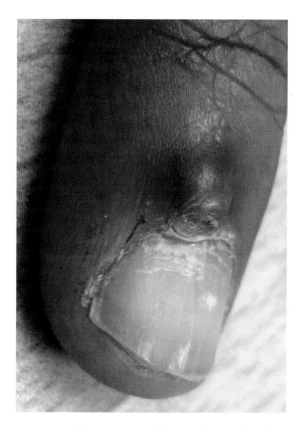

FIGURE 15.18 A solitary schwannoma of the proximal nail fold of an 8-year-old boy. (Courtesy of Zeegelaar JE.)

Schwann Cell Tumor, Plexiform Schwannoma, and Malignant Schwannoma

A Schwann cell tumor is a benign peripheral nerve tumor. Plexiform schwannoma is a rare variant of this tumor in which the Schwann cells are arranged in a plexiform pattern in the dermis and subcutis tissues. Peripheral nerve schwannomas are a diagnostic criterion for neurofibromatosis type 2. Schwannoma shows a predilection for the head and neck region and generally is asymptomatic. Solitary schwannoma of the nail unit may be seen in children (Figure 15.18), and also subungual plexiform schwannoma may arise in children.[74–76] Malignant transformation of schwannomas is very rare, and malignant transformation of plexiform schwannomas has not been reported. Yamamoto et al.[77] reported malignant schwannoma of the digital nerve in an 8-year-old boy without neurofibromatosis. The treatment of choice of lesions in fingers is amputation because of the difficulty of wide excision.

Soft Tissue Tumor of Uncertain Differentiation: Epithelioid Sarcoma

Epithelioid sarcoma is a sarcoma of unknown lineage. It is the most common soft tissue sarcoma of the wrist and hand.[78] Mainly, adolescents and young adults are involved but younger children have also been reported.[79,80] Metastases are found more often than in typical soft tissue sarcoma. Peripheral epithelioid sarcoma manifests as a painless, slow-growing dermal nodule that might have been present for a long time, often misdiagnosed as a benign lesion.[78] Local and plaque-like recurrences are common, but if it is completely excised with wide margins, it does not recur locally.

Cartilage and Bone Tumors

Osteochondroma and Exostosis

Osteochondromas or osteocartilaginous exostoses are thought to be the most common benign bone tumors, accounting for 35%–40% of all benign bone tumors and 10%–15% of all bone tumors. Subungual osteochondromas and subungual exostoses are discussed together because they share the same clinical picture, same biologic behavior, and benefit from the same treatment. Subungual osteochondromas and subungual exostoses share some radiographic features but pathologically represent a distinct entity.[81]

Osteochondromas are composed of cortical and medullary bone with an overlying hyaline cartilage cap and must demonstrate continuity with the underlying parent bone cortex and medullary canal. They result from the separation of a fragment of epiphyseal growth plate cartilage, which subsequently herniates through the periosteal bone cuff that normally surrounds the growth plate.[81] This process of separation of a fragment of epiphyseal growth plate cartilage may be assumed to be trauma induced but some authors believe osteochondromas have a congenital origin.[13] Osteochondromas may be solitary or multiple, the latter being associated with the autosomal dominant syndrome, hereditary multiple exostoses (see the section "Hereditary Multiple Exostoses"). Malignant transformation of osteochondromas in the direction of a chondrosarcoma is rare and occurs in adulthood. This is preceded by the sudden growth and increasing pain.[82] Malignant transformation occurs more often in hereditary multiple exostoses (3%–5%) than in isolated osteochondromas (1%).[81]

Subungual exostoses classically arise from the dorsal or dorsomedial aspect of the distal phalanx. Most consider it to be a reactive metaplasia resulting from microtrauma.[83] Contrary to osteochondromas, the bony excrescence usually appears in the tips of the phalanx, as opposed to the radiodense projection in subungual osteochondromas that appears in the union of the distal with the medium thirds of the phalanx.[84] Furthermore, there is typically no continuity with the underlying cortex and medullary canal, and the cartilage cap consists of fibrocartilage rather than hyaline cartilage. Malignant degeneration of exostoses has not been reported.

Osteochondromas mostly occur in the first two decades of life, subungual exostosis few years later. Pediatric cases of subungual osteochondromas have been reported frequently,[84–87] and 55% of exostosis patients are younger than 18 years of age,[83] making them typical pediatric nail tumors. The vast majority of exostoses involves the toes, with an obvious predilection for the great toe. Subungual exostoses are almost invariably solitary, with only rare reports of bilateral lesions.[81] Osteochondromas and subungual exostoses are painless but in patients with a subungual lesion they often present with pressure-inducible pain, which often is exacerbated while walking. Pain was mentioned in 93% of all patients with subungual osteochondromas,[84] and in 77% of all patients with subungual exostosis.[83] In typical periungual or subungual locations, osteochondromas appear as firm, shiny, yellowish papules or nodules that may deform the nail bed and nail plate (Figure 15.19). Exostoses may also present as firm and fixed tumors. Exostoses exhibit a white shiny hue with telangiectasia on their surface during the early stages but becomes more hyperkeratotic with time. Often, a collarette delineates the tumor (Figure 15.20). It usually lifts the nail plate, resulting in onycholysis or nail plate deformity. The overlying skin occasionally shows ulceration or infection, which might result in a subungual pyogenic-like outgrowth.[88]

On radiographs, the features of osteochondroma and exostoses often are pathognomonic: a lesion composed of cortical and medullary bone protruding from and, in the case of osteochondroma, continuous with the underlying bone. Unlike most osteochondromas in this region, subungual exostoses arise distal to the physeal scar and are not associated with growth deformities. The base of the lesion may be broad or narrow. The cartilage cap is typically larger than the base and may be either indistinct or well demarcated (Figure 15.20).[81]

Additional imaging modalities may be employed in the evaluation. CT scan demonstrates cortical and medullary continuity between the osteochondromas and host bone. MRI imaging is rarely indicated but the best modality for visualizing the effect of the lesion on surrounding structures and evaluating the hyaline cartilage cap.[81]

At histologic analysis, subungual exostosis is readily distinguishable from typical osteochondroma. Findings from a small preexcisional biopsy may lead to concern for chondrosarcoma.[81]

Complete surgical excision of the lesion should be considered if symptoms are present. The principle of treatment is to achieve complete excision of the lesion by curetting or burring down to normal trabecular bone while minimizing deformity to the nail plate.[83] There is often a postoperative discrete distal onycholysis.[88] The recurrence rate has varied between 11% and 53%.[89]

Enchondroma

Cartilaginous tumors involving bones of the hands and feet are not uncommon. Enchondromas are the most common, cartilage forming tumors. They usually occur as a single lesion, mainly in people aged

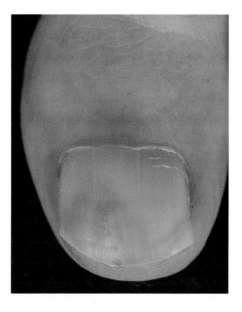

FIGURE 15.19 An osteochondroma presenting as a painful yellowish macule under the nail plate.

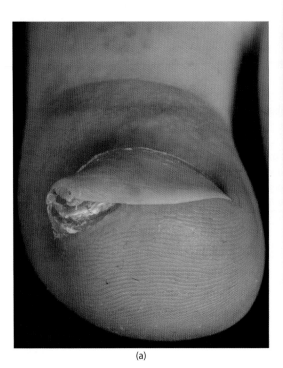
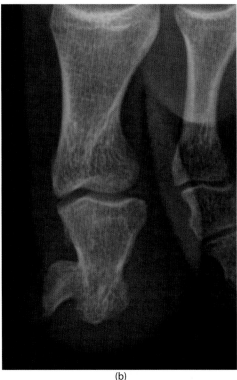

(a)   (b)

FIGURE 15.20 (a) An early exostosis exhibits a white shiny hue with telangiectasia on the surface but will become more hyperkeratotic with time. Often, a collarette delineates the tumor. (b) Typical radiography of an exostosis arising distal to the physeal scar. The cartilage cap is larger than the base.

10–40.[1,90] Occasionally, patients present with multiple enchondromas (enchondromatosis). Ollier disease and Maffucci syndrome are the most common enchondromatoses,[91] manifesting in early childhood.

Enchondromatas are usually asymptomatic but may enlarge and become painful. Located close to the nail unit pseudoclubbing often is present.

X-ray findings, including MRI and CT, may be diagnostic. Situated in the nail unit, histology might be the diagnostic procedure of choice. Although enchondromas of the hands and feet often show cytologic features suggestive of malignancy, the biologic behavior of these tumors is usually benign. The risk of developing a chondrosarcoma from a enchondroma is estimated to be about 4%, but it is more common in individuals with Ollier or Maffuci syndrome, where the risk approaches 25% and 100%, respectively.[91,92] Clinically, the presence of nonmechanical pain or night pain is a cause for concern and further immediate investigation is indicated. Located in the nail bed, pain will be present in most patients, also with benign enchondroma.[91] Therefore, treatment will be the rule. Surgical resection and curettage with cryotherapy are options.[90] Recurrences after surgical resection are rare.

Chondrosarcoma

While most cartilaginous tumors are benign, chondrosarcoma is the most common primary malignant bony tumor of the hand. Radiology and histology enable to differentiate chondrosarcoma from enchondroma.[93] The risk of developing a chondrosarcoma from a enchondroma is discussed in the previous paragraph. Chondrosarcomata of the nail unit are known to produce slow nail deformation that goes unrecognized for months until sudden pain and aggressive digit swelling develop. Also a case of pincer nail development due to a subungual chondrosarcoma was published.[94] It can present at any age, adolescent patients have also been described.[95] About 50% of hand chondrosarcomas affect phalangeal bone, but the involvement of the distal phalanx with its nail unit is rare with few reported cases.[94,95]

Phalangeal chondrosarcoma is resistant to chemotherapy and radiotherapy but has been categorized as a neoplasm different from classical hand chondrosarcoma with respect to the minimal metastatic potential, but has a high risk of both locally aggressive behavior.[93] Hence, treatment is indicated because of its locally destructive growth.

Chondromyxoid Fibroma

Chondromyxoid fibroma is a benign but locally aggressive bone tumor.[96] It presents in the second to third decade and is most often found around the knee. The clinical presentation is usually chronic pain (85%) and swelling (65%).

Histology differentiates these lesions from chondroblastoma and chondrosarcoma. A single pediatric case of chondromyxoid fibroma in the nail region has been reported.[97]

Osteoid Osteoma

Osteoid osteoma is a benign osteoblastic bone tumor most commonly found in long bones, such as the femur or tibia. Less commonly affected are the small bones of the hand and feet. Osteoid osteomas account for roughly 10%–15% of all benign bone tumors and characteristically present with pain. The pain is dull, unremitting, initially mild, and intermittent but increases in intensity and persistence over time. It tends to become increasingly severe at night and is usually relieved by salicylates and other nonsteroidal anti-inflammatory drugs (NSAIDs). They typically present in children and adolescents in a male to female ratio of 3:1.[98]

Osteoid osteomas of the distal phalanx of neonates and children commonly have a subtle clinical expression with swelling and tenderness.[99–102] Plain radiographs, CT, and MRI may be helpful diagnostic tools. Histology will reveal the true nature of the tumor.

Osteoid osteoma was traditionally treated with excision of the nidus. Nowadays destructive techniques are used as well.[98] The natural history is regression within 6–15 years without treatment; however, this can be reduced to 2–3 years with the use of aspirin and NSAIDs.[98]

Ewing's Sarcoma

Ewing's sarcoma are tumors assumed to be derived from primitive neuroectodermal cells or from a mesenchymal stem cell. They can occur anywhere in the body, but most commonly in the pelvis and proximal long tubular bones.[103] Ungual Ewing's sarcoma is very rare, but impressive case reports exist. In 2012, Baccari et al.[103] have summarized the literature and describe five pediatric patients with Ewing's sarcoma of the distal phalanx. Most present with pain and a fixed swelling of the digit. Another case report in a 13-year-old girl describes the lesions as painful and diffusely tender warm, cystic swelling of the tip of the finger.[104]

The radiological examination is highly abnormal in Ewing's sarcoma. The combination of excision and postoperative adjuvant chemotherapy has the best prognosis.

Aneurysmal Bone Cyst

Aneurysmal bone cysts (ABC) are benign osteolytic, expansive, and hemorrhagic bone lesions usually encountered in children and adolescents. The nature and histogenesis are still unclear; it is classified as an indeterminate tumor of intermediate malignancy, locally aggressive. They show characteristic translocations in 70%, the rest is secondary, without translocation and occur in reaction to other, usually benign, bone lesions.

ABCs may develop in all bones of the skeleton but ABC arising in the distal phalanx of the hand occur only occasionally.[105–108] They are revealed by pain, sometimes by swelling and nail clubbing over a relatively short duration of weeks to months. X-ray and MRI are the radiologic examinations of choice.[109] Biopsy is essential for diagnosing ABC and to rule out telangiectatic osteosarcoma and unicameral bone cysts.

The natural course is a resolution, spontaneously or within 4–6 weeks after simple biopsy. In other cases, the cyst may become aggressive, entirely destroying one end of the bone, raising fears of malignancy.[109] Real malignant transformation occurs only in case of irradiation. If spontaneous resolution does not occur, intralesional sclerotherapy with alcohol is an effective treatment option.[109] Also curettage has been described, particularly if the hand is involved.[110] Surgical resection or amputation of a digit guarantee against local recurrence but at the cost of reconstruction problems and of possible complications that the benign nature of ABC cannot justify.

Giant-Cell Tumor of the Bone

Giant-cell tumor of the bone is a benign but locally aggressive neoplasm with a tendency for local recurrence after curettage. Its appearance in the hand and foot is uncommon but involvement of the distal phalanxes of children and adolescents has been reported.[111–114] The most common complaint is pain that may be noted suddenly, following relatively mild trauma. Clinically a tender or painful swelling of the distal phalanx can be noted.

The radiographic appearance of giant-cell tumor in the tubular hand bones is variable and nonspecific; histologic examination of the tissue will be necessary for the definitive diagnosis. Surgical therapy is the most often used treatment for phalangeal giant-cell tumor.

Neural Tumors

Merkel Cell Carcinoma

Merkel cell carcinoma (MCC) is a highly aggressive neuroendocrine carcinoma of the skin demonstrating a high propensity of recurrence and metastasis. Its 5-year, disease-specific survival rate is only about 60%. Although MCC is still regarded as a very rare tumor entity, its incidence is rapidly increasing. The Merkel cell polyomavirus (MCV) has been found associated to 80% of MCC cases.[115] MCC occurs much more frequently in severely immunosuppressed populations and is often found on the sun-exposed skin of whites. Only one case of an MCC on a teenager's toe has been published.[116] The cornerstone for treatment is surgery.

Granular Cell Tumor

Granular cell tumors (GCT) are uncommon benign tumors, possibly arising from Schwann cells. They usually grow slowly, with benign behavior, with only a small minority showing malignant characteristics such as local infiltration or metastasis. GCT may occur in various sites and are infrequently seen in the pediatric population. Despite this, several pediatric and adult cases of benign but also malignant GCT on or around the nails of fingers and toes have been published.[117–120]

GCTs usually present as asymptomatic or pruritic, firm, dermal, or subcutaneous papulonodules. They are skin-colored or brownish-red and range in size from 0.5 to 3.0 cm in diameter. Occasionally, the overlying epidermis is verrucous or ulcerated. The clinical picture of GCT of the nail unit depends on the position of the tumor in relation to the nail matrix or nail bed but ungual GCTs often are painful.[118,119] Complete surgical resection is the treatment of choice. The recurrence rate after adequate local excision is low but with inadequate excision recurrence rates as high as 50% have been reported.[120]

Hematolymphoid Tumors

Langerhans Cell Histiocytosis

Langerhans cell histiocytosis (LCH) identifies a group of disorders characterized by clonal proliferation of Langerhans cells: Letterer–Siwe disease, Hand–Schüller–Christian disease, and eosinophilic granuloma of bone. More than 60% of LCH patients have single-system disease, which mostly involves bone, skin, or lymph nodes. Fingernails or toenails are rarely affected but occasionally may proceed as multi-organ LCH in infants by many months.[121,122]

The main sign of the nail involvement in LCH appears to be extensive asymptomatic subungual hyperkeratosis, involving several fingernails and toenails. Other signs are hemorrhages, pustules, longitudinal grooving, pitting, paronychia of the proximal or lateral nail folds, and onycholysis up to onychomade-sis.[121,123] The significance of nail changes as an independent (poor) prognostic indicator is controversial; nail changes in LCH mostly occur in patients with multisystem disease, which is known to be significantly related to mortality. In the scarce published cases in which nail changes were not associated with multisystem disease, the prognosis was excellent.[123,124] Patients with risk organ involvement and young age (<2 years) have a high mortality rate, ranging up to 66%.[125]

Juvenile Xanthogranuloma

Juvenile xanthogranuloma (JXG) is the most common form of non-Langerhans cell histiocytosis. It is a benign cutaneous histiocytic proliferation that is thought to represent a granulomatous reaction of histiocytes in response to undefined stimuli.

JXG generally occurs in infancy, with a peak incidence during the first year of life but may also appear in adolescents and adults. It appears as a well-demarcated, asymptomatic papule or nodule with a typical yellow-brown hue and some telangiectases on the surface. The head, neck, and the trunk are the most frequent locations but lesions of the nail unit have been described.[126–130] All patients described with nail involvement in JXG were less than 3 years old and presented with a wide range of clinical signs: lesions from the proximal nail fold may cover part of a finger, result in a hyperkeratotic cuticle, or in longitudinal depressions of the nail plate indicating nail matrix compression by the lesion.[129,130] Lesions arising from the nail bed may lift the nail plate and result in onychogryphosis.[126,127]

Histologic analysis is necessary for the diagnosis, especially to differentiate JXG from Langerhans cell granuloma. JXG regresses spontaneously within 2–6 years, often leaving a residual atrophy or discoloration. Surgical removal may be indicated to prevent permanent dystrophy but periodic follow-up may be sufficient to monitor evolution in order to prevent excessive growth of the lesion with a possible definitive nail matrix damage.[130] Although it is a benign condition and most patients only have a solitary lesion, it is important to rule out the presence of other possible skin, mucosal, or extracutaneous lesions in many organ systems.[126] In particular, intraocular involvement occurs relatively frequently. The possible association with neurofibromatosis type 1 should also be considered.

Acral Pseudolymphomatous Angiokeratoma of Children

Acral pseudolymphomatous angiokeratoma of children, known as APACHE, is a rare benign cutaneous pseudolymphomatous disorder of unknown etiology. It mostly affects children aged between 2 and 13, and is characterized by multiple (up to 40), small erythematous–violaceous papules and nodules, with a keratotic surface located unilaterally on the fingers, toes, and hands. The lesions can be asymptomatic but also painful and may tend to bleed. Located in the nail region longitudinal nail splitting, nail deformity, or onycholysis may be present.[131–133]Clinically, it is similar to an angiokeratoma, whereas histologically, it corresponds to a distinct type of pseudolymphoma.[131] Immunohistochemistry is required to distinguish APACHE from cutaneous lymphoma.[134]

The elective therapeutic choice is the total excision of lesions. Intralesional corticotherapy, cryotherapy, and radiotherapy are also described but recurrences are frequent.[134]

Congenital Nail Tumors and Nail Tumors in Inherited Syndromes

Epidermal Nevi

If linear patches or plaques develop early in life, the presence of an epidermal nevus should be considered, in particular, if both the nail fold and the corresponding nail are involved. They often follow Blaschko lines, which are believed to represent patterns of epidermal migration during embryogenesis.[135] In the nail unit inflammatory linear verrucous epidermal nevus,[136] and epidermal nevi in congenital hemidysplasia with ichthyosiform erythroderma and limb defects syndrome (CHILD syndrome) have been reported in pediatric patients.[137,138] Epidermal nevi are discussed in Chapter 9.

Hereditary Multiple Exostoses

Hereditary multiple exostoses (HME), also known as familial osteochondromatosis, multiple exostoses syndrome, or diaphyseal aclasis, are characterized by the development of multiple osteochondromas.[81] The disease shows an autosomal dominant inheritance pattern. Nail lesions will present as firm nontender nodules on the proximal two-thirds of the nail bed and the lunula, causing elevation of the proximal nail fold. Longitudinal dystrophy may be present due to pressure on the nail matrix. Also a shortened nail caused by onychoatrophy or nail plate malalignment have been reported.[139–143] The clinical relevance of early recognition of HME is stressed by the fact osteochondromas in HME have a higher rate of malignant transformation than isolated osteochondromas.[81]

Ollier Disease

Ollier disease is a rare condition, characterized by multiple enchondromas appearing in childhood. Most cases of Ollier disease have been sporadic. Maffucci syndrome combines the features of Ollier disease associated with angioma of the soft tissue. Ollier disease and Maffucci syndrome often are complicated by deformity, limb shortening, pathological fracture, and chondrosarcoma.[144] Malignant transformation of enchondromas to chondrosarcomas is common in individuals with multiple enchondromas as with Ollier or Maffuci syndrome, where the risk approaches 25% and 100%, respectively.[92] Juvenile patients with Ollier disease may present with onycholysis and nail dystrophy related to a subungual enchondroma,[145] or with thick fingers due to the enchondroma.[146]

Neurofibromatosis Type 1

Neurofibromatosis 1 (NF1) is a common inherited neurocutaneous disease that has a major impact on the nervous system, eye, skin, and bone.[147] Individuals with NF1 have a predisposition to benign and malignant tumor formation secondary to mutations in the tumor suppressor gene NF1. The hallmark lesion is the neurofibroma, a benign peripheral nerve sheath tumor (see the section "Nerve Sheath Tumors"). Neurofibromas in neurofibromatosis seldom occur in the nail region. This might be due to the fact that subungual neurofibromas are difficult to diagnose, particularly as they are often small and without obvious symptoms. Plexiform neurofibromas, which have the risk of malignant degeneration, have not been reported to occur in the nail unit. Glomus tumor is a subungual glomus tumor in young NF1 patients.[148–151] It is likely that the glomus tumor is the most frequent nail tumor in NF1 patients. Glomus tumors are described in the section "Pericytic (Perivascular) Tumors: Glomus Tumor"

Tuberous Sclerosis

Tuberous sclerosis is an autosomal dominant disorder characterized by multiple hamartomas of the skin, central nervous system, kidney, retina, and heart. Nail abnormalities in these patients are also discussed in Chapters 1 and 9. Ungual or periungual fibroma (≥2), which are called Koenen tumors, are one of the major diagnostic criteria of tuberous sclerosis complex. In children up to 18 years of age, the reported incidence is 15% but were completely absent under the age of 2 years.[152] In one case, the occurrence of Koenen tumors at the age of 12 years old was reported to be the only sign of tuberous sclerosis complex.[153] They appear as mostly asymptomatic, firm, smooth, skin-colored, or reddish papules around or under fingernails and toenails (Figure 15.21). Periungual fibroma are more common than subungual fibroma.[154] They frequently cause nail deformations and are discussed in more detail in the section "Fibrous, Fibrohistiocytic, and Histiocytic Tumors"

The indication for treatment of Koenen tumor is often pressure-induced pain or for cosmetic reasons. Malignant transformation has not been reported. Surgical excision from its very base is the treatment of choice in most patients. Also electrodesiccation, carbon dioxide laser vaporization, and shave and phenolization have been described.[155] Recently, Muzic et al.[156] reported the successful treatment of Koenen tumors with topical rapamycin under occlusion. Recurrences are common in tuberous sclerosis patients because they are prone to develop these tumors.

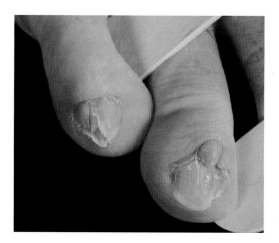

FIGURE 15.21 Koenen tumors appear as mostly asymptomatic, firm, smooth, skin-colored, or reddish papules around or under fingernails and toenails. Often multiple tumors can be seen.

Incontinentia Pigmenti

Incontinentia pigmenti is a rare genodermatosis that affects the skin, hair, teeth, nails, eyes, and central nervous system. Ungual alterations are observed in about 40% of incontinetia pigmenti patients and are discussed extensively in Chapters 1 and 9. Painful subungual dyskeratotic tumors (subungual tumors in incontinentia pigmenti) are one of the late manifestations, appearing after puberty (between the ages of 15 and 31 years).[157] They tend to destroy the distal phalanx by pressure necrosis of the underlying bone, and they displace the nail from the nail bed causing nail dystrophy. Partial onycholysis often precedes the appearance of keratotic crusted papules and nodules at the distal nail bed (Figure 15.22). Pain is initially intermittent but increases in intensity and duration as the tumor enlarges. In the proximal subungual tissue, the tumors may produce a paronychia-like lesion. Drainage of firm keratinaceous plugs or purulent debris secondary to bacterial infection may be present.

The initial treatment of the subungual tumors is surgical excision with bone curettage. Unfortunately, this does not prevent the occurrence of multiple new lesions appearing in other locations. Some success has been achieved with intralesional 5-fluorouracil injection, etretinate, and acitretin.[157]

Digitocutaneous Dysplasia

Digitocutaneous dysplasia, also known as terminal osseous dysplasia with pigmentary defects, is a rare X-linked, lethal male, dominant genetic syndrome. The digital fibromas of digitocutaneous dysplasia appear to be only histologically distinct from those that occur in patients with infantile digital fibromatosis (see the section "Fibrogenic/Fibroblastic/Myofibroblastic Tumors").

Juvenile Hyaline Fibromatosis

Juvenile hyaline fibromatosis syndrome (JHF) is an autosomal recessive condition characterized by abnormal growth of hyalinized fibrous tissue. Occurrence of digital nodules has been described as the first sign of JHF in some patients.[158] Excessively large periungual hyaline fibromas were reported.[159,160]

Congenital Hypertrophy of the Lateral Nail Folds of the Hallux

Congenital hypertrophy of the lateral nail folds of the hallux appearing at birth or shortly hereafter is not exceptional.[161–163] It is frequently associated with paronychia, inflammatory granulation tissue, and pain due to ingrowth of the nail (Figure 15.23). It will be discussed in Chapter 17.

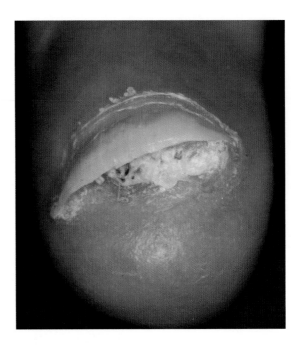

FIGURE 15.22 Painful subungual dyskeratotic tumors of incontinentia pigmenti tend to destroy the distal phalanx by pressure necrosis of the underlying bone, and they displace the nail from the nail bed, causing nail dystrophy.

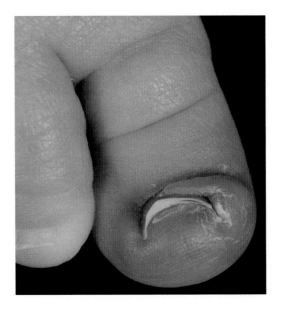

FIGURE 15.23 Congenital hypertrophy of the lateral nail folds of the hallux.

REFERENCES

1. Dominguez-Cherit J, Chanussot-Deprez C, Maria-Sarti H et al. Nail unit tumors: A study of 234 patients in the dermatology department of the "Dr Manuel Gea Gonzalez" General Hospital in Mexico City. *Dermatol Surg.* 2008; 34(10): 1363–1371.
2. Baek HJ, Lee SJ, Cho KH et al. Subungual tumors: Clinicopathologic correlation with US and MR imaging findings. *Radiographics.* 2010; 30(6): 1621–1636.

3. Herschthal J, McLeod MP, Zaiac M. Management of ungual warts. *Dermatol Ther.* 2012; 25(6): 545–550.

4. Kato M, Shimizu A, Hattori T et al. Detection of human papillomavirus type 58 in periungual Bowen's disease. *Acta Derm Venereol.* 2013; 93(6): 723–724.

5. Mammas IN, Sourvinos G, Spandidos DA. Human papilloma virus (HPV) infection in children and adolescents. *Eur J Pediatr.* 2009; 168(3): 267–273.

6. Tosti A, Piraccini BM. Warts of the nail unit: Surgical and nonsurgical approaches. *Dermatol Surg.* 2001; 27(3): 235–239.

7. Choi Y, Kim do H, Jin SY et al. Topical immunotherapy with diphenylcyclopropenone is effective and preferred in the treatment of periungual warts. *Ann Dermatol.* 2013; 25(4): 434–439.

8. Micali G, Dall'Oglio F, Nasca MR. An open label evaluation of the efficacy of imiquimod 5% cream in the treatment of recalcitrant subungual and periungual cutaneous warts. *J Dermatolog Treat.* 2003; 14(4): 233–236.

9. Schroeter CA, Kaas L, Waterval JJ et al. Successful treatment of periungual warts using photodynamic therapy: A pilot study. *J Eur Acad Dermatol Venereol.* 2007; 21(9): 1170–1174.

10. Salk RS, Grogan KA, Chang TJ. Topical 5% 5-fluorouracil cream in the treatment of plantar warts: A prospective, randomized, and controlled clinical study. *J Drugs Dermatol.* 2006; 5(5): 418–424.

11. AlGhamdi KM, Khurram H. Successful treatment of periungual warts with diluted bleomycin using translesional multipuncture technique: A pilot prospective study. *Dermatol Surg.* 2011; 37(4): 486–492.

12. Sardana K, Garg V, Relhan V. Complete resolution of recalcitrant periungual/subungual wart with recovery of normal nail following "prick" method of administration of bleomycin 1%. *Dermatol Ther.* 2010; 23(4): 407–410.

13. Sommer N, Neumeister MW. Tumors of the perionychium. *Hand Clin.* 2002; 18(4): 673–689, vii; discussion 691.

14. Chern E, Cheng YW. Treatment of recalcitrant periungual warts with cimetidine in pediatrics. *J Dermatolog Treat.* 2010; 21(5): 314–316.

15. Park HS, Choi WS. Pulsed dye laser treatment for viral warts: A study of 120 patients. *J Dermatol.* 2008; 35(8): 491–498.

16. Langdon RC. Erbium:YAG laser enables complete ablation of periungual verrucae without the need for injected anesthetics. *Dermatol Surg.* 1998; 24(1): 157–158.

17. Riddel C, Rashid R, Thomas V. Ungual and periungual human papillomavirus-associated squamous cell carcinoma: A review. *J Am Acad Dermatol.* 2011; 64(6): 1147–1153.

18. Wockel W, Meerbach W, Willnow U. [Metastasising squamous-cell carcinoma of the skin in a ten-year-old girl]. *Dtsch Med Wochenschr.* 1979; 104(31): 1104–1107.

19. Dominguez-Cherit J, Garcia C, Vega-Memije ME, Arenas R. Pseudo-fibrokeratoma: An unusual presentation of subungual squamous cell carcinoma in a young girl. *Dermatol Surg.* 2003; 29(7): 788–789.

20. Grundmeier N, Hamm H, Weissbrich B et al. High-risk human papillomavirus infection in Bowen's disease of the nail unit: Report of three cases and review of the literature. *Dermatology.* 2011; 223(4): 293–300.

21. Kim S, Sun GS, Wright TS. Periungual Bowen's disease in a 4-year-old girl. *Pediatr Dermatol.* 2014; 31(1): e22–e23.

22. Pena ZG, Brewer JD. Multiple subungual squamous cell carcinomas in a patient with incontinentia pigmenti. *Dermatol Surg.* 2014; 40(10): 1159–1161.

23. Mahmoud BH, Zembowicz A, Fisher E. Controversies over subungual tumors in incontinentia pigmenti. *Dermatol Surg.* 2014; 40(10): 1157–1159.

24. Lecerf P, Richert B, Theunis A, Andre J. A retrospective study of squamous cell carcinoma of the nail unit diagnosed in a Belgian general hospital over a 15-year period. *J Am Acad Dermatol.* 2013; 69(2): 253–261.

25. Jellinek NJ. Primary malignant tumors of the nail unit. *Adv Dermatol.* 2005; 21: 33–64.

26. Dalle S, Depape L, Phan A et al. Squamous cell carcinoma of the nail apparatus: Clinicopathological study of 35 cases. *Br J Dermatol.* 2007; 156(5): 871–874.

27. Baran R, Perrin C. Localized multinucleate distal subungual keratosis. *Br J Dermatol.* 1995; 133(1): 77–82.

28. Beggs S, Butala N, Heymann WR, Rubin AI. Onychopapilloma presenting as longitudinal erythronychia in an adolescent. *Pediatr Dermatol.* 2015; 32(4): e173–e174.

29. Criscione V, Telang G, Jellinek NJ. Onychopapilloma presenting as longitudinal leukonychia. *J Am Acad Dermatol*. 2010; 63(3): 541–542.

30. Miteva M, Fanti PA, Romanelli P et al. Onychopapilloma presenting as longitudinal melanonychia. *J Am Acad Dermatol*. 2012; 66(6): e242–e243.

31. Baran R, Perrin C. Longitudinal erythronychia with distal subungual keratosis: Onychopapilloma of the nail bed and Bowen's disease. *Br J Dermatol*. 2000; 143(1): 132–135.

32. Cohen PR. Longitudinal erythronychia: Individual or multiple linear red bands of the nail plate: A review of clinical features and associated conditions. *Am J Clin Dermatol*. 2011; 12(4): 217–231.

33. Calikoglu E. Pseudo-knuckle pads: An unusual cutaneous sign of obsessive-compulsive disorder in an adolescent patient. *Turk J Pediatr*. 2003; 45(4): 348–349.

34. Chen LH, Lin HC, Sheu HM, Chao SC. G59A mutation in the GJB2 gene in a Taiwanese family with knuckle pads, palmoplantar keratoderma and sensorineural hearing loss. *Clin Exp Dermatol*. 2012; 37(3): 300–301.

35. Hyman CH, Cohen PR. Report of a family with idiopathic knuckle pads and review of idiopathic and disease-associated knuckle pads. *Dermatol Online J*. 2013; 19(5): 18177.

36. Baran R, Kint A. Onychomatrixoma. Filamentous tufted tumour in the matrix of a funnel-shaped nail: A new entity (report of three cases). *Br J Dermatol*. 1992; 126(5): 510–515.

37. Tavares G, Di-Chiacchio N, Di-Santis E et al. Onychomatricoma: Epidemiological and clinical findings in a large series of 30 cases. *Br J Dermatol*. 2015; 173(5): 1305–1307.

38. Rashid RM, Swan J. Onychomatricoma: Benign sporadic nail lesion or much more? *Dermatol Online J*. 2006; 12(6): 4.

39. Piraccini BM, Antonucci A, Rech G et al. Onychomatricoma: First description in a child. *Pediatr Dermatol*. 2007; 24(1): 46–48.

40. Perrin C, Cannata GE, Bossard C et al. Onychocytic matricoma presenting as pachymelanonychia longitudinal. A new entity (report of five cases). *Am J Dermatopathol*. 2012; 34(1): 54–59.

41. Sass U, Kolivras A, Richert B et al. Acantholytic tumor of the nail: Acantholytic dyskeratotic acanthoma. *J Cutan Pathol*. 2009; 36(12): 1308–1311.

42. Saez-de-Ocariz MM, Dominguez-Cherit J, Garcia-Corona C. Subungual epidermoid cysts. *Int J Dermatol*. 2001; 40(8): 524–526.

43. Bukhari IA, Al-Mugharbel R. Subungual epidermoid inclusions. *Saudi Med J*. 2004; 25(4): 522–523.

44. Baran R, Bureau H. Two post-operative epidermoid cysts following realignment of the hallux nail. *Br J Dermatol*. 1988; 119(2): 245–247.

45. Telang GH, Jellinek N. Multiple calcified subungual epidermoid inclusions. *J Am Acad Dermatol*. 2007; 56(2): 336–339.

46. Keiler SA, Honda K, Bordeaux JS. Retiform hemangioendothelioma treated with Mohs micrographic surgery. *J Am Acad Dermatol*. 2011; 65(1): 233–235.

47. Londero M, Pastore S, Zanazzo GA et al. A child with pain after mild trauma. *J Pediatr*. 2010; 157(4): 693.

48. Kitagawa Y, Ito H, Iketani M et al. Epithelioid hemangioendothelioma of the phalanx: A case report. *J Hand Surg Am*. 2005; 30(3): 615–619.

49. Moss LA, Stueber K, Hafiz MA. Congenital hemangioendothelioma of the hand—Case report. *J Hand Surg Am*. 1982; 7(1): 53–56.

50. Oh ST, Kwon HJ, Lee JY, Cho BK. A case of lymphangioma circumscriptum developed on the finger. *Dermatol Surg*. 2007; 33(5): 648–649.

51. Kint A, Baran R, De Keyser H. Acquired (digital) fibrokeratoma. *J Am Acad Dermatol*. 1985; 12(5 Pt 1): 816–821.

52. Fetsch JF, Laskin WB, Miettinen M. Superficial acral fibromyxoma: A clinicopathologic and immuno-histochemical analysis of 37 cases of a distinctive soft tissue tumor with a predilection for the fingers and toes. *Hum Pathol*. 2001; 32(7): 704–714.

53. Goo J, Jung YJ, Kim JH et al. A case of recurrent superficial acral fibromyxoma. *Ann Dermatol*. 2010; 22(1): 110–113.

54. Hollmann TJ, Bovee JV, Fletcher CD. Digital fibromyxoma (superficial acral fibromyxoma): A detailed characterization of 124 cases. *Am J Surg Pathol*. 2012; 36(6): 789–798.

55. Muzaffar AR, Rafols F, Masson J et al. Keloid formation after syndactyly reconstruction: Associated conditions, prevalence, and preliminary report of a treatment method. *J Hand Surg Am.* 2004; 29(2): 201–208.

56. Tolerton SK, Tonkin MA. Keloid formation after syndactyly release in patients with associated macrodactyly: Management with methotrexate therapy. *J Hand Surg Eur Vol.* 2011; 36(6): 490–497.

57. Hu Z, Chou PM, Jennings LJ, Arva NC. Infantile fibrosarcoma—A clinical and histologic mimicker of vascular malformations: Case report and review of the literature. *Pediatr Dev Pathol.* 2013; 16(5): 357–363.

58. Ajitsaria R, Quinn E, Mew RC et al. Rare tumour presenting in a newborn infant. *Arch Dis Child.* 2013; 98(5): 362.

59. Inoue A, Hasegawa T, Ikata T, Hizawa K. Fibrosarcoma of the toe: A destructive lesion of the distal phalanx. *Clin Orthop Relat Res.* 1996; (333): 239–244.

60. Spingardi O, Zoccolan A, Venturino E. Infantile digital fibromatosis: Our experience and long-term results. *Chir Main.* 2011; 30(1): 62–65.

61. Taylor HO, Gellis SE, Schmidt BA et al. Infantile digital fibromatosis. *Ann Plastic Surg.* 2008; 61(4): 472–476.

62. Cabrera Gonzalez M, Perez Lopez LM, Gutierrez de la Iglesia D et al. Diagnosis and treatment of digitocutaneous dysplasia, a rare infantile digital fibromatosis: A case report. *Hand.* 2013; 8(4): 473–478.

63. Heymann WR. Infantile digital fibromatosis. *J Am Acad Dermatol.* 2008; 59(1): 122–123.

64. Bahnassy M, Abdul-Khalik H. Soft tissue chondroma: A case report and literature review. *Oman Med J.* 2009; 24(4): 296–299.

65. Ryu JH, Park EJ, Kim KH, Kim KJ. A case of congenital soft tissue chondroma. *J Dermatol.* 2005; 32(3): 214–216.

66. Eun YS, Kim MR, Cho BK et al. Subungual soft tissue chondroma with nail deformity in a child. *Pediatr Dermatol.* 2015; 32(1): 132–134.

67. Munk B, Kroner K. Dermal leiomyosarcoma of the right fifth finger. Case report. *Scand J Plast Reconstr Surg Hand Surg.* 1997; 31(2): 179–180.

68. Sironi M, Assi A, Pasquinelli G, Cenacchi G. Not all granular cell tumors show Schwann cell differentiation: A granular cell leiomyosarcoma of the thumb, a case report. *Am J Dermatopathol.* 1999; 21(3): 307–309.

69. Abbassi A, Amrani A, Dendane MA et al. [Glomus tumor of the finger pulp: An unusual pediatric case]. *J Mal Vasc.* 2012; 37(4): 219–221.

70. Kumar MG, Emnett RJ, Bayliss SJ, Gutmann DH. Glomus tumors in individuals with neurofibromatosis type 1. *J Am Acad Dermatol.* 2014; 71(1): 44–48.

71. Huajun J, Wei Q, Ming L et al. Solitary subungual neurofibroma in the right first finger. *Int J Dermatol.* 2012; 51(3): 335–338.

72. Niizuma K, Iijima KN. Solitary neurofibroma: A case of subungual neurofibroma on the right third finger. *Arch Dermatol Res.* 1991; 283(1): 13–15.

73. Stolarczuk Dde A, Silva AL, Filgueiras Fda M et al. Solitary subungual neurofibroma: A previously unreported finding in a male patient. *An Bras Dermatol.* 2011; 86(3): 569–572.

74. Altmeyer P. [Histology of a plexiform neuroma with Vater-Pacini-lamellar-corpuscle-like structures]. *Hautarzt.* 1979; 30(5): 248–252.

75. Posner MA, McMahon MS, Desai P. Plexiform schwannoma (neurilemmoma) associated with macrodactyly: A case report. *J Hand Surg Am.* 1996; 21(4): 707–710.

76. Bendon CL and Giele HP. Macrodactyly in the setting of a plexiform schwannoma in neurofibromatosis type 2: Case report. *J Hand Surg Am.* 2013; 38(4): 740–744.

77. Yamamoto T, Fujioka H, Mizuno K. Malignant schwannoma of the digital nerve in a child. A case report. *Clin Orthop Relat Res.* 2000; (376): 209–212.

78. Stein-Wexler R. Pediatric soft tissue sarcomas. *Semin Ultrasound CT MR.* 2011; 32(5): 470–488.

79. Theunis A, Andre J, Larsimont D, Song M. Epithelioid sarcoma: A puzzling soft tissue neoplasm in a child. *Dermatology.* 2000; 200(2): 179–180.

80. Stang F, Namdar T, Siemers F et al. Epithelioid finger-sarcoma in an 11 year old girl—A case report. *Ger Med Sci.* 2010; 8: 1–2.

81. Murphey MD, Choi JJ, Kransdorf MJ et al. Imaging of osteochondroma: Variants and complications with radiologic-pathologic correlation. *Radiographics.* 2000; 20(5): 1407–1434.

82. Steffner R. Benign bone tumors. *Cancer Treat Res.* 2014; 162: 31–63.

83. DaCambra MP, Gupta SK, Ferri-de-Barros F. Subungual exostosis of the toes: A systematic review. *Clin Orthop Relat Res.* 2014; 472(4): 1251–1259.

84. Vazquez-Flores H, Dominguez-Cherit J, Vega-Memije ME, Saez-De-Ocariz M. Subungual osteochondroma: Clinical and radiologic features and treatment. *Dermatol Surg.* 2004; 30(7): 1031–1034.

85. Eliezri YD, Taylor SC. Subungual osteochondroma. Diagnosis and management. *J Dermatol Surg Oncol.* 1992; 18(8): 753–758.

86. Schulze KE, Hebert AA. Diagnostic features, differential diagnosis, and treatment of subungual osteochondroma. *Pediatr Dermatol.* 1994; 11(1): 39–41.

87. Lee J, Kim SE, Park K, Son SJ. Subungual osteochondroma presenting as verruca vulgaris in a 6-year-old boy. *Pediatr Dermatol.* 2007; 24(5): 584–585.

88. Richert B, Lecerf P, Caucanas M, Andre J. Nail tumors. *Clin Dermatol.* 2013; 31(5): 602–617.

89. Letts M, Davidson D, Nizalik E. Subungual exostosis: Diagnosis and treatment in children. *J Trauma.* 1998; 44(2): 346–349.

90. Bauer HI, Kaatz M, Kluge WH, Elsner P. [Subungual chondroma, a case report]. *Z Rheumatol.* 2002; 61(1): 58–61.

91. Herget GW, Strohm P, Rottenburger C et al. Insights into enchondroma, enchondromatosis and the risk of secondary chondrosarcoma. Review of the literature with an emphasis on the clinical behaviour, radiology, malignant transformation and the follow up. *Neoplasma.* 2014; 61(4): 365–378.

92. Hsu CS, Hentz VR, Yao J. Tumours of the hand. *Lancet Oncol.* 2007; 8(2): 157–166.

93. Bovee JV, van der Heul RO, Taminiau AH, Hogendoorn PC. Chondrosarcoma of the phalanx: A locally aggressive lesion with minimal metastatic potential: A report of 35 cases and a review of the literature. *Cancer.* 1999; 86(9): 1724–1732.

94. Au S, Juhl ME, Emmadi R, Krunic AL. Nail dystrophy as a presenting sign of a chondrosarcoma of the distal phalanx—Case report and review of the literature. *Acta Derm Venereol.* 2015; 95(8): 1026–1027.

95. Ogose A, Unni KK, Swee RG et al. Chondrosarcoma of small bones of the hands and feet. *Cancer.* 1997; 80(1): 50–59.

96. De Mattos CB, Angsanuntsukh C, Arkader A, Dormans JP. Chondroblastoma and chondromyxoid fibroma. *J Am Acad Orthop Surg.* 2013; 21(4): 225–233.

97. Sharma H, Jane MJ, Reid R. Chondromyxoid fibroma of the foot and ankle: 40 years' Scottish bone tumour registry experience. *Int Orthop.* 2006; 30(3): 205–209.

98. Boscainos PJ, Cousins GR, Kulshreshtha R et al. Osteoid osteoma. *Orthopedics.* 2013; 36(10): 792–800.

99. Szabo RM, Smith B. Possible congenital osteoid-osteoma of a phalanx. A case report. *J Bone Joint Surg Am.* 1985; 67(5): 815–816.

100. Tsang DS, Wu DY. Osteoid osteoma of phalangeal bone. *J Formos Med Assoc.* 2008; 107(7): 582–586.

101. Ozturk A, Yalcinkaya U, Ozkan Y, Yalcin N. Subperiosteal osteoid osteoma in the hallux of a 9-year-old female. *J Foot Ankle Surg.* 2008; 47(6): 579–582.

102. Galdi B, Capo JT, Nourbakhsh A, Patterson F. Osteoid osteoma of the thumb: A case report. *Hand.* 2010; 5(4): 423–426.

103. Baccari S, Hamdi MF, Mabrouki Z et al. Ewing's sarcoma of the finger: Report of two cases and literature review. *Orthop Traumatol Surg Res.* 2012; 98(2): 233–237.

104. Jerome TJ, Varghese M, Sankaran B. Ewing's sarcoma of the distal phalanx of the little finger. *J Hand Surg Eur Vol.* 2008; 33(1): 81–82.

105. Fuhs SE, Herndon JH. Aneurysmal bone cyst involving the hand: A review and report of two cases. *J Hand Surg Am.* 1979; 4(2): 152–159.

106. Leeson MC, Lowry L, McCue RW. Aneurysmal bone cyst of the distal thumb phalanx. A case report and review of the literature. *Orthopedics.* 1988; 11(4): 601–604.

107. Katz MA, Dormans JP, Uri AK. Aneurysmal bone cyst involving the distal phalanx of a child. *Orthopedics.* 1997; 20(5): 463–466.

108. Sakka SA, Lock M. Aneurysmal bone cyst of the terminal phalanx of the thumb in a child. *Arch Orthop Trauma Surg.* 1997; 116(1–2): 119–120.

109. Mascard E, Gomez-Brouchet A, Lambot K. Bone cysts: Unicameral and aneurysmal bone cyst. *Orthop Traumatol Surg Res.* 2015; 101(1 Suppl): S119–S127.

110. Ropars M, Kaila R, Briggs T, Cannon S. [Aneurysmal bone cysts of the metacarpals and phalanges of the hand. A 6 case series and literature review]. *Chir Main.* 2007; 26(4–5): 214–217.

111. Averill RM, Smith RJ, Campbell CJ. Giant-cell tumors of the bones of the hand. *J Hand Surg Am.* 1980; 5(1): 39–50.

112. Kransdorf MJ, Sweet DE, Buetow PC et al. Giant cell tumor in skeletally immature patients. *Radiology.* 1992; 184(1): 233–237.

113. Yin Y, Gilula LA, Kyriakos M, Manske P. Giant-cell tumor of the distal phalanx of the hand in a child. *Clin Orthop Relat Res.* 1995; (310): 200–207.

114. Kiatisevi P, Thanakit V, Boonthathip M et al. Giant cell tumor of the distal phalanx of the biphalangeal fifth toe: A case report and review of the literature. *J Foot Ankle Surg.* 2011; 50(5): 598–602.

115. Schrama D, Ugurel S, Becker JC. Merkel cell carcinoma: Recent insights and new treatment options. *Curr Opin Oncol.* 2012; 24(2): 141–149.

116. Goldenhersh MA, Prus D, Ron N, Rosenmann E. Merkel cell tumor masquerading as granulation tissue on a teenager's toe. *Am J Dermatopathol.* 1992; 14(6): 560–563.

117. Urabe A, Imayama S, Yasumoto S et al. Malignant granular cell tumor. *J Dermatol.* 1991; 18(3): 161–166.

118. al-Qattan MM, Clarke HM. An isolated granular cell tumour of the thumb pulp clinically mimicking a glomus tumour. *J Hand Surg.* 1994; 19(4): 420–421.

119. Price MF, Paletta CE, Woodberry KM. Granular cell tumor in a child's finger. *Ann Plast Surg.* 2000; 44(4): 447–450.

120. Abraham T, Jackson B, Davis L et al. Mohs surgical treatment of a granular cell tumor on the toe of a child. *Pediatr Dermatol.* 2007; 24(3): 235–237.

121. Ashena Z, Alavi S, Arzanian MT, Eshghi P. Nail involvement in Langerhans cell histiocytosis. *Pediatr Hematol Oncol.* 2007; 24(1): 45–51.

122. de Berker D, Lever LR, Windebank K. Nail features in Langerhans cell histiocytosis. *Br J Dermatol.* 1994; 130(4): 523–527.

123. Mataix J, Betlloch I, Lucas-Costa A et al. Nail changes in Langerhans cell histiocytosis: A possible marker of multisystem disease. *Pediatr Dermatol.* 2008; 25(2): 247–251.

124. Uppal P, Bothra M, Seth R et al. Clinical profile of Langerhans cell histiocytosis at a tertiary centre: A prospective study. *Indian J Pediatr.* 2012; 79(11): 1463–1467.

125. Gadner H, Grois N, Arico M et al. A randomized trial of treatment for multisystem Langerhans' cell histiocytosis. *J Pediatr.* 2001; 138(5): 728–734.

126. Chang P, Baran R, Villanueva C et al. Juvenile xanthogranuloma beneath a fingernail. *Cutis.* 1996; 58(2): 173–174.

127. Frumkin A, Roytman M, Johnson SF. Juvenile xanthogranuloma underneath a toenail. *Cutis.* 1987; 40(3): 244–245.

128. Hughes DB, Hanasono MM, Nolan WB 3rd. Juvenile xanthogranuloma of the finger. *Pediatr Dermatol.* 2006; 23(1): 53–55.

129. Kim EJ, Kim MY, Kim HO, Park YM. Juvenile xanthogranuloma of the finger: An unusual localization. *J Dermatol.* 2007; 34(8): 590–592.

130. Piraccini BM, Fanti PA, Iorizzo M, Tosti A. Juvenile xanthogranuloma of the proximal nail fold. *Pediatr Dermatol.* 2003; 20(4): 307–308.

131. Ramsay B, Dahl MC, Malcolm AJ, Wilson-Jones E. Acral pseudolymphomatous angiokeratoma of children. *Arch Dermatol.* 1990; 126(11): 1524–1525.

132. Hara M, Matsunaga J, Tagami H. Acral pseudolymphomatous angiokeratoma of children (APACHE): A case report and immunohistological study. *Br J Dermatol.* 1991; 124(4): 387–388.

133. Gansz B, Stander S, Metze D. [Acral pseudolymphomatous angiokeratoma of children (APACHE)]. *Hautarzt.* 2005; 56(3): 270–272.

134. Lessa PP, Jorge JC, Ferreira FR et al. Acral pseudolymphomatous angiokeratoma: Case report and literature review. *An Bras Dermatol.* 2013; 88(6 Suppl 1): 39–43.

135. Brandling-Bennett HA, Morel KD. Epidermal nevi. *Pediatr Clin N Am.* 2010; 57(5): 1177–1198.

136. Landwehr AJ, Starink TM. Inflammatory linear verrucous epidermal naevus. Report of a case with bilateral distribution and nail involvement. *Dermatologica.* 1983; 166(2): 107–109.

137. Hashimoto K, Prada S, Lopez AP et al. CHILD syndrome with linear eruptions, hypopigmented bands, and verruciform xanthoma. *Pediatr Dermatol.* 1998; 15(5): 360–366.

138. Fedda F, Khattab R, Ibrahim A et al. Verruciform xanthoma: A special epidermal nevus. *Cutis*. 2011; 88(6): 269–272.

139. Baran R, Bureau H. Multiple exostoses syndrome. *J Am Acad Dermatol*. 1991; 25(2 Pt 1): 333–335.

140. Del-Rio R, Navarra E, Ferrando J, Mascaro JM. Multiple exostoses syndrome presenting as nail malalignment and longitudinal dystrophy of fingers. *Arch Dermatol*. 1992; 128(12): 1655–1656.

141. Hazen PG, Smith DE. Hereditary multiple exostoses: Report of a case presenting with proximal nail fold and nail swelling. *J Am Acad Dermatol*. 1990; 22(1): 132–134.

142. Schmitt AM, Bories A, Baran R. [Subungual exostosis of fingers in hereditary multiple exostosis. 3 cases]. *Ann Dermatol Venereol*. 1997; 124(3): 233–236.

143. Yanagi T, Akiyama M, Arita K, Shimizu H. Nail deformity associated with hereditary multiple exostoses. *J Am Acad Dermatol*. 2005; 53(3): 534–535.

144. Pansuriya TC, Kroon HM, Bovee JV. Enchondromatosis: Insights on the different subtypes. *Int J Clin Exp Pathol*. 2010; 3(6): 557–569.

145. Wilson CA, El-Khayat RH, Somerville J, McKenna K. Digitial endochondroma. *Dermatol Online J*. 2015; 21(2).

146. Fuessl HS. [Diagnostic quiz. A small girl with thick fingers. Enchondromatosis (Ollier disease)]. *MMW Fortschr Med*. 2000; 142(10): 45–46.

147. Ferner RE. Neurofibromatosis 1 and neurofibromatosis 2: A twenty first century perspective. *Lancet Neurol*. 2007; 6(4): 340–351.

148. Brems H, Park C, Maertens O et al. Glomus tumors in neurofibromatosis type 1: Genetic, functional, and clinical evidence of a novel association. *Cancer Res*. 2009; 69(18): 7393–7401.

149. Leonard M, Harrington P. Painful glomus tumour of the thumb in an 11-year-old child with neurofibromatosis 1. *J Hand Surg Eur Vol*. 2010; 35(4): 319–320.

150. Stewart DR, Sloan JL, Yao L et al. Diagnosis, management, and complications of glomus tumours of the digits in neurofibromatosis type 1. *J Med Genet*. 2010; 47(8): 525–532.

151. Dahlin LB, Muller G, Anagnostaki L et al. Glomus tumours in the long finger and in the thumb of a young patient with neurofibromatosis-1 (Nf-1). *J Plast Surg Hand Surg*. 2013; 47(3): 238–240.

152. Jozwiak S, Schwartz RA, Janniger CK et al. Skin lesions in children with tuberous sclerosis complex: Their prevalence, natural course, and diagnostic significance. *Int J Dermatol*. 1998; 37(12): 911–917.

153. Unlu E, Balta I, Unlu S. Multiple ungual fibromas as an only cutaneous manifestation of tuberous sclerosis complex. *Indian J Dermatol Venereol Leprol*. 2014; 80(5): 464–465.

154. Aldrich CS, Hong CH, Groves L et al. Acral lesions in tuberous sclerosis complex: Insights into pathogenesis. *J Am Acad Dermatol*. 2010; 63(2): 244–251.

155. Mazaira M, del Pozo Losada J, Fernandez-Jorge B et al. Shave and phenolization of periungual fibromas, Koenen's tumors, in a patient with tuberous sclerosis. *Dermatol Surg*. 2008; 34(1): 111–113.

156. Muzic JG, Kindle SA, Tollefson MM. Successful treatment of subungual fibromas of tuberous sclerosis with topical rapamycin. *JAMA Dermatol*. 2014; 150(9): 1024–1025.

157. Young A, Manolson P, Cohen B et al. Painful subungual dyskeratotic tumors in incontinentia pigmenti. *J Am Acad Dermatol*. 2005; 52(4): 726–729.

158. Denadai R, Raposo-Amaral CE, Bertola D et al. Identification of 2 novel ANTXR2 mutations in patients with hyaline fibromatosis syndrome and proposal of a modified grading system. *Am J Med Genet A*. 2012; 158A(4): 732–742.

159. Cam B, Kurkcu M, Ozturan S et al. Juvenile hyaline fibromatosis: A case report follow-up after 3 years and a review of the literature. *Int J Dermatol*. 2015; 54(2): 217–221.

160. Schaller M, Stengel-Rutkowski S, Sollberg S, Kind P. [Juvenile hyaline fibromatosis]. *Hautarzt*. 1997; 48(4): 253–257.

161. Hammerton MD, Shrank AB. Congenital hypertrophy of the lateral nail folds of the hallux. *Pediatr Dermatol*. 1988; 5(4): 243–245.

162. Cambiaghi S, Pistritto G, Gelmetti C. Congenital hypertrophy of the lateral nail folds of the hallux in twins. *Br J Dermatol*. 1997; 136(4): 635–636.

163. Piraccini BM, Parente GL, Varotti E, Tosti A. Congenital hypertrophy of the lateral nail folds of the hallux: Clinical features and follow-up of seven cases. *Pediatr Dermatol*. 2000; 17(5): 348–351.

16

The Painful Nail

Marie Caucanas and Bertrand Richert

Onychalgia comes from the rich innervation of the terminal phalanx, with 60% of digital nerve axons. Ungual pain develops in the context of a unique anatomic configuration: the absence of subcutaneous tissue between the plate and the underlying bony phalanx, added to the presence of fibrous collagenic fibers firmly attaching the plate to the terminal phalanx, thus making the subungual space virtual, without possible dilation. With the help of the parents, the anamnesis aims to qualify the pain: its way of development (quick, progressive, insidious); its type (continuous, repetitive, throbbing); its intensity (acute, moderate, mild); its rhythm (diurnal, nocturnal); and the existence of precipitating, aggravating, or relieving factors (pressure, temperature, elevation of the limb, drug). A history of trauma of the nail apparatus should always be searched for. First-choice workup remains X-rays. Magnetic resonance imaging (MRI) may be helpful to precise a diagnosis and detail the anatomic boundaries of any solid tumor, facilitating the surgical approach. Avulsion allows biopsy or excision of the lesion.

In infancy, pain causes vary from that of adults.[1] By decreasing order, the most common reasons for onychalgia are trauma, infections, inflammatory disorders, tumors, congenital and hereditary conditions, and finally, iatrogenic disorders.

Traumas

Nail bed injuries are the commonest pediatric hand injuries presented to the emergency department. These injuries are often underestimated and, consequently, delegated to the most junior and inexperienced staff. Failure to adequate management can result in devastating complications.[2] Acute nail traumas are very painful and not seen in routine consultation. This is mainly their sequelae that are a frequent cause of pediatric nail consultation. Too often, patients ask for help for late dystrophies resulting from inadequate management of a nail trauma in early childhood. A nail trauma in a child should never be minimized. Radiographs should always be performed and hand surgeons involved if necessary (Figure 16.1a and b). Great care should be taken in their management, as initial care and treatment are vital for the best patient outcome.[3] A nail always regrows if the matrix is spared. This painful experience still remains too frequent in toddlers for a home accident that can be often prevented by the acquisition of cheap specific protective devices.[4]

Hematomas

Subungual hematomas are common, very painful, and result most commonly form finger crushing. The diagnosis is obvious. There is still no consensus regarding the optimal mode of managing the acute traumatic subungual hematoma in the hand.[5] The acutely painful subungual hematoma should be decompressed, whether this is done by trephining or nail removal and nail bed repair. There is no difference in cosmetic outcome when comparing nail bed repair with simple decompression.[5,6]

Foreign Bodies

Due to its role in gripping, the nail unit is exposed to penetration of foreign bodies, especially in children who are keen to explore their new surroundings. These are most commonly wood splinter, thorn, glass,

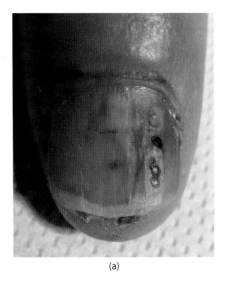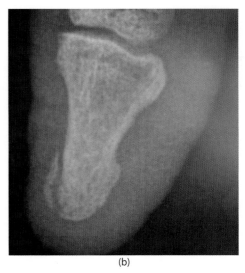

(a)   (b)

FIGURE 16.1   (a) The painful subungual hematoma was drained by trephining the plate with a hot paper clip. (b) X-ray demonstrates a bony fracture.

metal, or plastic fibers. Pain is acute, increased by pressure, but the foreign body cannot be seen in most instances. Bedside ultrasound has become increasingly important to identify and characterize the foreign body before removal and then to evaluate for any residual foreign body after removal.[7]

Pyogenic Granuloma

Nail pyogenic granuloma (PG) is a relatively common acquired benign vascular tumor that frequently involves the nail, including the periungual tissues and the nail bed. In most instances, it is slightly tender only on pressure. Nail PGs are due to different causes that act through different pathogenetic mechanisms. There are three main causes for PG which are as follows:

1. PGs most commonly appear after local trauma: nail ingrowing, retronychia,[8] and frictional PG after a long walk[9] (Figure 16.2a and b). Among self-induced nail trauma, onychotillomania, onychophagia may be responsible for the arising of PG.[10] PGs can also occur after penetration of a foreign body within the nail tissue or after an acute mechanical trauma.

2. Different conditions, all sharing peripheral nerve injury, are associated with the development of nail changes and PGs of the proximal nail fold. Cast immobilization has been reported as a possible cause of periungual PG[11]: an improper cast application may induce peripheral nerve damage, probably by mechanical compression. Patients, almost solely teenagers and young adults, complain of moderate paraesthesia and pain during cast wearing and develop painful onychomadesis, periungual swelling and a PG from the proximal nail fold a few days after cast removal, very similar to retronychia (Figure 16.3). Similar nail changes are observed in reflex sympathetic dystrophy.[12]

3. A main characteristic of *drug-induced PGs* is the involvement of multiple nails, both of the fingers and of the toes. Several cases have been reported during treatment by retinoids (systemic acitretin, systemic isotretinoin, systemic etretinate, topical retinoic acid, topical tazarotene).[13–17] The new generation of antineoplastic therapies are prone to develop multiple PGs: epidermal growth factor receptor (EGFR) inhibitors (cetuximab, gefitinib),[13] agents of the fluoropyrimidine family (capecitabine),[18–20] and agents of the taxan family (docetaxel, paclitaxel).[13,21,22] These drugs are fortunately not frequently used on children.

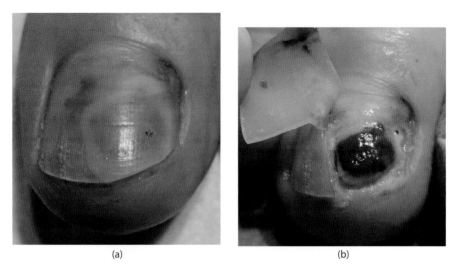

(a)   (b)

FIGURE 16.2 (a) Painful great toenail with subungual oozing following a long walk with improper footwear. (b) Partial avulsion reveals a frictional pyogenic granuloma.

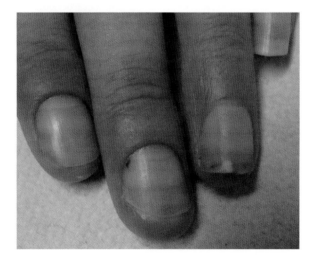

FIGURE 16.3 This girl complained of finger dysesthesia during her cast wearing for a broken arm. A few days after its removal, she developed a periungual swelling, with loss of the cuticle and xanthonychia on two nails that also stopped growing. This is a post-cast removal retronychia.

Infections

Bacterial

Bacterial acute paronychia generates pain and throbbing. It results from direct or indirect trauma to the cuticle or nail fold allowing penetration of pathogens, such as *Staphylococcus aureus* and β-hemolytic *Streptoccocus.*[23] It is precipitated by finger-sucking and onychophagia.[24] Pus collects under the proximal nail fold and/or extends to the lateral nail folds, sometimes with blisters (Figure 16.4). Involvement of the proximal nail fold is of concern, as the nail matrix in children is very fragile and that pressure and inflammation may precipitate matrix necrosis with subsequent permanent nail dystrophy.[25] As oral antibacterial have not been proved better or worse than drainage,[26] the following approach should be

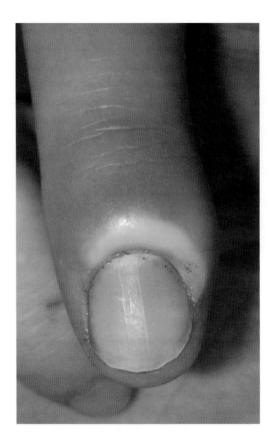

FIGURE 16.4   Acute paronychia.

proposed: if empiric antibacterial treatment fails after 48 hours, surgical drainage should be undertaken along with smears. Bacterial acute paronychia should not be confused with parakeratosis pustulosa, affecting most commonly the thumb or the index finger, typically in girls around the age of 7 years and considered as a symptom of an inflammatory disease of the nail apparatus such as psoriasis, contact dermatitis, or atopic dermatitis.[27]

Viral

- Herpetic whitlow starts with a prodromal phase of burning, pruritus and/or tingling of the affected finger and evolves to clinical signs of pain, swelling, erythema, and nonpurulent vesicle formation.[28] It is due to herpes simplex virus (HSV) type 1 or 2 infection of a distal phalanx of the digits, occasionally the toes. HSV-1 will be more often identified in children, either after a primary oral herpes infection or less frequently through person-to-person transmission from family members with herpes labialis.[29] In adolescents, herpetic whitlow tends to be caused by autoinoculation of HSV-2. Diagnosis is readily confirmed by Tzanck test. Specific diagnosis can be made by polymerase chain reaction, culture,[28] or direct fluorescent antibody testing. Herpetic whitlow is often misdiagnosed as a bacterial felon and thus improperly treated. Early diagnosis should allow prescription of oral antivirals with rapid alleviation of the painful symptoms. Recurrences occur frequently (23%) in adults too.[29]
- Warts are the most common tumors involving the nail unit. They are caused by various human papillomavirus. They present as hyperkeratotic papules showing a rough surface. Most commonly they are located on the nail folds (proximal and lateral) but sometimes extend to the nail bed with associated onycholysis (Figure 16.5). Fissuring of the hyperkeratosis causes pain.

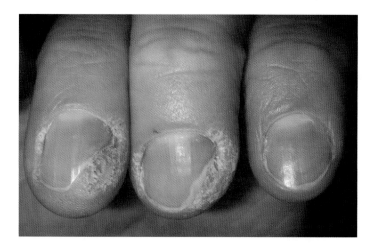

FIGURE 16.5 Subungual warts. Cracks and fissure may induce pain.

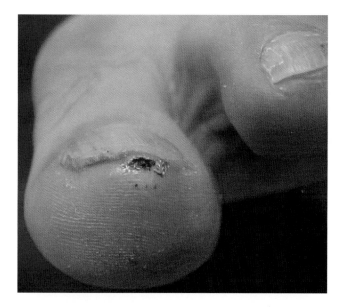

FIGURE 16.6 Tungiasis in a teenager. (Courtesy of di Chiacchio N.)

Distorsion of the nail plate is exceptional. Nail-biting enhances spreading to other fingernails. Although spontaneous regression is reported in 30% of the cases, treatment is advisable when the lesion causes pain and to avoid spreading of the same.[30] Warts are hard to treat in the immunosuppressed, particularly in organ-transplant recipients.[31]

Parasitic

Tungiasis diagnosis should be evoked in front of painful toe lesions in children able to walk, either in countries where it represents a public health concern or in family travelers coming back from endemic regions (Figure 16.6). Tungiasis is an infestation caused by the penetration in the skin of the gravid female of the flea *Tunga penetrans*. A cross-sectional study on tungiasis was conducted in Northern Tanzania in more than 60 infected schoolchildren (6–14 years) with 865 lesions. The first and the fifth toes were especially involved; pain was reported in 42 children, itching in 39, and trouble walking in 28. One child presented with fever, which was considered to be caused by superinfected tungiasis. Complications were nail dystrophy (48 patients), deformity of the fingers or toes (12 patients), scarring (4 patients), and nail loss (4 patients). Thirteen children needed oral antibiotic therapy because of bacterial superinfections.[32]

Inflammatory Nail Disorders

Chronic Paronychia

Finger-sucking is mainly responsible for a tender chronic paronychia in infants, affecting almost exclusively the thumb (Figure 16.7). The proximal nail fold appears erythematous, swollen, and the cuticle is absent. It might be precipitated by teeth growth. Thumb-sucking represents a predisposing factor for chronic candida paronychia. Treatment is difficult as it is almost impossible to prevent this habit. It should be attempted to dry the digit, either with topical clindamycin (bitter taste) or with a combination of topical corticosteroids and antibiotics under occlusive dressing.[30]

Congenital Hypertrophic Folds

Congenital hypertrophy of the lateral nail folds was reported as the most common nail alteration (2.5%) on a series of 250 toddlers.[33] It mainly happens in big toenails and manifests as a hypertrophic lip that partially covers the nail plate (Figure 16.8). The lateral, the medial, the distal, or several folds may be involved. The condition may be present at birth or develops shortly thereafter. It has been attributed to an asynchronism between the growth of the nail plate and that of the soft tissues.[34]

It is frequently associated with inflammation and moderate-to-severe pain due to an ingrown nail. The child refuses to wear shoes or socks. The only series on the follow-up of patients demonstrates a spontaneous or partial improvement in 40%, no improvement in 30%, and worsening in 30% of cases.[35] Conservative treatment is recommended first and consists of disinfection and vigorous massaging with topical corticosteroids. Taping may be of some help.[36] Surgical excision (shaving of the excess tissue) should be reserved for long-standing and unresponsive cases.

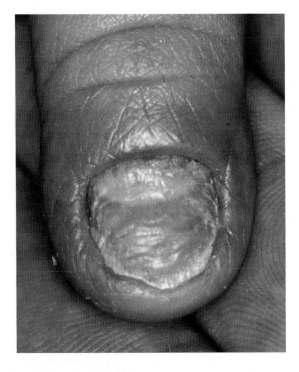

FIGURE 16.7 Chronic paronychia from thumb-sucking.

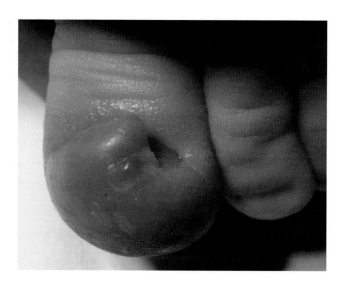

FIGURE 16.8   Impressive hypertrophy of the distal nail fold in a toddler. Here surgery was mandatory.

Ingrowing Toenails

Juvenile ingrown nails are a common complaint in teenagers. The nail is usually embedded laterally, but both sides may be affected. The condition is often precipitated by improper trimming of the nails in the corners and hyperhidrosis induced by sport shoes. Some patients like to play with their softened nails and tear them off. All these conditions provoke an irregular, jagged lateral nail edge that irritates or breaks the epidermis of the lateral groove with subsequent inflammatory reaction and pain. With time, granulation tissue may develop with concomitant oozing, bleeding, and secondary infection (Figure 16.9). Early stages may benefit from conservative measures such as removal of the nail spicule, disinfection, and topical corticosteroids. Taping, acrylic nails, as well as gutter splints, in association with curettage or silver nitrating of the PG, are useful conservative treatments in the early stages. In more advanced cases, phenolization of the matrix lateral horns is the first choice treatment.[37]

Multiple ingrown fingernails in newborns (around the sixth day after birth) are the consequence of the grasp reflex. The condition regresses spontaneously in the newborn as the reflex disappears around the fourth month.[38]

Retronychia

The term retronychia, derives from the word *retro*, Latin for backward, and the Greek term *onychia*, meaning nail. It is characterized by a triad associating arrest of the growth of the nail plate, proximal paronychia, and xanthonychia. The most probable etiology is distal trauma from footwear. It mostly affects women (>80%) and the great toenails (>90%) confirming the probable role of poorly fitting, or tight-toed footwear. In men, sports where running plays a major role may explain its arising. For some reason, the distal edge of the nail plate adheres very firmly to its bed and does not move forward. A newly formed nail grows beneath the old one and gets stuck again distally. Another new nail may grow again beneath the former one and so on. This lifts up the proximal nail fold that becomes inflamed and irritated from the proximal stacked thin sharp nails, resulting in paronychia.[8] With time, a PG may develop under the proximal nail fold and the oozing will induce a yellowish discoloration (Figure 16.10). Another clue for the diagnosis is the shortening of the distal nail bed due to the excessive pressure of the distal plate onto the bed and the lifting of the proximal part of the plate from the successive superposed nails.[39]

This underestimated condition that mostly affects adults, may also occur in children, adolescents, and young adults. The main complaint is a chronic stabbing pain at the base of the nail. Fingernails may be affected, but in this case, it always follows an acute injury that the patient remembers. Treatment is

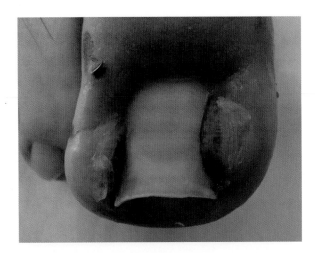

FIGURE 16.9   Ingrowing toenail, bilateral.

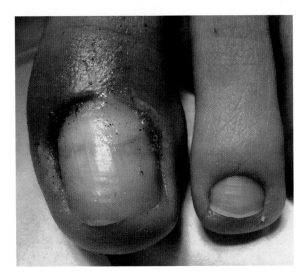

FIGURE 16.10   Typical appearance of retronychia.

avulsion of the superposed nails. Even after an adequate surgical treatment, a permanent nail dystrophy may be observed in about 30% of teenager cases.[40]

Hereditary Pincer Nail

Pincer nail is due to an overcurvature of the plate, inducing variable degrees of pain, which can occasionally develop during childhood or adolescence. It may present with[41] or without hereditary features.[42]

Pernio

Pernio, also called chilblains, is a localized inflammatory lesion of the skin resulting from an abnormal response to cold.[43] Single or multiple erythematous, reddish to purplish, edematous lesions appear on the digits and/or the toes, accompanied by intense pain, itching, or burning.[44] Chilblains are not uncommon in the pediatric population, as shown in an epidemiologic prospective study conducted over 51 patients: 49% were aged 0–18 years. Primary or idiopathic chilblains is more frequent in children, compared to the secondary form, associated with connective tissue disease and hematologic disorders.[45] Familial autosomal-dominant chilblain lupus develops in early childhood, is rare, and is caused by a mutation in *TREX1*.[46]

In a recent large pediatric case series of 33 patients presenting chronic digital chilblains, the mean age reached 13.5 years and there was a clear female predisposition (sex ratio 4.5:1). Capillary refill time was prolonged in 100% and modified Allen test was abnormal in 75.6%. Beside finger swelling and proximal interphalangeal joint swelling, skin ulceration was observed in more than half of the cases (54.5%). All patients had normal nail fold capillaroscopy. Antinuclear factor (ANA) was positive in 25%.[43]

The major differential diagnoses include Raynaud's phenomenon, (sharply demarcated cutaneous pallor and cyanosis, followed by far shorter duration of the erythemic phase), frostbite (freezing of tissue, with resultant tissue necrosis). Predisposing factors among children are the presence of cryoproteins,[47] excessive cold exposure, and anorexia nervosa.[44]

Biological investigation is not mandatory unless persistence of the symptomatology beyond the cold seasons and presence of photosensitivity.[45]

Better than symptomatic treatment and rewarming the extremities, prevention with cold protection measures is a must. If needed, nifedipine, which produces vasodilation, has been demonstrated to be effective in reducing pain, facilitating healing, and preventing new lesions of pernio.[44]

Tumors

Exostosis

The pain from subungual exostoses may vary from nil to severe, whatever the size of the tumor. When present, it is induced either by pressure during clinical examination or from footwear. The authors have observed an extremely painful exostosis, associated with an infection with septic shock in a child (Figure 16.11a and b). Subungual exostosis is an osteocartilaginous tumor that affects the distal phalanx of the toes or fingers. It was for a long time considered as a reactive dermal metaplasia resulting from microtrauma.[48] It is now considered a true neoplasm harboring a pathognomonic translocation *t(X;6)(q22;q13-14)*,[49] instead of being a reactive process in response to trauma. Other lesions of the bone surface such as bizarre parosteal osteochondromatous proliferation (BPOP or Nora lesion), once thought to be a related proliferative process to subungual exostoses, have unique chromosomal rearrangements, and represent a distinct molecular pathogenesis.[50] A recent review of the literature[51] showed that subungual exostoses are not uncommon in teenagers' toenails, as 55% of all cases appeared in children aged under 18 years. The female : male ratio was approximately equal. The hallux was the most common location of the exostoses (80%) followed by the second toe (6%), third toe (7%), fourth toe (5%), and the fifth toe (2%). Pain was the most common complaint (77%) followed by a swelling mass under the nail (31%), nail dystrophy (15%), or other complaints such as shoe wear rubbing or stiffness (3%). The duration of symptoms ranged widely from 2 to 48 months. A history of toe trauma before diagnosis was present in one-third of the cases. The bony proliferation usually elevates the nail plate, mostly at its distolateral part, sometimes mimicking a subungual wart.[52,53] Erosion and infection of the nail bed may give rise to an ingrown toenail. The skin overlying the lesion may be normal, ulcerated, or hyperkeratotic.[54] It may often exhibit a porcelain white hue with telangiectasia running on its surface (Figure 16.12). Radiographs demonstrate a pediculated exophytic lesion of the distal phalangeal bone. Treatment is by resection of the outgrowth under full aseptic conditions.[55]

Osteoid Osteoma

Osteoid osteomas are benign bone-forming tumors that typically occur in children, particularly adolescents. They account for approximately 10% of all benign bone lesions, and there is a male predilection (male : female 2–4:1).[56] About 3% of cases occur in children younger than 5 years.[57] Most osteoid

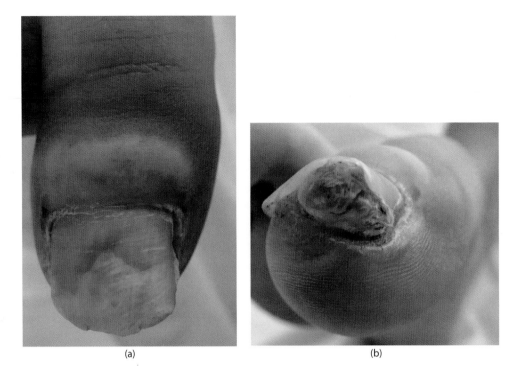

(a)   (b)

FIGURE 16.11   (a) This child was referred to us for an acute paronychia, almost in septic shock. (b) Clinical examination revealed an infected exostosis.

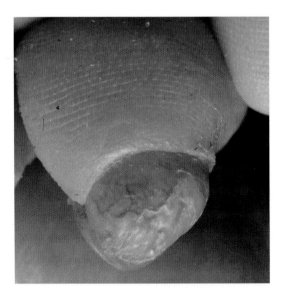

FIGURE 16.12   Typical aspect of a subungual exostosis, lifting up the nail plate. Note the collarette at its base and the telangiectasia running on its surface.

osteomas occur in long tubular bones of the limbs (especially proximal femur), but essentially any bone may be involved. Phalanges are rarely affected (8%) and if so, there is an index predominance.[58]

Osteoid osteoma is a small tumor usually measuring less than 1.5 cm, composed of a central zone named nidus, which is an atypical bone completely enclosed within a well-vascularized stroma. Prostaglandins are found in the nidus at levels of 100 to 1 000 times than that of normal tissue. The nidus releases prostaglandins (via Cox-1 and Cox-2), which in turn induce vasodilation. The resultant increased capillary permeability in the surrounding tissues is believed to mediate tumor-related pain, classically described as night nagging pain relieved by salicylates. However, some osteoid osteomas have been reported to be totally painless.[59–61] Medical imaging supports diagnosis. Plain films may be normal or may show a solid periosteal reaction with cortical thickening. The nidus is sometimes visible as an ovoid well-circumscribed lucent region, occasionally with a central sclerotic dot. Computed tomography (CT) scan is excellent at characterizing the lesion and is the modality of choice. It typically shows a focally lucent nidus within surrounding sclerotic reactive bone. A central sclerotic dot may also be seen. Although MRI is certainly sensitive, it is nonspecific and often unable to identify the nidus.[56]

The location at the distal phalanx is rare and the radiological appearance is peculiar. It most commonly demonstrates a lytic lesion rather than the classic appearance of reactive sclerosis surrounding a central lucent nidus. CT scan is of considerable value when there is no evidence on plain films to localize the nidus. At that location, osteoid osteoma causes swelling of the distal phalanx or even enlargement of the entire tip and clubbing. The skin is either normal in color or faintly violaceous. Increased sweating of the area has been described.

Because of persisting pain, treatment is usually surgical, but spontaneous remission could be achieved in some patients following long-term treatment with nonsteroidal anti-inflammatory drugs.[62] In some cases, the digital enlargement persisted after removal of the lesion.

Subungual Neurofibroma

Exceptionally, a subungual neurofibroma may induce moderate tenderness and deform the distal phalanx, as reported in an adolescent female.[63]

Giant Cell Tumor of the Bone

Giant cell tumor may be responsible for sudden pain, sometimes following relatively mild trauma. It usually occurs in the distal bony phalanx of young adults. Curettage appears to be ineffective with a high rate of recurrence. Local resection or amputation in extreme cases are recommended. Since there is an 18% incidence of multicentric foci of giant cell tumors of the hand, bone scan is advised when they occur in that location.[64]

Chondroma

Chondroma is a benign cartilaginous tumor that is classified into three types in accordance with the area of occurrence: enchondroma (within the medullary cavity), periosteal (juxtacortical) chondroma, and soft tissue chondroma.

Enchondroma is the most common benign cystic lesion in the phalanges. They probably develop slowly during childhood and are often revealed by a fracture in young adults (20–40 years old). Pain is very mild from the progressive swelling. On plain X-rays, it invariably presents with a calcified chondroid matrix, except in phalanges. Multiple enchondromatosis is a rare condition appearing in early childhood. It tends to be unilateral. When the bone alone is affected, it is named Ollier's disease. Pain is present only during periods of rapid growth. Once the individual stops growing, then, in general, so do the enchondromas. If growth occurs afterward, this should suggest a potential malignant transformation (chondrosarcoma).[65] Association with soft tissue and visceral hemangiomas represents Maffuci's syndrome.

Juxtacortical chondroma is a rare benign bone lesion in children. It usually presents with a mildly painful mass, which prompts diagnostic imaging studies. Hopefully, it has characteristic features on plain radiographs, CT and MRI. The rarity of this condition often presents a diagnostic challenge. It mainly affects long bones (humerus, femur) and may rarely be observed in the distal phalanx.[66]

Soft tissue chondroma is a tumor of cartilage without any connection to the underlying bone. It is usually asymptomatic and grows slowly. It can occur in patients of any age, but is most common in middle-aged patients. Only one case was reported in a child.[67]

Implantation Cyst

Implantation cysts are common in the vicinity of a scar. They result from the implantation of epidermal tissue in deeper tissue from heavy or penetrating trauma or during surgery via the blade, skin hooks, or the suturing needle. At the nail unit, their occurrence is estimated around 5.5% after Emmert surgery (surgical removal of the lateral horn of the matrix) for ingrowing toenail.[68] Intraosseous implantation is possible and mostly results from an old trauma that may have occurred very long ago (up to decades). The three dominant digits are electively affected. From its slow arising, only one case has been reported in a child.[69] Tenderness or pain are of late onsets and result from pressure of the bone. Clinically, there might be some swelling of the distal extremity, a pincer nail,[70] or a paronychia.[71]

Plain X-rays will demonstrate the lytic bony lesion. Treatment is surgical with curettage of the cyst and its lining.

Aneurysmal Bone Cyst

Aneurysmal bone cyst may be responsible for digit pain, although it rarely occurs on digits[72] and exceptionally on toes.[73] MRI and biopsy prior to surgery are recommended. Curettage with or without bone graft are advised in most cases. An aggressive treatment approach will be reserved to advanced situations where the articular surface is involved, in case of full bone invasion or after more than one recurrence.[74]

Congenital and Genetic Disorders

Eccrine Angiomatous Hamartoma

Eccrine angiomatous hamartoma (EAH) is a rare benign cutaneous tumor characterized by the proliferation of eccrine glands and capillaries. Sudden enlargement can happen, sometimes associated with pain and hyperhidrosis. The lower extremities were affected in 61.5% in a 26-case series[75] and Sezer et al.[76] described a case of EAH of the fingers with nail destruction. In case of pain, functional or cosmetic impairment, the treatment remains surgical.[77]

Epidermolysis Bullosa

Nail dystrophies due to repeated blistering are frequently encountered in congenital epidermolysis bullosa.[78,79] However, they are not specific to the different subtypes.[80,81] Nail abnormalities are more frequent in epidermolysis bullosa junctionalis and dystrophica. In late-onset, junctional epidermolysis bullosa and pretibial, dystrophic epidermolysis bullosa, nail abnormalities precede skin blistering. In some rare instances of dominant dystrophic epidermolysis bullosa, the nail abnormalities may be the only sign of epidermolysis bullosa over several generations.[82] The diagnosis remains obscure until a family member develops bullae revealing the disease.[83,84]

Incontinentia Pigmenti and Distal Digital Tumors

The arising of multiple subungual painful keratotic tumors in a young adult should always raise the diagnosis of incontinentia pigmenti (IP). These tumors are indistinguishable from keratoacanthomas on histology. From 15 to 30 years of age, painful subungual tumors or warty periungual tumors can appear as a manifestation of IP.[85,86] The keratotic mass produces dystrophy or onycholysis. Erythema and swelling of the fingertip may be observed. Location under the proximal nail fold is unusual and induces paronychia. The tumors destroy the underlying phalanx (scalloped bone deformities on X-rays), which is the reason for the acute pain. Self-healing is possible, but the patient begs for treatment because of the intense pain. Surgery is the best option. In case of recurrence, acitretin 1 mg/kg/d is an excellent alternative. There is only one report of a prepubertal child (10 years old) with such lesions. The digital subungual lesions

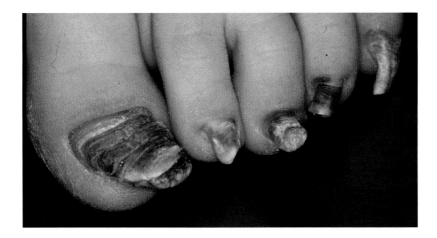

FIGURE 16.13 Pachyonychia congenita.

were mild, probably, because it was an early stage of the disease. However, it was difficult to correlate the severity of the fingertip pain with the absence of true tumoral swelling.[87]

Pachyonychia Congenita

Pachyonychia congenita is usually inherited as an autosomal-dominant disease, although an autosomal recessive form has also been described. It is due to mutations of four keratin genes (*KRT6A*, *KRT6B*, *KRT16*, and *KRT17*) responsible for a distal prominent thickening of the nails and abnormal keratinization of the skin and mucous membranes. Nail and skin changes are present at birth in only 50% of patients, but, by 5 years of age, they are seen in more than 75% of the children.[88] By the age of 10, pain is a common associated symptom and greatly impairs quality of life. Toenail thickening is the most common finding, with severe subungual keratosis (hoof-like nails) and difficulty in trimming nails (Figure 16.13). A review of the clinical findings of pachyonychia congenita in a large series of patients with genetically confirmed pachyonychia congenita, showed that the most suggestive symptoms for the condition are toenail dystrophy associated with plantar keratoderma and plantar pain in children older than 3 years.[89]

In all types of pachyonychia congenita, systemic retinoid should be attempted even during early childhood as some positive results may be obtained.[90] If the nails severely impair domestic life, chemical or surgical nail ablation may be suggested.[91]

Iatrogenic

Photo-onycholysis

Photo-onycholysis is believed to be a rare manifestation of phototoxicity. A few cases have been reported among the pediatric population[92–94] while under oral doxycycline treatment. Clinical signs include nail pain, subungual hemorrhages, and/or distal onycholysis. Self-resolution occurs within several months.[92]

Chemotherapy

See the section "Pyogenic Granuloma" for drug-induced pyogenic granulomas.

REFERENCES

1. Richert B, Baran R. L'ongle douloureux. In Richert B, Baran R, (eds.), *L'ongle de la Clinique au Traitement*, Second Edition. Med' Com, Paris, France; 2009. pp. 91–94.
2. Fairbairn N. No such thing as "just" a nail bed injury. *Pediatr Emerg Care*. 2012; 28(4): 363–365.
3. Hart RG, Kleinert HE. Fingertip and nail bed injuries. *Emerg Med Clin North Am*. 1993; 11(3): 755–765.
4. Claudet I, Toubal K, Carnet C et al. When doors slam, fingers jam! *Arch Pediatr*. 2007; 14(8): 958–963.
5. Dean B, Becker G, Little C. The management of the acute traumatic subungual haematoma: A systematic review. *Hand Surg*. 2012; 17(1): 151–154.
6. Gellman H. Fingertip-nail bed injuries in children: Current concepts and controversies of treatment. *J Craniofac Surg*. 2009; 20(4): 1033–1035.
7. Teng M, Doniger SJ. Subungual wooden splinter visualized with bedside sonography. *Pediatr Emerg Care*. 2012; 28(4): 392–394.
8. de Berker DA, Richert B, Duhard E et al. Retronychia: Proximal ingrowing of the nail plate. *J Am Acad Dermatol*. 2008; 58(6): 978–983.
9. Richert B. Frictional pyogenic granuloma of the nail bed. *Dermatology*. 2001; 202(1): 80–81.
10. Colver GB. Onychotillomania. *Br J Dermatol*. 1987; 117(3): 397–399.
11. Tosti A, Piraccini BM, Camacho-Martinez F. Onychomadesis and pyogenic granuloma following cast immobilization. *Arch Dermatol*. 2001; 137(2): 231–232.
12. Tosti A, Baran R, Peluso AM et al. Reflex sympathetic dystrophy with prominent involvement of the nail apparatus. *J Am Acad Dermatol*. 1993; 29(5 Pt 2): 865–868.
13. Piraccini BM, Bellavista S, Misciali C et al. Periungual and subungual pyogenic granuloma. *Br J Dermatol*. 2010; 163(5): 941–953.
14. Piraccini BM, Iorizzo M. Drug reactions affecting the nail unit: Diagnosis and management. *Dermatol Clin*. 2007; 25(2): 215–221, vii.
15. Campbell JP, Grekin RC, Ellis CN et al. Retinoid therapy is associated with excess granulation tissue responses. *J Am Acad Dermatol*. 1983; 9(5): 708–713.
16. Teknetzis A, Ioannides D, Vakali G et al. Pyogenic granulomas following topical application of tretinoin. *J Eur Acad Dermatol Venereol*. 2004; 18(3): 337–339.
17. Dawkins MA, Clark AR, Feldman SR. Pyogenic granuloma-like lesion associated with topical tazarotene therapy. *J Am Acad Dermatol*. 2000; 43(1 Pt 1): 154–155.
18. Piguet V, Borradori L. Pyogenic granuloma-like lesions during capecitabine therapy. *Br J Dermatol*. 2002; 147(6): 1270–1272.
19. Piqué-Duran E, Pérez-Díaz MJ, Pérez-Cejudo JA. Pyogenic granuloma-like lesions caused by capecitabine therapy. *Clin Exp Dermatol*. 2008; 33(5): 652–653.
20. Vaccaro M, Barbuzza O, Guarneri F, Guarneri B. Nail and periungual toxicity following capecitabine therapy. *Br J Clin Pharmacol*. 2008; 66(2): 325–326.
21. Paul LJ, Cohen PR. Paclitaxel-associated subungual pyogenic granuloma: Report in a patient with breast cancer receiving paclitaxel and review of drug-induced pyogenic granulomas adjacent to and beneath the nail. *J Drugs Dermatol*. 2012; 11: 262–268.
22. Minisini AM, Tosti A, Sobrero AF et al. Taxane-induced nail changes: Incidence, clinical presentation and outcome. *Ann Oncol*. 2003; 14(2): 333–337.
23. Rigopoulos D, Larios G, Gregoriou S, Alevizos A. Acute and chronic paronychia. *Am Fam Physician*. 2008; 77(3): 339–346.
24. Balighian E, Tuli SY, Tuli SS et al. Index of suspicion. Case 1: Persistent fever and cough following episodes of emesis in a 7-year-old girl. Case 2: Blurry vision and unilateral dilated pupil in a 14-year-old girl. Case 3: Swelling, pain, and erythema of the thumb in a 10-year-old girl with habits of nail biting and thumb sucking. *Pediatr Rev*. 2012; 33(1): 39–44.
25. de Berker D. Childhood nail diseases. *Dermatol Clin*. 2006; 24(3): 355–363.
26. Shaw J, Body R. Best evidence topic report. Incision and drainage preferable to oral antibiotics in acute paronychial nail infection? *Emerg Med J*. 2005; 22(11): 813–814.
27. Tosti A, Peluso AM, Zucchelli V. Clinical features and long-term follow-up of 20 cases of parakeratosis pustulosa. *Pediatr Dermatol*. 1998; 15(4): 259–263.
28. Wu IB, Schwartz RA. Herpetic whitlow. *Cutis*. 2007; 79(3): 193–196.

29. Szinnai G, Schaad UB, Heininger U. Multiple herpetic whitlow lesions in a 4-year-old girl: Case report and review of the literature. *Eur J Pediatr*. 2001; 160(9): 528–533.

30. Piraccini BM, Starace M. Nail disorders in infants and children. *Curr Opin Pediatr*. 2014; 26(4): 440–445.

31. Tosti A, Richert B, Pazzaglia M. Tumors of the nail apparatus. In Scher RK, Daniel CR (eds.), *Nails: Diagnosis, Therapy, Surgery*, Third Edition. Philadelphia, PA: Elsevier Saunders; 2005. pp. 195–204.

32. Dassoni F, Polloni I, Margwe SB, Veraldi S. Tungiasis in Northern Tanzania: A clinical report from Qameyu village, Babati District, Manyara Region. *J Infect Dev Ctries*. 2014; 8(11): 1456–1460.

33. Sarifakioglu E, Yilmaz AE, Gorpelioglu C. Nail alterations in 250 infant patients: A clinical study. *J Eur Acad Dermatol Venereol*. 2008; 22(6): 741–744.

34. Martinet C, Pascal M, Civatte J, Larrègue M. Lateral nail-pad of the big toe in infants. A propos of 2 cases. *Ann Dermatol Venereol*. 1984; 111(8): 731–732.

35. Piraccini BM, Parente GL, Varotti E, Tosti A. Congenital hypertrophy of the lateral nail folds of the hallux: Clinical features and follow-up of seven cases. *Pediatr Dermatol*. 2000; 17(5): 348–351.

36. Arai H, Arai T, Nakajima H, Haneke E. Formable acrylic treatment for ingrowing nail with gutter splint and sculptured nail. *Int J Dermatol*. 2004; 43(10): 759–765.

37. Eekhof JA, Van Wijk B, Knuistingh Neven A, van der Wouden JC. Interventions for ingrowing toenails. *Cochrane Database Syst Rev*. 2012; 4: CD001541.

38. Matsui T, Kidou M, Ono T. Infantile multiple ingrowing nails of the fingers induced by the grasp reflex—A new entity. *Dermatology*. 2002; 205(1): 25–27.

39. Richert B, Caucanas M, André J. Retronychia. *Ann Dermatol Venereol*. 2014; 141(12): 799–804.

40. Piraccini BM, Richert B, de Berker DA et al. Retronychia in children, adolescents, and young adults: A case series. *J Am Acad Dermatol*. 2014; 70(2): 388–390.

41. Mimouni D, Ben-Amitai D. Hereditary pincer nail. *Cutis*. 2002; 69(1): 51–53.

42. Lee JI, Lee YB, Oh ST et al. A clinical study of 35 cases of pincer nails. *Ann Dermatol*. 2011; 23(4): 417–423.

43. Padeh S, Gerstein M, Greenberger S, Berkun Y. Chronic chilblains: The clinical presentation and disease course in a large paediatric series. *Clin Exp Rheumatol*. 2013; 31(3): 463–468.

44. Simon TD, Soep JB, Hollister JR. Pernio in pediatrics. *Pediatrics*. 2005; 116(3): e472–e475.

45. Takci Z, Vahaboglu G, Eksioglu H. Epidemiological patterns of perniosis, and its association with systemic disorder. *Clin Exp Dermatol*. 2012; 37(8): 844–849.

46. Günther C, Berndt N, Wolf C, Lee-Kirsch MA. Familial chilblain lupus due to a novel mutation in the exonuclease III domain of 3' repair exonuclease 1 *(TREX1)*. *JAMA Dermatol*. 2015; 151(4): 426–431.

47. Weston WL, Morelli JG. Childhood pernio and cryoproteins. *Pediatr Dermatol*. 2000; 17(2): 97–99.

48. Haneke E. Bone and cartilage tumours. In Krull EA, Zook EG, Baran R et al. (eds.), *Nail Surgery. A Text Atlas*, First Edition. Philadelphia, PA: Lippincott Williams & Wilkins; 2001. pp. 287–291.

49. Storlazzi C, Wozniak A, Panagopoulos I et al. Rearrangement of the *COL12A1* and *COL4A5* genes in subungual exostosis: Molecular cytogenetic delineation of the tumor-specific translocation *t(X;6) (q13-14;q22)*. *Int J Cancer*. 2006; 118(8): 1972–1976.

50. Zambrano E, Nosé V, Perez-Atayde A et al. Distinct chromosomal rearrangements in subungual (Dupuytren) exostosis and bizarre parosteal osteochondromatous proliferation (Nora lesion). *Am J Surg Pathol*. 2004; 28(8): 1033–1039.

51. DaCambra MP, Gupta SK, Ferri-de-Barros F. Subungual exostosis of the toes: A systematic review. *Clin Orthop Relat Res*. 2014; 472(4): 1251–1259.

52. Van der Burg JM, van Leeuwen RL. A boy with a wart-like lesion of the toe. *Ned Tijdschr Geneeskd*. 2014; 158: A7417.

53. Bach DQ, McQueen AA, Lio PA. A refractory wart? Subungual exostosis. *Ann Emerg Med*. 2011; 58(5): e3–e4.

54. Davis DA, Cohen PR. Subungual exostosis: Case report and review of the literature. *Pediatr Dermatol*. 1996; 13(3): 212–218.

55. De Berker DA, Langtry J. Treatment of subungual exostoses by elective day case surgery. *Br J Dermatol*. 1999; 140(5): 915–918.

56. Greenspan A, Jundt G, Remagen W. *Differential Diagnosis in Orthopaedic Oncology*. Philadelphia, PA: Lippincott Williams & Wilkins; 2007. pp. 458–480.

57. Frassica FJ, Waltrip RL, Sponseller PD et al. Clinicopathologic features and treatment of osteoid osteoma and osteoblastoma in children and adolescents. *Orthop Clin North Am.* 1996; 27(3): 559–574.

58. Di Gennaro GL, Lampasi M, Bosco A, Donzelli O. Osteoid osteoma of the distal thumb phalanx: A case report. *Chir Organi Mov.* 2008; 92(3): 179–182.

59. De Smet L, Spaepen D, Zachee B, Fabry G. Painless osteoid osteoma of the finger in a child. Case report. *Chir Main.* 1998; 17(2): 143–146.

60. Rex C, Jacobs L, Nur Z. Painless osteoid osteoma of the middle phalanx. *J Hand Surg Br.* 1997; 22(6): 798–800.

61. Walker LG, Meals RA. Answer please. Painless osteoid osteoma of the phalanx. *Orthopedics.* 1989; 12(5): 774–776.

62. Hedrich CM, Fiebig B, Sallmann S et al. Osteoid osteomas of the fingers: An atypical localization? Two case reports and a review of the literature. *Z Rheumatol.* 2008; 67(2): 145–148, 150.

63. Niizuma K, Iijima KN. Solitary neurofibroma: A case of subungual neurofibroma on the right third finger. *Arch Dermatol Res.* 1991; 283(1): 13–15.

64. Averill RM, Smith RJ, Campbell CJ. Giant-cell tumors of the bones of the hand. *J Hand Surg Am.* 1980; 5(1): 39–50.

65. Kumar A, Jain VK, Bharadwaj M, Arya RK. Ollier disease: Pathogenesis, diagnosis, and management. *Orthopedics.* 2015; 38(6): e497–e506.

66. Miller SF. Imaging features of juxtacortical chondroma in children. *Pediatr Radiol.* 2014; 44(1): 56–63.

67. Eun YS, Kim MR, Cho BK et al. Subungual soft tissue chondroma with nail deformity in a child. *Pediatr Dermatol.* 2015; 32(1): 132–134.

68. Wadhams PS, McDonald JF, Jenkin WM. Epidermal inclusion cysts as complication of nail surgery. *J Am Podiatr Med Assoc.* 1990; 80(11): 610–612.

69. Hensley CD. Epidermoid cyst of the distal phalanx occurring in an eight-year old-child. A case report. *J Bone Joint Surg Am.* 1966; 48(5): 946–948.

70. Baran R, Broutart JC. Epidermoid cyst of the thumb presenting as a pincer nail. *J Am Acad Dermatol.* 1988; 19(1 Pt 1): 143–144.

71. Connolly JE, Ratcliffe NR. Intraosseous epidermoid inclusion cyst presenting as a paronychia of the hallux. *J Am Podiatr Med Assoc.* 2010; 100(2): 133–137.

72. Tarazona-Velutini P, Romo-Rodríguez R, Saleme-Cruz J. Aneurysmatic bone cyst in the proximal phalanx of a finger. Case report and literature review. *Acta Ortop Mex.* 2012; 26(4): 245–249.

73. El-Khoury GY, Seaman RW. Case report 125: Aneurysmal bone cyst terminal phalanx of the first toe. *Skeletal Radiol.* 1980; 5(3): 201–203.

74. Ropars M, Kaila R, Briggs T, Cannon S. Aneurysmal bone cysts of the metacarpals and phalanges of the hand. A 6 case series and literature review. *Chir Main.* 2007; 26(4–5): 214–217.

75. Sanusi T, Li Y, Sun L et al. Eccrine angiomatous hamartoma: A clinicopathological study of 26 cases. *Dermatology.* 2015; 231(1): 63–69.

76. Sezer E, Koseoglu RD, Filiz N. Eccrine angiomatous hamartoma of the fingers with nail destruction. *Br J Dermatol.* 2006; 154(5): 1002–1004.

77. Yun JH, Kang HK, Na SY et al. Eccrine angiomatous hamartoma mimicking a traumatic hemorrhage. *Ann Dermatol.* 2011; 23(Suppl 1): S84–S87.

78. Baran R, Dawber RPR, de Berker DAR. The nail in childhood and old age. In Baran R, Dawber RPR, de Berker DAR et al. (eds.), *Diseases of the Nail and Their Management*, Third Edition. Oxford, United Kingdom: Blackwell Scientific Publications; 2001. pp. 104–128.

79. Tosti A, Piraccini BM. Nail disorders. In Harper J, Oranje A, Prose N (eds.), *Textbook of Pediatric Dermatology*, Second Edition. Oxford, United Kingdom: Blackwell Scientific Publications; 2006. pp. 1790–1798.

80. Tosti A, Peluso AM, Piraccini BM. Nail diseases in children. *Adv Dermatol.* 1997; 13: 353–373.

81. Fine JD, Eady RA, Bauer EA et al. The classification of inherited epidermolysis bullosa (EB): Report of the Third International Consensus Meeting on Diagnosis and Classification of EB. *J Am Acad Dermatol.* 2008; 58(6): 931–950.

82. Tosti A, de Farias DC, Murrell DF. Nail involvement in epidermolysis bullosa. *Dermatol Clin.* 2010; 28(1): 153–157. Erratum in *Dermatol Clin.* 2010; 28(2): 443.

83. Tosti A, Piraccini BM, Scher RK. Isolated nail dystrophy suggestive of dominant dystrophic epidermolysis bullosa. *Pediatr Dermatol.* 2003; 20(5): 456–457.

84. Dharma B, Moss C, McGrath JA et al. Dominant dystrophic epidermolysis bullosa presenting as familial nail dystrophy. *Clin Exp Dermatol.* 2001; 26(1): 93–96.

85. Mascaro JM, Palou J, Vives P. Painful subungual keratotic tumors in incontinentia pigmenti. *J Am Acad Dermatol.* 1985; 13(5 Pt 2): 913–918.

86. Adeniran A, Townsend PL, Peachey RD. Incontinentia pigmenti (Bloch-Sulzberger syndrome) manifesting as painful periungual and subungual tumours. *J Hand Surg Br.* 1993; 18(5): 667–669.

87. Abimelec P, Rybojad M, Cambiaghi S et al. Late, painful, subungual hyperkeratosis in incontinentia pigmenti. *Pediatr Dermatol.* 1995; 12(4): 340–342.

88. Shah S, Boen M, Kenner-Bell B et al. Pachyonychia congenita in pediatric patients: Natural history, features, and impact. *JAMA Dermatol.* 2014; 150(2): 146–153.

89. Eliason MJ, Leachman SA, Feng BJ et al. A review of the clinical phenotype of 254 patients with genetically confirmed pachyonychia congenita. *J Am Acad Dermatol.* 2012; 67(4): 680–686.

90. Hoting E, Wassilew SW. [Systemic retinoid therapy with etretinate in pachyonychia congenita.] *Hautarzt.* 1985; 36(9): 526–528.

91. Baran R, Haneke E. Matricectomy and nail ablation. *Hand Clin.* 2002; 18(4): 693–696, viii; discussion 697.

92. Nag S, Weinstein M, Greenberg S. 14-year-old boy with painful nail changes. *Pediatr Rev.* 2015; 36(3): e8–e10.

93. Pazzaglia M, Venturi M, Tosti A. Photo-onycholysis caused by an unusual beach game activity: A pediatric case of a side effect caused by doxycycline. *Pediatr Dermatol.* 2014; 31(1): e26–e27.

94. Atiq N, van Meurs T. [A boy with nail abnormalities.] *Ned Tijdschr Geneeskd.* 2013; 157(27): A6429.

17

Pediatric Ingrown Toenails

Robert Baran

Most of the changes of the great toenails are relatively common at birth,[1] and the "redundant tissue around the great toenails is a variation of normal. Any persistence is due to partial ingrowing of the great toenail setting up a chronic inflammatory state."

"Infantile ingrowing toenails presents with several variants. The age distribution shows two peaks: 0–3 years old and 9–13 years old. Ingrown nails develop in different patterns at different ages. In the first 2 years of life, there can be problems with distal ingrowing. Then, the sharp, leading edge of the big toenail embeds into the hypertrophic dorsal aspect of the pulp. This ingrown can be a pattern in the very first months of life, when the nail has never grown over the digital pulp."[2]

Conservative measures are always suggested. Also, they are best combined with educating the family.

It is essential to avoid constricting clothes. The use of an antiseptic shaving soap under occlusion is certainly helpful as well as a cotton wool or steri-strip insert. Finally, appropriate nail care is essential. The multiple anchor-taping method for the ingrowing nail is also a useful method for appropriate nail care (as discussed in Chapter 18).

The etiology of infantile ingrown toenail may have a congenital origin: intrauterine positioning, inherited factors, and normal variations in the development of the great toe. However, acquired factors may also play a role: prone position, constricting garments, unsuitable shoes, and improper nail care.[3]

Distal Embedding with Normally Directed Nail

This infantile type of ingrowing toenail presents a rim of tissue at the distal edge of the nail and some hypertrophy of the lateral nail fold. This prominent ridge of skin at the extremity of the big toe forms an anterior nail wall, which encourages ingrowing and prevents the free margin of the nail from growing normally (Figure 17.1a and b). Owing to the elevation of the hallux pulp, the nail may even pierce through the distal nail groove, producing a painless skin bridge over the nail plate (NP) (Figure 17.2).[4] At 6 months, spontaneous healing occurs despite the necrosis of the hypertrophic tissue above the perforation.[5]

Surgical avulsion or spontaneous nail shedding resulting from tennis toe, for example, may be responsible for the heaping up of the distal subungual tissues that have lost their physiological counterpressure, and the newly formed NP abuts this distal wall.

Whenever feasible, other conservative treatment modalities are indicated for treating early-stage ingrowing nails where erythema and edema are associated with pain or pressure on the distal nail plate. Conservative treatment may start with taping, a very effective long-lasting procedure, but tedious, if more than one nail is involved.

After nail shedding, good preparation is obtained with a preformed plastic artificial nail applied on the whole nail bed and fixed with a micropore that is changed every day (Figure 17.3a and b). It prevents the lifting of the distal tissues.

As an alternative, premixed gel nails are applied to the defective distal plate as a prosthesis extending beyond the heaped-up tissues. This procedure is very helpful if the bulge is not pronounced.

Where the previously mentioned options are ineffective, surgery remains the logical treatment.[1–4,6] The foot is prepared and draped in the usual sterile manner. A crescent wedge-shaped excision is

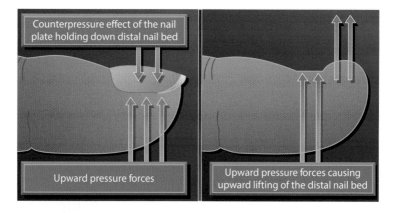

FIGURE 17.1 (Left) Normal toe; (right) toe after nail plate avulsion; formation of the distal heaping up of tissue.

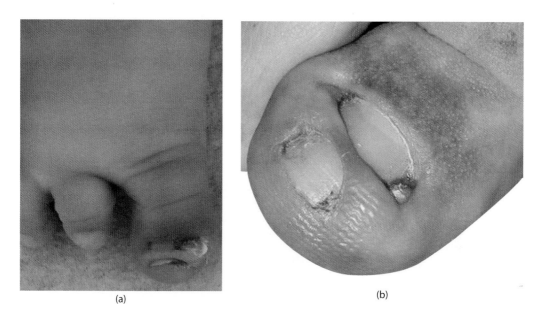

(a)

(b)

FIGURE 17.2 Skin bridge in (a) infancy and (b) adolescence over the nail plate. ([a] Courtesy of Goettman S [b] courtesy of Camacho F.)

carried out all around the distal phalanx (Figure 17.4a through e). The wedge is 4–5 mm at its greatest width and is dissected from the bone. The defect is closed with 5-0 monofilament sutures, removed after 12–14 days.

Congenital Hypertrophic Lip of the Hallux

When hypertrophic lips appear at birth, they are generally bilateral and symmetrical, most often affecting the medial nail fold of the hallux. They present as erythematous lateral pads, firm and tender on pressure. They enlarge progressively, forming a skin bridge, sometimes covering one-third of the NP (Figure 17.5a).[4,5,7–10]

The treatment is conservative because this condition, which resembles the digital fibrous tumor of childhood Rey's fibromatosis, usually disappears spontaneously after 1 or 2 years (Figure 17.5b). Surgery

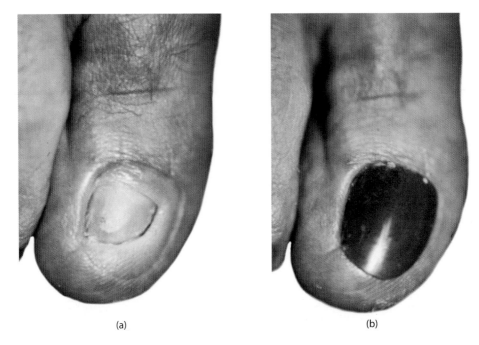

FIGURE 17.3 (a) The nail plate starts to abut the distal tissue. (b) Preformed plastic nail lowers the periungual tissue.

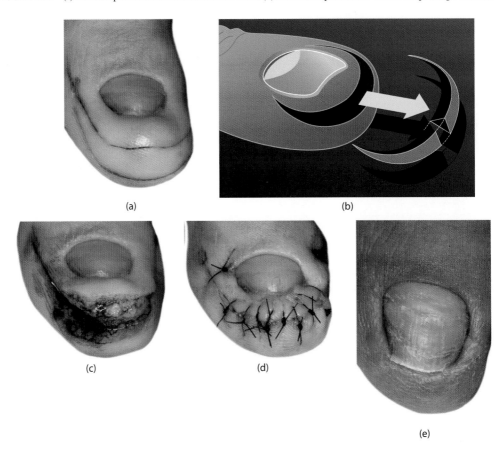

FIGURE 17.4 (a–e) Crescent wedge-shaped excision carried out around the distal phalanx (different stages).

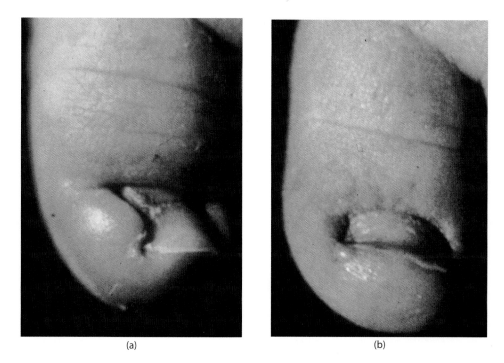

(a)   (b)

FIGURE 17.5   (a) Congenital hypertrophic lip. (b) Spontaneous healing 1 year later. (Courtesy Ceccolini E.)

is restricted to cases in which (1) inflammation is unresponsive to conservative measures, (2) there is a dense condensation of tissue crossing the nail surface, or (3) there is a significant hypertrophy persisting past 1 year of age with no sign of evolution.[11]

The main clinical differential diagnoses include pyogenic granuloma as a consequence of ingrowing toenails, recurring digital fibrous tumor of childhood, which usually spares the great toes, and Koenen's tumor, which is a periungual fibrokeratoma associated with tuberous sclerosis.

Distal Lateral Ingrown Nails

Lateral ingrown nails are most commonly seen in adolescents. They usually occur in the great toes. The nail may be embedded medially, but both sides may also be affected. In an effort to relieve the pain, the offending corner under the inflamed swollen soft tissue can be cut off. The remaining portion will give rise to a nail spicule piercing through the epithelium of the lateral nail groove, which produces secondary infection and excessive granulation tissue.

First Stage

The treatment of the early stage (Figure 17.6a) must be conservative but demands a high degree of compliance. This explains why the recurrence rate found with conservative treatment is high.

Pushing the offending nail edge away from the adjacent soft tissue with a cotton collodion insert[12,13] immediately alleviates pain. Bathing is allowed and the foot is soaked daily in lukewarm water with povidone iodine soap or with potassium permanganate (1/10,000 solution). In fact, it is essential to remove the lateral nail spike acting as a foreign body. Under local anesthesia, a gutter splint[14] may be affixed with formable acrylics or a vinyl intravenous drip infusion tube, 1–2 cm long and 2–3 mm in diameter, the tube split from top to bottom with one end cut diagonally for smooth insertion, and placed around the offending nail edge. However, sufficient nail size and shape for accepting the gutter are needed.

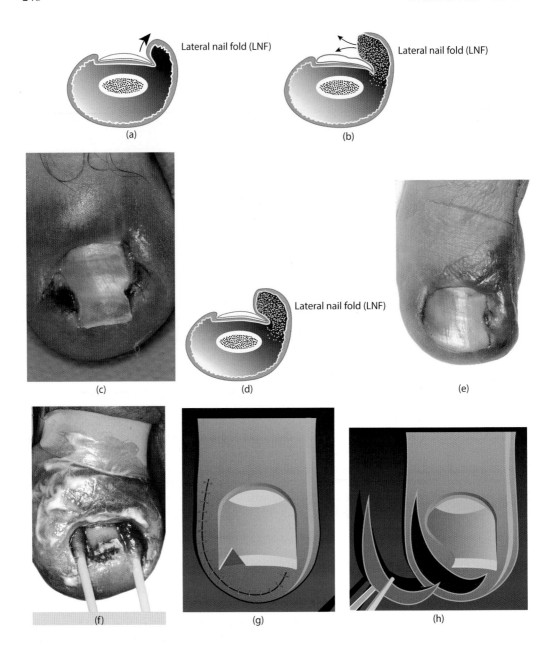

FIGURE 17.6 (a) Schematic slight embedding of the nail. (b) Development of granulation tissue. (c) Clinical presentation of the second stage. (d) Epithelialization of the granulation tissue. (e) Epithelialization of the granulation tissue (third stage). (f) Cauterization of the lateral horns of the matrix with phenol. (g and h) Half fishmouth excision. ([a,b,d] Adapted from Zaias N.)

Good results have been obtained with formable acrylic resin made up of mixing together powder polymer and liquid monomer, which during polymerization is quickly molded for use as a prosthesis and also as a suitable fixation for gutter splints. The requirements are "primer" (with acrylate acid) brushes, a nail platform (i.e., negative film) coarse nail file, and punch plastic cutters. It is easier to use premixed polymer and monomer. The polymerization is carried out under ultraviolet (UV) light.

In squeamish patients, the "taping" method is advised (see Chapter 18). It is a simple and effective method. A strip of adhesive tape is stuck to the lateral wall and gently held with the index fingertip, which also pushes the nail wall away from the nail margin. The tape is pulled obliquely around the toe in a proximal-plantar direction, thus separating the skin of the sulcus from the nail edge. This procedure is easily repeated by the patient on a daily basis and gives quick relief from pain. Again, taping has to be performed till the nail has grown normally. Taping and packing may be combined to enhance the efficacy of this method.

Second Stage

If the treatment is not sufficient, the lateral nail groove may be affected along its entire length, developing excess granulation tissue (Figure 17.6b). The lateral groove becomes filled with "proud flesh" extending beneath the NP, and pus may exude from the nail groove (Figure 17.6c). Systemic antibiotics and 50% trichloracetic acid applied on granulation tissue and repeated at 2-weeks intervals are useful to treat pseudopyogenic granuloma. Intralesional injection of triamcinolone acetonide associated with mupirocine can improve recalcitrant cases.

Third Stage

In this late stage characterized by the epithelialization of the granulation tissue (Figure 17.6d and e), with exceptional transformation into epithelized fibrous tissue and skin bridging (harpoon nail),[15] there are usually two options for a complete cure: chemical cauterization of the lateral horn of the nail matrix, which permanently narrows the nail, and surgically performing half a fishmouth involving the soft tissues.

In the first option, the lateral fifth of the NP is freed with a nail elevator from the proximal nail fold (PNF) and the subungual tissues. It is then cut longitudinally with an English nail splitter or nail-splitting scissors and extracted with a sturdy hemostat.

A better alternative to a surgical approach is when the lateral matrix horn is cauterized with a freshly made solution of liquefied phenol (88% solution). This requires a bloodless field since blood inactivates phenol. Hemostasis is therefore accomplished with a tourniquet, and the blood is carefully cleaned from the space under the PNF using a sterile gauze. The surrounding skin is protected with petroleum jelly. The phenol is rubbed onto the matrix epithelium for 90 seconds with a cotton-tipped small hemostat, three times for 30 seconds each (Figure 17.6f).

Postoperative pain is minimal since phenol has a local anesthetic action and is an antiseptic. The matrix epithelium is sloughed off, and oozing usually occurs for 2–6 weeks. However, the effect of 20% ferric chloride after phenol chemical matricectomy[4] results in a significant reduction in oozing from the operation site. Daily warm foot baths with povidone iodine soap accelerate healing.

Half a fishmouth, the second option, is sometimes preferred for girls, because it does not narrow the NP, but systemic antibiotics (e.g., pristinamycin) may be necessary. An elliptical wedge-shaped tissue excision is carried out from the lateral wall of the toe and limited to its distal lateral portion around the distal phalanx to a distance of about 4 mm from the nail (Figure 17.6g and h). The wedge is 5 mm at its greatest width and is dissected from the bone. The defect is closed with 5-0 monofilament sutures that are removed after 14–21 days.

Pincer Nails

The dystrophic condition called pincer nails is characterized by transverse overcurvature that increases along the longitudinal axis of the nail and reaches its greatest extent at the distal part, leading to trumpet nails.[16,17] The edges constrict the nail bed tissue and dig into the lateral nail grooves. Overcurvature of the nails may affect the great toe or all the digits. This condition may be so painful that even the use of a bedsheet may become unbearable in adulthood. There are several different variants of pincer nails, both hereditary (Figures 17.7a and b) and acquired (Figure 17.7c).

The hereditary pincer nail is almost always symmetrical. Similar nail changes may be seen in other family members. The great toes are usually affected but the smaller toes may also be involved. The great toe

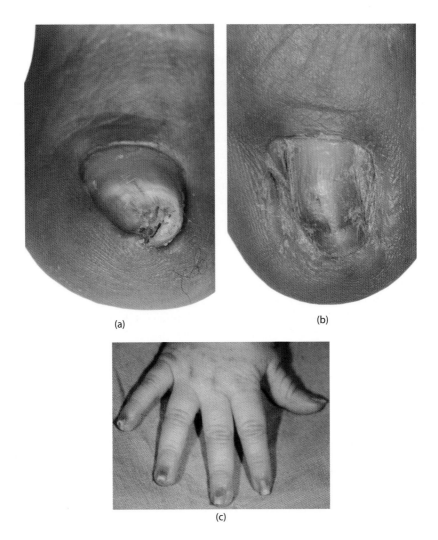

(a)   (b)

(c)

FIGURE 17.7 (a) Hereditary pincer nail in an adolescent. (b) Same patient after phenol cauterization. (c) Acquired pincer nail deformity in Kawasaki disease.

commonly shows a lateral deviation of the long axis of the distal phalanx, but the overcurved nails are deviated even more laterally. When the lesser toes are involved they exhibit a medial deviation. This anomaly may be congenital or observed in adolescents. Of interest, epidermolysis bullosa simplex (Dowling-Meara type) may be associated with pincer nail abnormality, with a slight thickening, in both finger and toenails. Pincer nail deformity has also been reported as a manifestation of Clouston syndrome.

Acquired pincer nails are not symmetrical, though fingernail involvement may be extensive and appears to be fairly symmetrical. Acquired pincer nails may be due to a number of different dermatoses, of which psoriasis is the most frequent. Tumors of the nail apparatus such as exostosis and implantation cyst may lead to pincer nails, a condition reversible after the treatment of cause.

Tinea ungium due to *Trichophyton rubrum*, affecting equally the great toenail and thumb nail, has been shown to be responsible for pincer nails. The nails gradually return to normal after the systemic antifungal treatment.

Acquired pincer nail deformity in infants with Kawasaki disease may affect all digits of the hands (Figure 17.7c) and, to a lesser extent, the toes. Given the absence of pain, the nails were left undisturbed and the overcurvature spontaneously resolved as the nails grew out.

Congenital Malalignment of the Hallux

Congenital malalignment of the big toenail may present with gross nail deformation, greenish-gray discoloration, thickening, and oyster shell-like appearance (Figure 17.8a).[18–20] The deviation is almost always to the lateral side, and the nail usually grows faster on its medial side, adding to the lateral deviation. The obliquely positioned nail usually has sharply downward-bent lateral margins, often digging into the lateral nail fold and distal nail bed (Figure 17.8b). There is no attachment to the nail bed; therefore, counterpressure to the forces acting on the tip of the toe during gait is lacking, allowing the tip and pulp tissue to be dislocated dorsally to form a distal nail wall. The lack of attachment to the nail bed epithelium can readily be shown by placing a blunt-tipped probe under the nail. The ridged skin of the pulp of the toe is constantly dislocated under the free end of the nail obscuring the hyponychium. The thickened NP easily breaks into slightly curved pieces. It is only adherent to the matrix, and repeated trauma from inadequate shearing forces to the matrix is most probably the cause for the oyster shell-like NP growth. The PNF commonly covers just a short portion of the proximal NP, which, however, has lateral matrix horns reaching deep proximally.

About 50% of patients experience spontaneous improvement leading to an almost normal-looking yet still malaligned nail with a good nail bed attachment before the age of 10 years. The existence of a ligamentous structure corresponding to a dorsal expansion of the lateral ligament of the distal interphalangeal joint appears to be connected with the nail matrix. Its physical properties may change with the passage of time, and this therefore explains spontaneous cures.

If the deviation is marked and the nail buried in the soft tissues, the surgical rotation of the misdirected matrix associated with the simple section of the dorsal expansion of the lateral ligament is essential to prevent permanent nail dystrophy (Figure 17.8c).

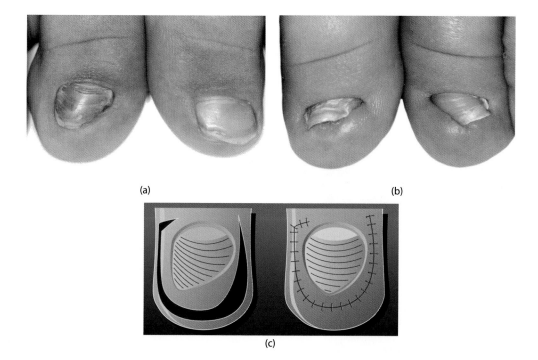

(a)

(b)

(c)

FIGURE 17.8 (a) Oystershell-like appearance of misdirected nail. (b) Bilateral nail malalignment. (c) Surgical rotation of the misdirected subungual tissues (matrix and nail bed).

Retronychia or Proximal Embedding

The discovery of this condition is very recent. It involves a big toe but the involvement of fingernails has been reported. There is a thickening of the proximal portion of the yellowish NP and painful paronychia (Figure 17.9a).

Instead of embedding of the NP into the distal or lateral periungual skin, retronychia involves embedding of the nail into the proximal nail groove following an acute insult of fingers or toes.[21–27] Retronychia produces a characteristic triad: disruption of the linear nail growth, subacute paronychia with lifting at the rear of the nail due to a double- or triple-layered proximal plate (Figure 17.9b), and frequent xanthonychia; often a longitudinal overcurvature is also produced. In addition, proximal granulation tissue, inflammatory subungual exudate, and onycholysis are very often observed and play an important role in the maintenance of retronychia.[28]

The transitory growth arrest produces a Beau's line. If this arrest lasts 4–6 weeks, the NP separates from the subungual tissue, leading to latent onychomadesis with secondary nail shedding. But after a trauma, a complete onychomadesis may not develop as the NP is still held in the lateral wings of the nail matrix. This is due to the curvature of those areas. With the growth of a new NP, the old one is pushed upward and backward, leading to embedding of the top nail into the ventral aspect of the PNF, leading consequently to secondary paronychia.

In early cases, a conservative treatment with an adhesive technique is a valid option.

If the clinical diagnosis is doubtful, an ultrasound shows the pathognomonic sign: the shortening of the distance between the proximal edge NP and the distal interphalangeal joint.[26,27]

The surgical treatment consists of avulsing the nail that may show many generations of superimposed layers of nail keratin when viewed proximally.

Grasp Reflex Multiple Ingrowing Fingernails

There is a new clinical entity of ingrowing fingernails of infants being associated with the grasp reflex, inducing paronychia (Figure 17.10).[29] Twenty-six cases were published and the median age was 1 month (age range: 6 days to 4 months). Since "ossification of the distal phalanx has not developed in infants, the NP can easily penetrate into the surrounding soft tissue under pressure." Because the grasp reflex causes

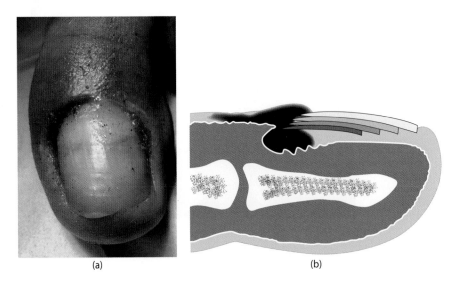

(a)   (b)

FIGURE 17.9   (a) Typical presentation of retronychia. (b) The pathophysiological process. (Courtesy of Richert B.)

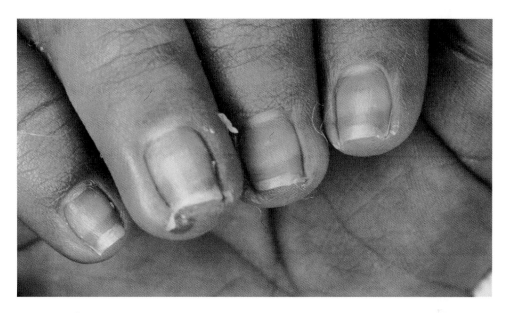

FIGURE 17.10 Clinical presentation of grasp reflex of ingrowing fingernails. (Courtesy of Matsui T et al.)

pressure on the fingernails, due to a foreign-body reaction to the buried nail, the soft tissue swells and encourages the condition of ingrowing nails.

A grasp reflex may be elicited by the stimulation of the palm of the hand by firm pressure to produce flexion of the fingers. It usually disappears by about 3 months of age.

Although in severe cases, the administration of antibiotics or drainage was needed to treat abscess formation around the NP, the mild cases have a good prognosis with the advice to reduce stresses on the fingernails.

Differential diagnosis includes paronychia induced by finger sucking.

REFERENCES

1. Honig PJ, Spitzer A, Berstein R et al. Congenital ingrown toenails: Clinical significance. *Clin Pediatr.* 1982; 21: 424–426.
2. De Berker DAR. Childhood nail diseases. *Dermatol Clin.* 2006; 24: 355–363.
3. Hendricks WM. Congenital ingrown toenails. *Cutis.* 1979; 24: 393–394.
4. Mazuecos J, Peres-Bernal A, Camacho FM. Skin bridge on a nail plate caused by distal onychocryptosis. *Eur J Dermatol.* 2015; 25: 185–186.
5. Kraft B, Marsch WC, Wohlnab J. Kongenitale und post partale Ungues incarnate. *Hautarzt.* 2003; 54: 1083–1086.
6. Bentley-Phillips B, Coll I. Ingrowing toenails in infancy. *Int J Dermatol.* 1983; 22: 115–116.
7. Rufli Th, von Schulthess A, Itin P. Congenital hypertrophy of the lateral nail folds of the hallux. *Dermatology.* 1992; 184: 296–297.
8. Hammerton MD, Shrank AB. Congenital hypertrophy of the lateral nail folds of the hallux. *Pediatr Dermatol.* 1988; 5: 243–245.
9. Ceccolini E, Neri I, Balducci A et al. Cilindretto latero-ungueale del primo dito del piede del neonata. *G Ita Dermatol Venereol.* 1988; 123: 551–552.
10. Piraccini BM, Parente GL, Varotti E et al. Congenital hypertrophy of the lateral nail folds of the hallux: Clinical features and follow-up of seven cases. *Pediatr Dermatol.* 2000; 17: 348–351.
11. Exton R, Smith G. Surgical intervention for congenital nail fold hypertrophy. *J Foot Ankle Surg.* 2012; 51: 69–70.
12. Ilfeld FW. Ingrown toenail treated with cotton collodion insert. *Foot Ankle.* 1991; 11: 312–313.

13. Gutierrez-Mendoza D, De Anda Juarez M, Fonte Avalos et al. "Cotton nail cast": A simple solution for mild and painful lateral and distal embedding. *Dermatol Surg.* 2015; 41: 411–414.

14. Taheri A, Mansoori P, Alinia H et al. A conservative method to gutter splint ingrowing toenails. *JAMA Dermatol.* 2014; 150: 1359–1360.

15. Richert B, Caucanas M, Di Chiacchio N. Surgical approach to harpoon nail: A new variant of ingrowing toenail. *Dermatol Surg.* 2014; 40: 700–701.

16. Baran R, Haneke E, Richert B. Pincer nails. Definition and surgical treatment. *Dermatol Surg.* 2001; 27: 261–266.

17. Haneke E. Ingrown and pincer nails: Evaluation and treatment. *Dermatol Ther.* 2002; 15: 148–158.

18. Baran R, Bureau H. Congenital malalignment of the big toenail as a cause of ingrowing toenail in infancy. Pathology and treatment (a study of thirty cases). *Clin Exp Dermatol.* 1983; 8: 619–623.

19. Guéro S, Guichard S, Freitag SR. Ligamentary structure of the base of the nail. *Surg Radiol Anat.* 1994; 16: 47–52.

20. Baran R, Haneke E. Etiology and treatment of nail malalignment. *Dermatol Surg.* 1998; 24: 719–721.

21. De Berker DAR, Rendall JR. Retronychia—Proximal ingrowing nail. *J Eur Acad Dermatol Venereol.* 1999; 12: S126.

22. De Berker DAR, Richert B, Duhard E et al. Retronychia: Proximal ingrowing of the nail plate. *J Am Acad Dermatol.* 2008; 58: 978–983.

23. Piraccini BM, Richert B, de Berker DAR et al. Retronychia in children, adolescents and young adults: A case series. *J Am Acad Dermatol.* 2014; 70: 388–390.

24. Dahdah MJ, Kibbi AG, Ghosn S. Retronychia: Report of 2 cases. *J Am Acad Dermatol.* 2008; 58: 1051–1053.

25. Richert B, Caucanas M, André J. La Rétronychie. *Ann Dermatol Vénéréol.* 2014; 141: 799–804.

26. Ventura F, Correia O, Duarte AF et al. Retronychia—Clinical and pathophysiological aspects. *J Eur Acad Dermatol Venereol.* 2016; 30: 16–19.

27. Wortsman X, Wortsman J, Guerrero R et al. Anatomical changes in retronychia and onychomadesis detected using ultrasound. *Dermatol Surg.* 2010; 36: 1–6.

28. Wortsman X, Calderon P Baran R. Finger retronychias detected early by 3D ultrasound examination. *J Eur Acad Dermatol Venereol.* 2012; 2: 254–256.

29. Matsui T, Kidou M, Ono T. Infantile multiple ingrowing nails of the fingers induced by the grasp reflex—A new entity. *Dermatology.* 2002; 205: 25–27.

18

Noninvasive Treatment for Ingrown Nails: Anchor Taping, Acrylic Affixed Gutter Splint, Sculptured Nail, and Others

Hiroko Arai and Eckart Haneke

Introduction

Ingrown nail is a common disorder in children and adults. The treatment of choice for ingrown nail has long been surgical due to the misunderstanding of its pathophysiology. Currently, discussion regarding the controversies of invasive vs. noninvasive treatment is a hot topic in pediatric ingrown nails.[1] Now is the time to uncover and reconsider some of these issues.

Definition

Ingrown nail is defined as a nail plate digging into the periungual soft tissue, which is the lateral nail folds, the proximal nail fold, the nail bed, or distal nail fold.

Frequency

Ingrown nails are one of the most frequent nail disorders of children and young adults, severely interfering with daily activities and sports.

Age and Gender

Ingrown nails are observed at any age, from neonates to very old age. There is a slight to marked male predominance in the most common, adolescent type of lateral ingrowing. To the contrary, retronychia is, at least in our experience, slightly more frequent in girls and young women.[1]

Etiology and Pathomechanism

The etiology of ingrown nail is multifactorial, with the primary cause being improper nail cutting by patients, caregivers, and even doctors (Figures 18.1 and 18.2),[2,3] small nail trauma, and nail breakages (picking or biting). Cutting the nail too short, diagonally, round, or pointed can leave behind hidden spicules or offending lateral nail edges and partial nail loss. These irregular nail edges pierce the epidermis of the surrounding soft tissue causing pain, inflammation, and granulation tissue due to a chronic foreign-body reaction elicited by the nail digging into the dermis. Ill-fitting footwear compressing the distal nail bed with its too-short nail further compounds the problem.

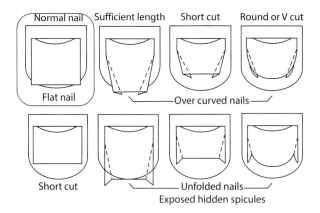

FIGURE 18.1   Improper nail cutting. (From Arai H et al., *Rinsho Hifuka*, 57, 110–119, 2003. With permission; Arai H et al., *Int J Dermatol*, 43, 759–765, 2004. With permission.)

1. Improper nail cutting
   by patients, parents, caregivers, doctors

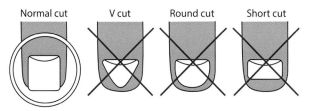

2. Nail breakage/trauma

3. Ill-fitting footwear

4. Sports, walking, foot deformity, disability, etc.

FIGURE 18.2   Causes of ingrown nails. (From Arai H et al., *Rinsho Hifuka*, 57, 110–119, 2003. With permission; Arai H et al., *Int J Dermatol*, 43, 759–765, 2004. With permission.)

In response to the upward pressure forces from the ground (when walking), a normal-sized nail plate creates a counterpressure effect and protects and holds all underlying tissues. However, these upward pressure forces from the ground on partial or entire nail loss caused by improper nail cutting, nail trauma, or nail avulsion gives rise to the development of a distal nail fold and distal–lateral bulging as there is no pulp support, often with resulting bone changes such as the development of a distal dorsal exophytic growth or—in the very young—an upward deformation of the distal phalanx (Figure 18.3). Hypertrophy and hyperkeratosis of the nail folds may occur. Hypertrophic distal bulging disturbs nail regrowth, leading to ingrown nails and onychogryphosis[4–6] (Figure 18.3). All these events are results of the vicious cycle of ingrown nails.

The secondary cause of ingrown nail is improper footwear, which can occur with shoes that have inadequate toe-box room (too small or big) and socks that apply external pressure at the sides, top, or front.

Other factors include overcurved or pincer nails, hallux valgus, and other foot deformations, inward rotation of the big toe, gait abnormalities, age-associated changes, lack of walking and exercise, obesity, systemic illness, hyperhidrosis, diabetes, onychomycosis, drug side effects, neoplastic conditions of the nail apparatus, and participation in sports activities.[1–3,7–13]

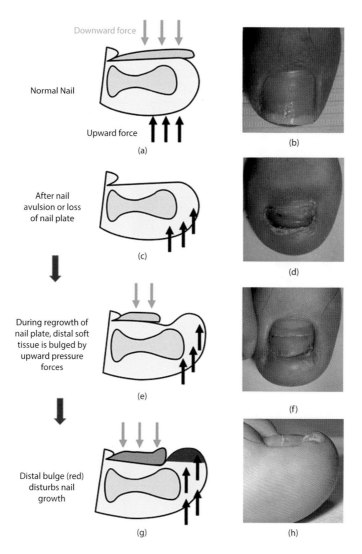

FIGURE 18.3 Mechanism of distal bulge formation: ingrowing nail/onychogryphosis[6]: (a and b) Normal nail; (c) after nail avulsion or loss of nail plate; (d) nail loss after trauma; (e) during regrowth of nail plate, distal soft tissue is bulged by upward forces; (f) distal nail embedding; (g) distal bulger (red) disturbs nail growth; (h) distal bulging.

Clinical Features of Ingrown Nail in Children

Ingrown nails occur at every age (Figure 18.4), even in babies and infants who are yet to walk or wear shoes. They are a significant problem in pediatric patients and, in particular, adolescents and youth (school children and young adults, ages 6–18).[9] Severe cases are very frequent among adolescents (ages 12–15) who are physically active (Figures 18.5 and 18.6). Among our study population, although ingrown nails were seen in all age groups, over one-third (35.3%) were found in youth and young adults (ages 10–29), presumably because they are more active[2,3,9] (Figure 18.4).

Characteristics of ingrown nails in children depend on age (Figure 18.6), nail plate thickness (thin, easily breakable, and rapidly growing), body weight, and level of physical activity. Newborns and infants tend to go barefoot, have thin nail plates, light body weight, and low physical and walking activity. Toddlers begin to wear shoes and have increased physical activity. Young adults have higher physical activity levels, such as sports, dancing, and afterschool activities.

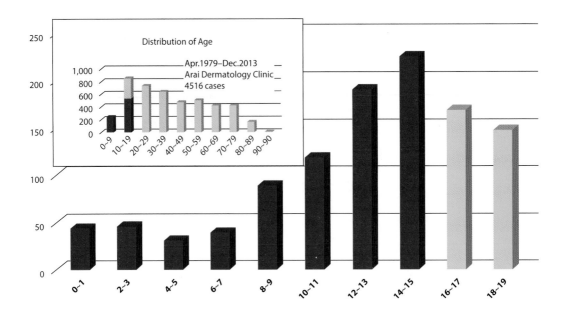

FIGURE 18.4 Ingrown nails in children: distribution of age. (786 cases, age 0–15, 318 cases, age 16–19; Inset: distribution of age in 4516 cases, from two months to 94 years, 1979–2013, Arai Dermatology Clinic.)

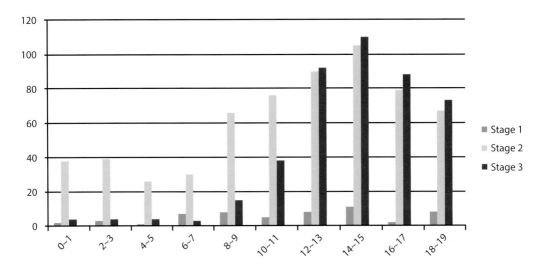

FIGURE 18.5 Breakdown by age group and stage in children and young adults. (786 cases, age 0–15, 318 cases, age 16–19, 1979–2013, Arai Dermatology Clinic.)

Signs of ingrown nail include redness, swelling, pus discharge, granulation tissue formation, hypertrophy of the nail folds, and swollen toes and fingers.

The pathologic stages of ingrown nails are classified as follows[14]: the first or early inflammatory stage is characterized by erythema, slight edema, and pain upon pressure; the second by pus discharge; and the third by granulation tissue formation with chronic inflammation, hypertrophy, and/or induration of the nail fold (Figure 18.6).

Ingrown nails mainly occur at distal–lateral or lateral nail folds,[1–3] but may involve each nail fold: distal nail fold (distal nail embedding, distal or anterior ingrown nail) and proximal nail fold (retronychia[15] or posterior ingrown nail).

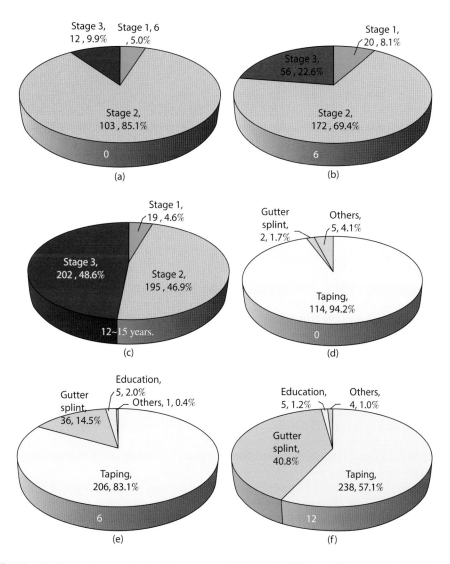

FIGURE 18.6 Distribution by stage (a–c) and treatment modalities (d–f) (786 cases, 1979–2013): (a, d) 0–5 years; (b, e) 6–11 years; (c, f) 12–15 years.

In children, ingrown nails occur mainly on the lateral nail folds of the toes (92.6% or 728/786), mostly on big toes (91.0%). Most incidents are confirmed on the distal–lateral nail fold (96.2%), followed by distal nail folds (2.1%) and retronychia (1.8%). Some occur on fingers (7.4% or 58/786) or lesser on toenails (9.0%).

Symptoms include tenderness, limited movement, discomfort, or worsening of pain from tight footwear and sensitivity to pressure of any kind, even the weight of bed sheets or comforters. Children may hide their ingrown nail from their parents, even though the condition can cause significant pain. Parents should carefully observe their children's actions to detect ingrown nail problems.

Natural Course

If left untreated, most ingrown toenails worsen with time and the overgrowth of the inflamed nail folds, including distally, may occur. Constant pain, granulation tissue, and oozing are the main features.

Treatment

The treatment principle of ingrown nails is to eliminate the cause of ingrown nails, protect the nail fold, and help normal nail regrowth. Since it is the nail plate that grows into the nail fold, the latter has to be protected against the former by pulling it away (taping), by inserting a buffer between them (packing and gutter), or by combining these methods. They offer quick reduction of pain, inflammation and granulation tissue, and nail fold protection with promising results. Anchor taping and acrylic affixed gutter splint are effective on their own or in combination.[2,3,7–13]

Treatment selection depends on the condition and should be tailored to the individual's condition. Foot care with soaking, proper nail trimming and footwear, antibiotics, and steroids can be considered in combination. Preventive education should be conducted as part of the treatment. Furthermore, these methods are also effective for paronychia and ingrown nails that have undergone chemotherapy or biologics. Almost all ingrown nails can be treated noninvasively using these methods.

Anchor Taping

Anchor taping is highly effective, child and patient friendly, and inexpensive. The basic taping method for an ingrown nail was already described by Nishioka.[16] Taping was improved into anchor taping in 2002,[8] using additional multiple layers of tapes for foundation (stay cloth) and fixation.[2,3,8–13]

Anchor taping separates the nail fold from the nail edge, reducing pain, inflammation, and granulation tissue. It is even useful for oozing lesions such as a pus-discharging infection or granulation tissue with slippery surface.[2,3,8–13] The mechanisms of anchor taping are the overlapping tapes that offer increased dynamics of taping in terms of traction, pressure (push), protection and fixation, and also prevent shifting, slipping, and peeling off of main tapings, while providing increased adequate support.[2,3,8–13]

Medical elastic gauze tapes such as Elastopore®, and those from Germany or the United States, are preferred, although any tape is suitable for primary care. Tape sizes are approximately 20 mm × 80 mm, or 20 mm × 60 mm for the main tape, and 10–20 mm × 30–60 mm for the foundation tape, but can be varied. Fixation tapes (6–12 mm × 30–40 mm surgical paper tapes such as 3M Micropore® or Nichiban Skinagate®) are used as anchor tapes to attach the tapes and skin.

Anchor taping is the first choice treatment for all types of ingrown nail, particularly finger nails, lesser toenails, and especially for children with ingrown nails. Based on experience, taping should be continued for approximately 6 months after the site is cured, during athletic activities, and when walking long distances.

Patients and caregivers are instructed how to apply taping themselves. Duration depends on the condition of ingrowing nail and length of nail loss. Taping is applied all day in case of inflamed stages especially with granulation tissue, but only during daytime hours in cases without inflammation. Tapes with a low incidence of contact dermatitis are chosen.

Applying the Anchor-Taping Method

Fixation Anchor-Taping Method (Arai's Method)

Basic anchor taping is indicated for mild ingrown nail cases.[2,3,8–13] It consists of placing the tape edge slightly onto the nail plate at the affected distal–lateral or lateral nail fold where the offending nail edges are supposed to be present (Figure 18.7). The tapes are placed slightly overlapping the nail edge, so that when the tape is pulled, it comes right against the edge of the nail or underneath the nail plate. The tape is wound around the toe or finger diagonally toward the ventral side, thereby pulling the nail fold away from the offending nail edges while fixing the other tape end on the dorsal toe or finger side. Surgical paper fixation tapes are used as anchor tapes and applied by attaching them onto the previously applied tape, by the nail edge as well as the adjacent skin. The fixation tape is pulled in a manner that separates the nail from the nail fold. When taping, tourniquet effects and binding over two joints are avoided to prevent the impairment of blood supply and movement (Figure 18.7).

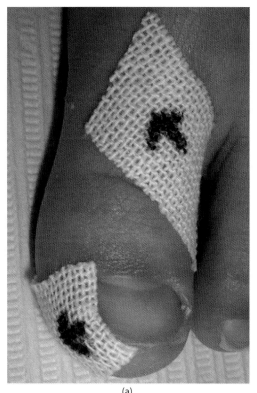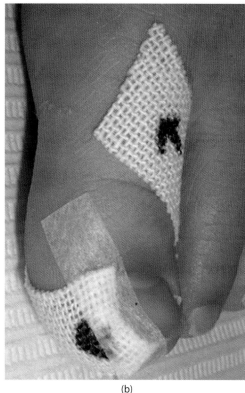

(a)   (b)

FIGURE 18.7   (a) Taping; (b) basic fixation anchor taping (male, 3 years).

Foundation Anchor-Taping Method—Multiple Anchor Taping for Lateral Ingrown Nail (Arai's Method)

Multiple anchor tapings using two or three pieces of main tape and paper fixation tape are recommended mainly for lateral and distal–lateral ingrown nail in any type and its prevention (Figure 18.8).[2,3,8–13] It is especially effective in cases with oozing granulation tissue and swollen and hypertrophic nail folds.[2,3,8–13] It is done by first applying the anchor tape (10–20 mm × 20–50 mm) as a foundation, parallel to and around the affected nail fold (lateral, distal, or proximal), including the granulation tissue and even the hidden portions of the nail edge. The foundation tape for granulation tissue is wider and much longer than the granulation tissue, covering the entire affected area.

Next, the usual anchor taping mentioned above is followed in a perpendicular manner on top of the first anchored tape. When the tape is placed at the right angle, a portion is held down to prevent moving, and slowly and gently one end of the tape is pulled and wound around the toe or finger. The tape placed directly on the granulation tissue/hidden portion is tucked or adhered inward as much as possible, covering the granulation. Two or three pieces of surgical paper tape are used to secure the tape and skin in place.

Multiple Anchor Taping for Distal Nail Embedding and Retronychia and Their Prevention (Arai's Method)

Two or three pieces of main tapes are used and have the size of 20–15 mm and 50–60 mm.[2,3,8–13] First, the tape end is attached at the distal nail fold or nail bed with vertical nail loss and is pulled distally toward the ventral side. Then the basic anchor taping is applied at the lateral or distal–lateral nail fold, diagonally, as mentioned above. Furthermore, the surgical tape is applied by the same method for increased fixation (Figure 18.9). The foundation tape technique[2,3,8–13] (Figure 18.10) is applied to maximize the

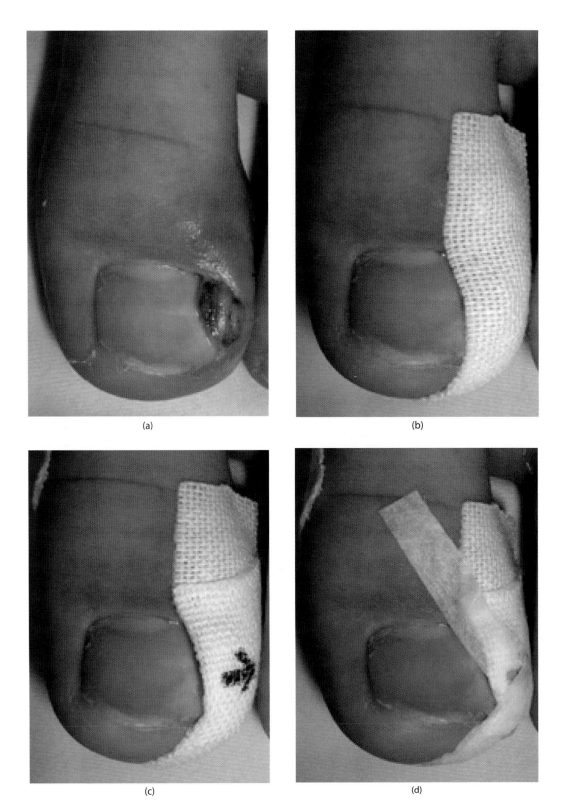

(a) (b)

(c) (d)

FIGURE 18.8 Multiple anchor taping for lateral ingrown nail (Arai's method): (a) before treatment; (b) foundation anchor tape applied; (c) additional basic taping; (d) tape fixation (male, 14 years).

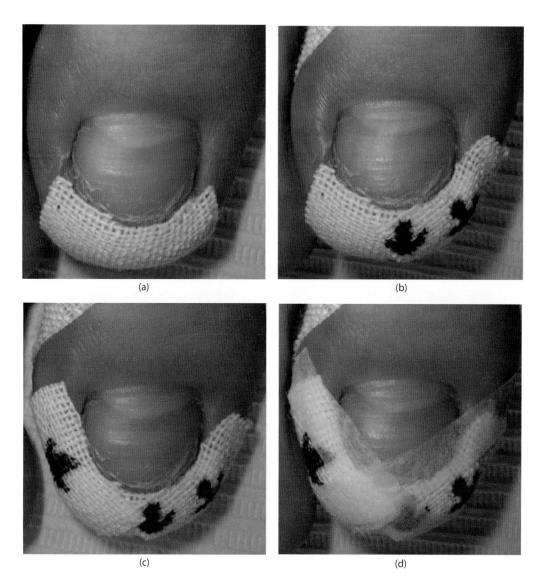

(a)   (b)

(c)   (d)

FIGURE 18.9 Multiple anchor taping for distal nail embedding (three pieces of main tape): (a) vertical taping; (b) diagonal taping; (c) further diagonal taping; (d) tape fixation (male, 19 years).

effect. The number of tapes may vary depending on the condition. For retronychia as posterior ingrown nail, two or three pieces of tapes are applied at the proximal and proximal-lateral nail folds (Figure 18.11). The tape is pulled proximally. If necessary, the proximal nail edge, matrix horn, and other foreign objects are removed. The nail plate is often preserved using anchor taping.

Multiple anchor taping for distal ingrown nail offers stronger pulp support especially for distal nail embedding (anterior ingrown nail), partial/entire nail loss or nail avulsion, extremely short-cut nail, partial nail removal of onychomycosis-affected part, and disappearing nail bed, while preventing distal bulging.

Window-Taping Method: Improved by Arai

The Onagawa method, where a slit is made on a tape, was described in 2011.[17] It has since been improved by Arai as a window-taping method to accommodate the patient's comfort and effectiveness and is done by making a circular hole in the tape as opposed to cutting the tapes apart (Figure 18.12). The size and direction of the medical elastic gauze tape as well as the size and shape of the hole are tailored to the patient's needs. The basic tape size is around 40 mm long, 30 mm wide. An approximately 10–15 mm

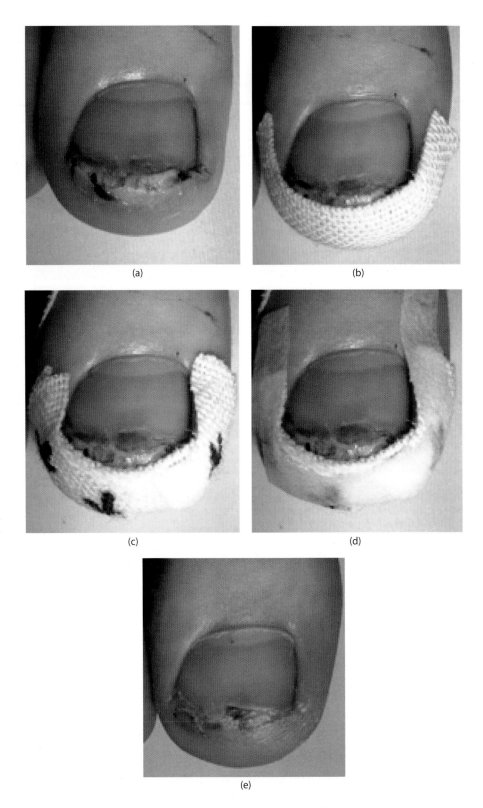

(a)

(b)

(c)

(d)

(e)

FIGURE 18.10 Foundation anchor tape technique for distal nail embedding (four pieces of main tape): (a) before treatment; (b) anchor tape applied; (c) additional taping; (d) tape fixation; (e) after 1 week (female, 15 years).

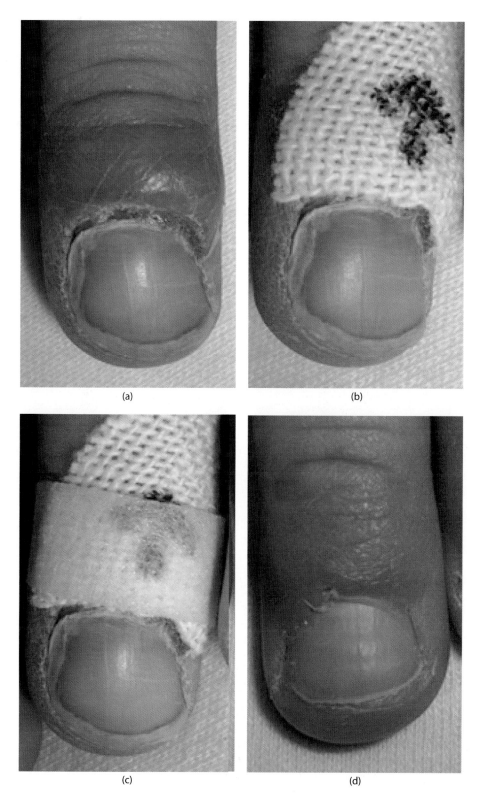

FIGURE 18.11 Anchor taping for retronychia: (a) before treatment; (b) anchor tape applied and pulled proximally; (c) paper tape fixation; (d) after 9 months (female, 4 years).

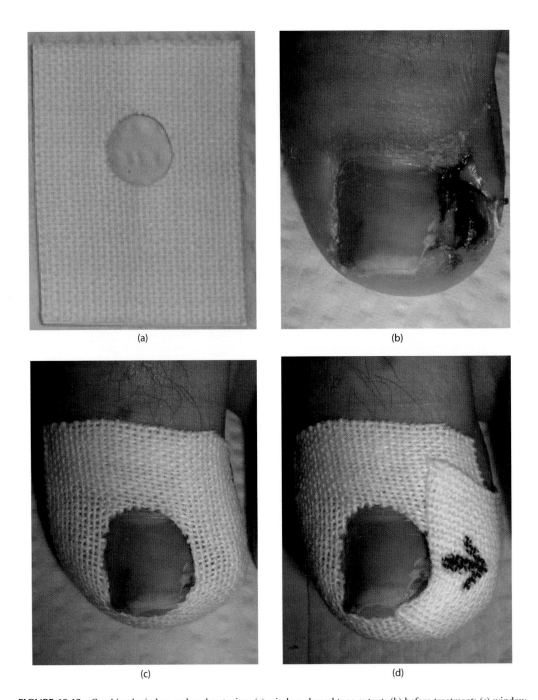

FIGURE 18.12 Combined window and anchor taping: (a) window-shaped tape cutout; (b) before treatment; (c) window taping as a foundation tape; (d) additional anchor taping on top of the window taping (female 13 years).

diameter circle is cut out, 10 mm down from the top, with 10 mm on each side (Figure 18.12). The edge of the window is attached on top of the nail plate, slightly overlapping over the nail, and for distal–lateral ingrown nail, it is hooked under the nail edge and pulled toward proximal as well as laterally. For retronychia, it is pulled with a focus on the proximal edge and perpendicularly toward proximal. For distal nail embedding, nail loss, or disappearing nail bed, the longer end of the tape is placed on the ventral side of the digit, and the edge is pulled distally. The window-taping method is helpful for elevating the buried distal nail edges, especially in the case combined with pincer nail. This window tape is an effective foundation tape in the anchor-taping method (Figure 18.12).

Treatments with Formable Acrylics

In the treatment of ingrown nail and nail trauma, formable acrylics are very helpful materials for acrylic affixed gutter splints[2,3,7–13] and sculptured nails.[2,3,7–13] Acrylic artificial sculptured nails are created by mixing acrylic liquid and powder, essentially the same ingredients used in dentures and readily purchased at outlets such as nail salons and drug stores. The odorless type is strongly recommended (O.P.I. Clarite®). This formable acrylic resin is easily molded into any shape of the artificial nail in replacing nail loss and they strongly glue the round gutter to flat nails. Possible adverse effects of formable acrylic resin are allergic contact dermatitis, eye and respiratory allergy from the meta-acrylate monomer liquid.[18,19] Therapists can avoid this allergy with appropriate caution of use. Prerequisite is absence of fungal infection.

Materials required for preparing acrylic nails are brushes, acrylic powder, acrylic solution, primer, a piece of nail platform for sculptured nail (a piece of negative film may be used), and a coarse nail file.

Acrylic Affixed Gutter-Splint Method

Gutter treatment was described by Wallace (Figure 18.13).[20] It is attached by suture[20,21] and later improved into acrylic affixed gutter splint using formable acrylics as adhesive material.[2,3,7–13] Its mechanism is nail fold protection by round gutter tubes covering the nail edges and supporting normal nail regrowth. It helps to immediately reduce pain, inflammation, granulation tissue, and hypertrophic nail fold. The tube compressed the granulation inhibiting blood flow, decreasing the granulation and inflammation. While gutter tubes can be affixed with suture or surgical paper tapes or acrylic glue, formable acrylic is the best adhesive material[2,3,7–13] in terms of taking away pain and affixing the gutter to the nail (Figures 18.15 and 18.16).

Prerequisites for gutter splints are sufficient nail size and shape to accept the gutter. In this case, taping and other treatments are applied first for 1–2 weeks.

Preparation

The gutter splint is made of a sterilized plastic tube, such as a vinyl intravenous drip infusion tube, 1.5–2.5 cm long and 2.0–3.0 mm in diameter, slit from top to bottom with one end cut diagonally for smooth insertion (Figure 18.13). The nail plate surface is cleaned using 70% alcohol. The patient is

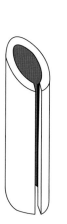
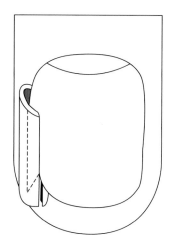

FIGURE 18.13 Gutter treatment; the offending spicule or nail edge is included in the gutter. (From Arai H et al., *Jpn J Clin Dermatol*, 71: 31–35, 2002.)

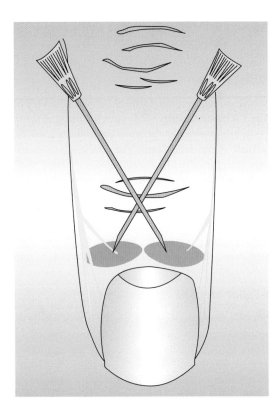

FIGURE 18.14   Distal wing block anesthetizes the three branches of the palmar proper digital nerve. (From Haneke E, *Dermatol Clin*, 24, 291–296, 2006. With permission.)

under anesthesia, e.g., distal wing block[22] (Figure 18.14) and or local anesthesia, using 2% mepiva-caine or 2% lidocaine buffered with sodium bicarbonate (7:3) to diminish injection pain by acidity control.[23]

Method

The offending nail edge is elevated and separated from the nail bed using mosquito forceps. The nail plate is splint along the lateral nail margin with the prepared plastic gutter tube (Figures 18.15 and 18.16).

When the inserted tube is open, the offending nail edge should be visible in the tube. It is very important to preserve the spicule of the ingrowing nail in order to provide a supportive platform for the gutter and nail plate.

The acrylic bonding agent (primer) is applied onto the nail and plastic tube with a brush. Formable acrylics are mixed by first dipping the tip of the brush into acrylic liquid followed with a light touch of acrylic powder, creating an acrylic ball on the tip. This acrylic ball is applied to the inside upper portion of the tube and the tube is closed. Next, the acrylics are applied to the outside of the tube to seal the tube onto the nail plate. A spatula is used to shape the acrylic so that it does not overhang. Polymerization is for 10 minutes. The affixed tube is then trimmed with pinch cutters for plastics.

Most patients experience pain relief within 24 hours. Granulation tissue usually disappears in a few weeks and sometimes as early as several days. Combined anchor taping helps to accelerate granulation tissue reduction. Intralesional corticosteroid injection, curettage, electrodesiccation, and excision are also available. The gutter is left in place until the disappearance of granulation tissue or sufficient nail growth is achieved (2 weeks–3 months). If the gutter is dislodged, it is easily slipped back on, often without the need for anesthesia. Cyanoacrylate medical or nail bond is helpful in improving fixation in such cases. However, if the granulation tissue disappears, anchor taping or sculptured nail is applied instead

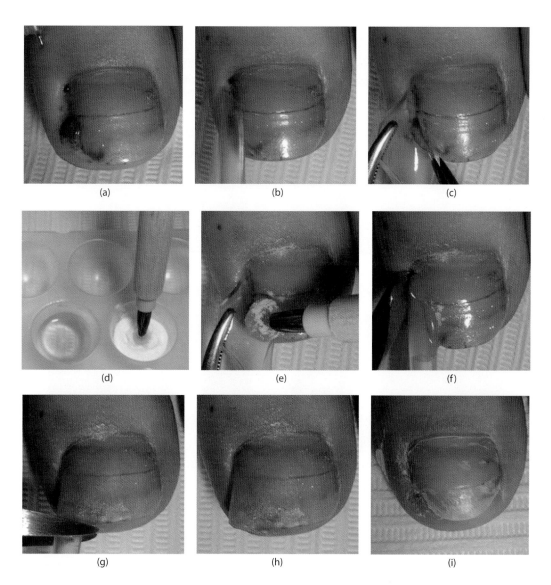

FIGURE 18.15 Acrylic fixed gutter splint: (a) wing block; (b) gutter tube inserted; (c) gutter tube opened up; (d) acrylic ball formation; (e) formable acrylic applied; (f) gutter tube closed; (g, h) polymerization and gutter tube trimmed by pinch cutter; (i) after 2 weeks (female, 14 years).

(Figure 18.17). Daytime taping is applied for continued protection of the fragile nail fold. Taping prevents recurrence and leads to a complete cure.

When the gutter is used, patients have little or no discomfort and return to most of their daily activities. Perioperative antibiotic prophylaxis is prescribed if needed.

Sculptured Nail[2,3,6–13]

The sculptured nail method for the treatment of ingrown nail was introduced by Higashi.[6] The indication for sculptured acrylic nails is an ingrown nail with nail plate loss, acting as a prosthetic nail for the defective part. A sculptured nail is easily made and indicated for small or no granulation tissue after gutter splint and/or taping (Figure 18.17). When granulation tissue is present, nail loss is important and the gutter method alone is not feasible, the sculptured-nail method is used together with the gutter-splint method

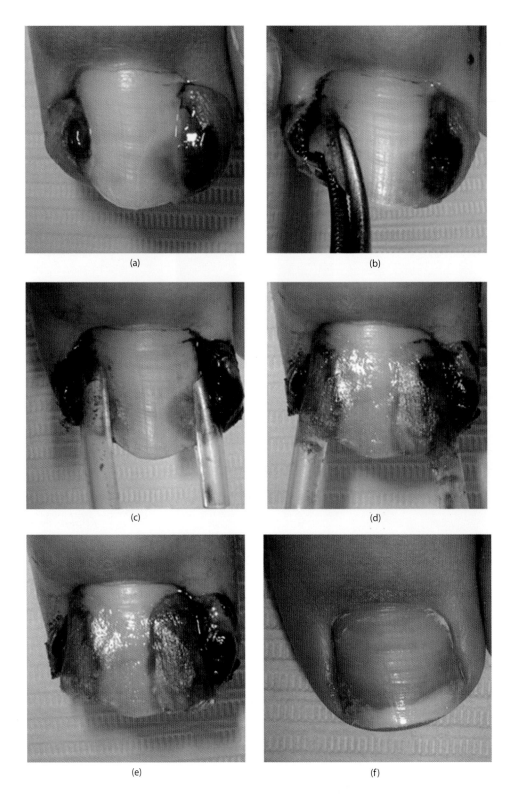

FIGURE 18.16   Acrylic affixed gutter splint: (a) before treatment, (b) spicule lifting, (c) plastic gutter insertion, (d) acrylics application, (e) polymerization /trimming, (f) after 5 months. sculptured nail, (female, 13 years) (From Arai H et al., *Int J Dermatol*, 43, 759–765, 2004. With permission.)

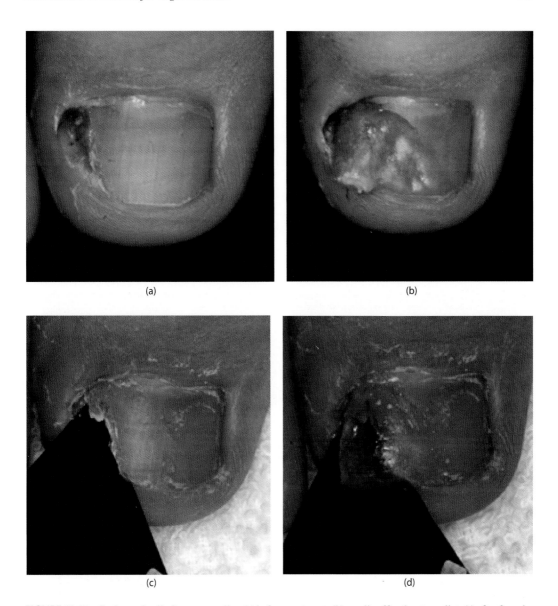

FIGURE 18.17 Sculptured nail after gutter splint: (a) before treatment; (b) acrylic affixed gutter splint; (c) after 2 weeks, plastic film insertion; (d) sculptured nail application (male, 11 years).

(Figure 18.18). Anchor taping can be used to supplement this method to move the granulation tissue to insert the splint and to expedite the healing of the granulation tissue. The treatment mimics normal nail functions, where patients achieve faster recovery with better quality of life (QOL).

A piece of plastic film or nail platform is placed under the nail and fixed with adhesive tape. After cleaning the nail plate surface with 70% alcohol, a primer is applied. Formable acrylic balls are made by mixing acrylics (as described above). The formable acrylic is then placed on the nail and platform, where it is molded into a nail shape to cover a portion or the entire nail area surface. After complete polymerization, the artificial nail is shaped with a nail file. The treatment duration depends on the time required for the normal nail to grow over the tip of the toe (2–12 weeks). Sculptured nails and gutter splint are removed, if required, by soaking in acetone.

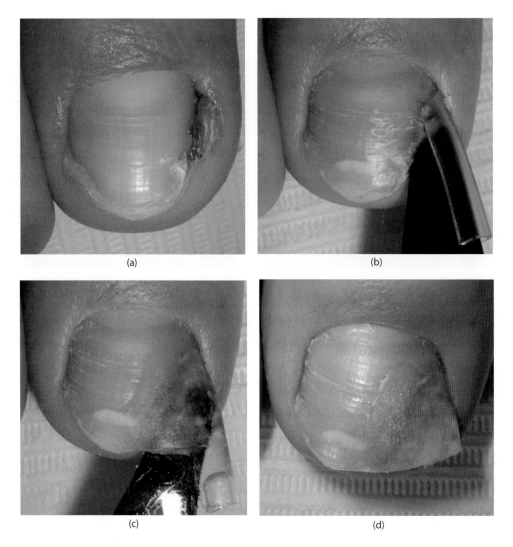

(a)   (b)

(c)   (d)

FIGURE 18.18   Acrylic affixed gutter splint combined with sculptured nail: (a) Before treatment; (b) gutter tube and plastic film inserted; (c) formable acrylic applied; (d) gutter tube combined with sculptured nail (female, 24 years).

Other Treatment Methods Used Together with Anchor-Taping or the Gutter-Splint Method

Other methods used in combination with anchor taping and the gutter splint methods are packing,[1,2,7,24] nail ironing,[2,12,25] plastic nail braces[12,26] (Figure 18.19), and shape memory alloy nail wire[12] (Figure 18.19) or clips.[12,27] Packing in combination with anchor taping uses antibiotic impregnated gauze[2,7,24] or cotton[1] to prevent the nail margin from digging in. For nail ironing, the upper working tip of a mosquito forceps is heated using an alcohol lamp[27] or a beads sterilizer (e.g., Steri 350® [Swiss made])[2,12] to prevent any possible burn. The unheated tip of the mosquito forceps is inserted underneath the nail plate. The nail edge is gripped and flattened using the forceps in a hair ironing motion, allowing the heat to flatten the nail. Then the flatness is cooled and secured with liquid nitrogen spray. Nail braces and clips are used at times for ingrown nail with overcurvature, though hardly seen in younger children. Use of braces alone is not recommended. They might be considered by the body as a foreign object.

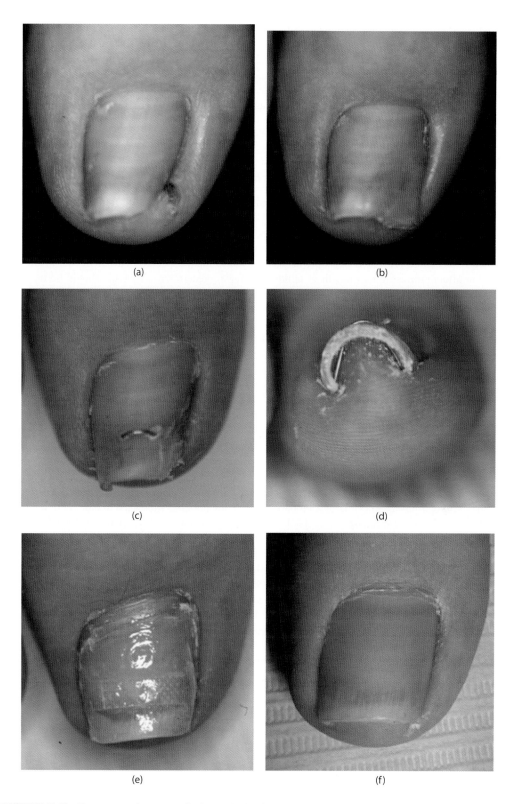

FIGURE 18.19 Treatment cycle: gutter splint/super elastic wire/plastic nail brace. (a) Before treatment; (b) acrylic affixed gutter treatment; (c, d) after 8 weeks, elastic wire; (e) after 10 months with plastic nail brace; (f) after 2 years (female, 18 years).

Other methods include antibiotics for cases with severe infection, topical application, or injection of corticosteroids (e.g., Kenalog® injection) to reduce granulation tissue. CO_2 and other lasers are used in the same manner as the nail iron method (not nail matrix-destructive)[28] to lift and flatten the piercing nail edges. Cauterization of granulation tissue with electric/laser appliances/available tools or chemicals is also done. Mohs' paste is effective in granulation tissues for its tissue hardening effect.[12,29] However, this procedure is not recommended for small children as they are more sensitive to pain from heat.

Prevention of and Education about Ingrown Nail

To prevent recurrence, taping is strongly recommended for several months to protect fragile nail folds during walking and athletic activities.

Prevention depends on the parent/guardians' and the child's (patients') understanding of the causes of ingrown nail, changes made in their nail trimming habits, and the choice of footwear and activities. Ingrown nails can be prevented if people are properly informed, especially earlier in life. Preventive education offers promising nail health of children in future generations. Toenails should be trimmed straight across, without curves or angles, and not cut too short (Figures 18.1 and 18.2). Fingernails should be trimmed long enough to cover the fingertip, especially at the distal–lateral nail edge.

Children should wear proper fitting footwear. The shoe width and toe-box size and shape are most important. The fit of the shoe should be based on the shape of the toe-box, the widest part of the child's foot, not only the length.

Statistics at Arai Dermatology Clinic

The total ingrown nail cases observed at Arai Dermatology Clinic between 1979 and 2013 were 4516 (2238 patients), of which 786 ingrown nails (380 patients) were pediatric cases (17.4%) (15 and under). Of the total number in children, 92.62% (728 lesions) occurred in toes and 7.38% (58 lesions) occurred in finger nails. Of the ingrown toenail cases (728 lesions) 95% occurred in the big toe. The majority of ingrown nails (96.98%) concerned the lateral nail fold, followed by distal nail embedding (1.51%) and proximal nail fold/retronychia (1.51%). Compared by age, the numbers increased in older children (adolescents), with the highest occurrence in 14–15-year-olds, followed by 12–13-year-olds, schoolchildren (6–11-year-olds), and toddlers and infants (0–5) (Figures 18.4 through 18.6).

Treatment outcome was observed by stages of disease and treatment methods. Of the total 786 lesions, the average treatment duration was 30.86 days, 4.00 visits, with a cure rate of 93.64%. Of the cases that were treated mostly with taping (520 lesions, 520/786, 91.6%), the average treatment duration was 22.90 days, 3.15 visits, with a cure rate of 93.19%. In cases treated mostly with gutter splint method (202 lesions, 202/786 or 25.70%), the average treatment duration was 56.61 days, 6.70 visits, with a cure rate of 97.12%. The recurrence rate of the 786 lesions was 12.21% (96/786).

In regards to the length and shape of the nails, of the 620 lesions with descriptions, 334 nails (53.87%) were cut short or extremely short. Meanwhile, in regards to the nail shape, 247 (39.84%) were round-cut, 169 (27.26%) were corner dropped cut, 104 (16.77%) were in an angle/steps/blade/V shape cut (16.77%), 30 (4.84%) were longitudinal/rectangular cut with 70 (11.29%) unknown. The nails in most cases (88.71%) were cut in problematic ways.

Discussion

Ingrowing nails are mechanical, external injuries caused either naturally (nail breakage, trauma) or artificially (improper nail cutting, treatment). Doctors often employ "simple" methods such as the removal of spicules, nail avulsion, and wedge-shaped excisions without taping, which are considered types of iatrogenic external injuries.[2,3,5–13] This pushes back the corner, forming new corners in areas closer to the proximal nail fold that aggravate the situation, causing the patient to endure pain over a longer period. Other treatments that destruct the nail matrix, such as partial matricectomy (phenol, other chemicals, laser, etc.), and remove nail folds make the nail plate narrower, adversely affecting the ability of the nail to support body weight.[5,6,11] Invasive treatment methods for ingrowing nails can be considered as iatrogenic injuries possibly leading to other iatrogenic nail disorders, ensuing chronic pain, difficulty walking, and interference with social life.[5,6,11]

Ingrown toenails surgery carries a significant recurrence and reoperation rate.[30] Of a total of 880 procedures performed on 414 patients (median age 8.5), almost half (48%) of the children underwent two or more procedures. The high recurrence rates and their expected cosmetic end results are important details influencing parents and patients to discuss surgical options prior to treatment.

Although the short-term outcomes of surgery are positive, the long-term results of recurrent ingrown nails may create multiple problems for children and adults at a time when restricting their movement is not only inconvenient but also harmful for their growing bodies.

The benefit of conservative treatment methods is that the shape, size, and width of the nail plate are maintained. The nail heals naturally without deformation. Conservative treatment methods are outstanding from a physiological, functional, and aesthetic aspect, and inexpensive for patients. Both the gutter and taping methods are easy to perform and positive results are almost always guaranteed.

Conclusions

As shown, most ingrown nail cases are noninvasively cured by the combination of anchor-taping and acrylic affixed gutter splint methods and do not require invasive surgeries. Anchor taping and acrylic affixed gutter splint are recommended as the first-line treatment for ingrown nail before considering invasive surgical treatment, as they cure nails naturally without disfigurement or complication. Taking into account the long-term prognosis, it is desirable to select noninvasive conservative methods to treat these painful nail disorders.

REFERENCES

1. Haneke E. Controversies in the treatment of ingrown nails. *Dermatol Res Pract.* 2012; 2012: 1–12.
2. Arai H, Arai T, Nakajima H, Haneke E. Improved conservative treatment of ingrowing nail-acrylic affixed gutter treatment, sculptured nail, taping, antibiotic impregnated gauze packing, plastic nail brace, and nail ironing. *Rinsho Hifuka.* 2003; 57(Suppl 5): 110–119 (Japanese).
3. Arai H, Arai T, Nakajima H, Haneke E. Formable acrylic treatment for ingrowing nail with gutter splint and sculptured nail. *Int J Dermatol.* 2004; 43: 759–765.
4. Fowler AW. Excision of the germinal matrix: A unified treatment for embedded toe-nail and onychogryphosis. *Br J Surg.* 1958; 45: 382–387.
5. Higashi N, Matsumura T. The etiology of onychogryphosis of the great toenail and of ingrowing nail. *Skin Res.* 1988; 30: 620–625 (Japanese).
6. Higashi N, Kume A, Ueda K. Treatment of nail deformity with sculptured nail. *Skin Res.* 1996; 38: 296–300 (Japanese).
7. Arai H, Arai T, Nakajima H. Conservative outpatient treatment of ingrowing nail—Gutter treatment combined with the application of acrylic resin for sculptured nail and sculptured artificial nail. *Hifubyoh-Shinryoh.* 1999; 21: 1159–1166 (Japanese).
8. Arai H, Arai T, Nakajima H, Haneke E. Simple and highly effective treatment for ingrowing nail—Gutter treatment with acrylic fixation, acrylic artificial nail and taping. *Jpn J Clin Dermatol.* 2002; 71: 31–35 (Japanese).
9. Arai H, Arai T, Nakajima H, Haneke E. Treatment of ingrowing nail in children, acrylic affixed gutter splint, sculptured nail and taping. *J Pediatr Dermatol.* 2004; 23: 67–72 (Japanese).
10. Arai H, Arai T. Anchor taping for ingrown nail. *J Jpn Hair Sci Assoc.* 2008; 40: 72–77 (Japanese).

11. Arai H, Arai T. We recommend conservative treatment methods for ingrown nails. Stop invasive surgery now! *J Visual Dermatol*. 2008; 7: 1052–1054 (Japanese).

12. Arai H, Arai T, Haneke E. Simple and effective non-invasive treatment methods for ingrown nail and pincer nail including acrylic affixed gutter splint, anchor taping, sculptured nails, shape memory alloy and plastic nail braces as well as 40% urea paste. *JKMA*. 2011; 16(1): 37–56 (Japanese).

13. Arai H, Arai T, Haneke E. Anchor taping method for the treatment of ingrown nail, nail trauma and other nail disorders. *Jpn J Clin Dermatol*. 2012; 29 (1): 007–0013 (Japanese).

14. Heifetz CJ. Ingrown toe-nail. *Am J Surg*. 1937; 38: 298–315.

15. de Berker DA, Richert B, Duhard E et al. Retronychia: Proximal ingrowing of the nail plate. *J Am Acad Dermatol*. 2008; 58: 978–983.

16. Nishioka K, Katayama I, Kobayashi Y et al. Taping for embedded toenails. *Br J Dermatol*. 1985; 113: 246–247.

17. Watabe A, Hasegawa S, Hashimoto A et al. Treatment of ingrown nail using new taping method. *Hifubyoshinryo*. 2011; 33: 303–306 (Japanese).

18. Kanerva L, Estlander T, Alanko K et al. Allergy from acrylics. *J Eur Acad Dermatol Venereol*. 1999; 12: S6.

19. Fisher AA, Franks A, Glick H. Allergic sensitization of the skin and nails to acrylic plastic nails. *J Allergy*. 1957; 28: 84.

20. Wallace W, Milne DD, Andrew T. Gutter treatment for ingrowing toenails. *Br Med J*. 1979; 21: 168–171.

21. Schulte KW, Neumann NJ, Ruzicka T. Surgical pearl: Nail splinting by flexible tube—A new noninvasive treatment for ingrown toenails. *J Am Acad Dermatol*. 1998; 39: 629–630.

22. Haneke E. Surgical anatomy of the nail apparatus. *Dermatol Clin*. 2006; 24: 291–296.

23. Mackay W, Morris R, Mushlin P. Sodium bicarbonate attenuates pain on skin infiltration with lidocaine, with or without epinephrine. *Anesth Analg*. 1987; 66: 572–574.

24. Nakajima A. Non-invasive treatment for ingrown nail. *Rinsho Derma (Tokyo)*. 1977; 19: 153 (Japanese).

25. Narita H. Radical operation of pincer nail. *Rinsho Hifuka*. 2001; 55(Suppl 5): 154–159 (Japanese).

26. Effendy I, Ossowski B, Happle R. Zangennagel, Konservative Korrektur durch Aufkleben einer Kunststoffspange. *Hautarzt*. 1993; 44: 800–802.

27. Ishibashi M, Tabata N, Suetake T et al. A simple method to treat an ingrowing nail with a shape-memory alloy device. *J Dermatol Treat*. 2008; 19: 291–292.

28. Kuwana R. New treatment for ingrowing nail using CO_2 laser. *Rinsho Derma (Tokyo)*. 2010; 52: 365–370 (Japanese).

29. Takahashi M, Ogata M, Urushibata M, Hino H. Case reports: Four cases treated with Mohs' ointment. *Rinsho Derma* (Tokyo). 2012; 54(2):287–291 (Japanese).

30. Mitchell S, Jackson CR, Wilson-Storey D. Surgical treatment of ingrown toenails in children: What is best practice? *Ann R Coll Surg Engl*. 2011; 93: 99–102.

19

Biopsy of Pediatric Nails

Bertrand Richert and Marie Caucanas

Performing a nail biopsy in a child is not always easy, as many factors may interfere with the procedure. Pain tolerance, especially during the local anesthesia, is the cornerstone of any surgical procedure. The second essential point is the immobility of the child during the procedure. Postoperative pain should be managed adequately. Renewal of the dressing is also a source of anxiety for the child.

The main technical difficulty for the surgeon is the reduced nail size.

There are no specific surgical procedures for children. Fortunately, the indications of a nail biopsy in a child are very limited and should be done only for specific purposes.

Indications of Nail Biopsy in Children

Contrary to adults, nail biopsy is rarely performed in children, unless necessary. Indeed, the scope of nail conditions in children is different from the one in adults and hopefully, many pediatric nail diseases are clinically recognizable. Nail biopsy is required mainly in three conditions:

1. In case of inflammatory nail disorders, especially when a lichen planus (LP) is suspected. The latter is aggressive and should be diagnosed as soon as possible to avoid any permanent scarring.[1] Treatment consists in systemic steroids and therefore, a confirmation of the diagnosis with histology is mandatory[2,3] before embarking into such a therapy that may interfere with the child's growth. Nail psoriasis is much less often biopsied as there are in most cases clues to help the diagnosis, such as plaques on the body or scalp or a familial history of psoriasis. Moreover, there are no dystrophic sequelae from the disease and the treatment mostly remains topical. If a systemic treatment is planned (retinoids, methotrexate, biologic, etc.), histological confirmation is advised.[4]

2. When a tumor is suspected in the patient. In this instance, it is almost always a benign tumor. The lesion is biopsied because it has an unusual location or an unusual presentation[5] (Figure 19.1) or an unusual presentation (juvenile xanthogranuloma at the nail unit) (Figure 19.2).[6–8]

3. In the case of longitudinal melanonychia (LM). A series of 40 consecutive LM in children was excised, and demonstrated that more than three-fourths of LM in children are due to benign melanocytic hyperplasia (nevus or lentigo), the rest being melanocytic activation.[9] These results were confirmed very recently in another study on 30 young patients.[10] However, some exceptional cases of melanoma in situ (some of which had a histological diagnosis that remains debatable) were described[11–13] and some LM should be excised in children (see Chapter 13) as well.

In some rare instances of dominant dystrophic epidermolysis bullosa, the nail abnormalities may be the only sign of the condition over several generations.[14] The diagnosis remains obscure until a family member develops bullae, revealing the disease.[15,16] Biopsy of the subungual bullae usually gives very little information and is not specific.

Preparing the Child for the Biopsy

Preparing the child starts with explaining to the parents the reasons for the biopsy and the sequence of events. Preparation will, of course, depend on the age of the patient. For toddlers and infants, full information will be given to the parents. One should remember that the stress of the parents is very easily transmitted to the child. Older children should be included in the discussion and a simple, clear, and reassuring explanation should be given to them. Drawings are worth a thousand words.

There are no specific studies on nail surgery procedures in children, but one may get good information from publications on venous puncture and dental procedures in this age group.

Management of young children with behavior problems may need premedication. Several studies compared different regimens: those with midazolam, chloral hydrate, hydroxyzine, and mepiridine, respectively.[17] Oral midazolam was found to be useful, but not effective in all cases.[18] This was confirmed by a Cochrane study demonstrating that there is some weak evidence that oral midazolam is an effective sedative agent for children undergoing dental treatment.[19] However, a recent study showed that orally given midazolam optimized the children's behavior during skin laser treatment (more similar to skin and nail procedures) with no serious adverse effects.[20]

Children are mostly afraid of the needle. For this, application of lidocaine–prilocaine emulsion (EMLA: eutectic mixture of lidocaine 2.5% and prilocaine 2.5%) is highly effective in preventing pain from the puncture.[21] To be effective, parents should be instructed on how to apply the cream adequately. It is amazing to discover how parents are unable to carry out this kind of dressing. A demonstration on how to perform an adequate occlusion (with any cream) during the preoperative consultation is of great help. Time of occlusion should be respected, too, at least 2 hours prior to the procedure for fingers or toes. Review of the literature shows disparity on the efficacy of EMLA cream for reducing pain from a nerve block for ingrowing toenail.[22] One should understand that EMLA cream may suppress pain from the puncture if applied adequately and that pain from the block not only comes from the needlestick but also from the dilation of the soft tissue and the acidity of the anesthetic. A recent study showed that there was an age-related response to EMLA cream with preventing pain from venipunctures in the youngest patients, the group that is most in need of pain prevention.[23]

For very young children and for kids with behavior problems, nitrous oxide analgesia is the best option. It is a cost-effective and efficacious alternative to conscious sedation or general anesthesia for minor pediatric surgical procedures. It may be performed in an outpatient setting. The technique provides

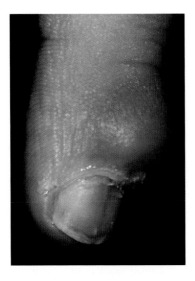

FIGURE 19.1 Swelling of the proximal nail fold. Biopsy revealed a subungual wart. (Courtesy of Lateur N.)

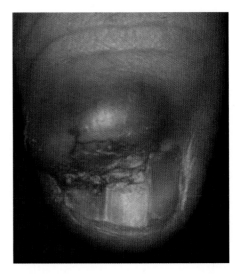

FIGURE 19.2 Swelling of the proximal nail fold. Biopsy revealed a juvenile xanthogranuloma. (Courtesy of Piraccini B-M.)

almost a painless and anxiety-free surgery, no postoperative monitoring, and a high degree of satisfaction for the patients, parents, and staff.[24,25] It needs a well-trained staff, able to perform child resuscitation.

Managing the Child during the Biopsy

Pain from the Needle

As previously mentioned, children mostly fear the needle. EMLA cream works very well for preventing pain from the needle. However, it is sometimes impossible to apply before the procedure (parents forgot, waited too long, did not do it properly) and other tips should be used to overcome the discomfort from the needle insertion. Pain is highly subjective, and it is neurologically proven that stimulation of large diameter fibers using cold, rubbing, pressure, or vibration can close the neural "gate" so that the central perception of pain is reduced. This is called the "gate control" theory. The mother (or the nurse) may be asked to firmly press on the point of injection for at least 5 minutes before the needle prick. Another option is to use a vibrating tool for several minutes, at the location of the future injection, until the child finds that the area is becoming numb (Figure 19.3). This was demonstrated as an effective method to decrease pain during local anesthesia.[26–28] Interestingly, it was shown that the ethnic group is an important factor in the pain response and that special effort should be made to customize approaches to pain management in children.[28]

Using very thin needles (30G) will also minimize the concurrent pain from the needle prick.

Pain from Dilation

Once the needle is inserted painlessly, the infusion of the anesthetic may start. At that moment, pain will emerge from dilation. The subungual space is very limited, and excessive pressure on the Vater-Pacini corpuscules within the distal soft tissue will trigger pain. The injection should be extremely slow, thus performing a very slowly progressive swelling. Using a very small needle will also limit the anesthetic flow.

It is not unusual to spend more time performing the anesthesia than the surgical procedure itself. If the child moves a little bit, showing some discomfort from the infusion, the surgeon should stop injecting for a few seconds, then start again. Usually older children are asked to inform the doctor when they feel some ache.

Pain from Acidity

Lidocaine is acid. Buffering it (1 volume of bicarbonate for 9 volumes of lidocaine) dramatically reduces pain during infusion.[29,30] Addition of too much sodium bicarbonate will result in a milky solution secondary to flocculation. This may impair the flow through the needle and may even get blocked.

Keeping the anesthetic out of the fridge or at body temperature in a water bath will render the infusion less painful.

The best way to reduce pain from infusion is to inject warmed, buffered lidocaine.[31]

Immobility during the Procedure

Immobility during the procedure is a must, as the surgeon is performing a precise work on a very small area. For this, multiple tips that have demonstrated efficacy should be tried.

Distraction is a very commonly used trick, called talkesthesia, which was known to work well with children. A Cochrane database showed that there is strong evidence supporting the efficacy of distraction for needle-related pain and anxiety in children and adolescents (Figure 19.4). However, there is no evidence that any one technique among the ones used (parents coaching, blowing out air, memory alteration, distraction, and suggestion) is superior to another.[32] A more recent publication investigated three different distraction methods (distraction cards, listening to the music of a cartoon, and balloon inflation). All forms of distraction significantly reduced pain and anxiety perception. The distraction card group had lower pain levels.[33]

Several trials attempted to evaluate the effect of tasting sweets for reduction of needle-related pain. There is insufficient evidence of the analgesic effects of sweet-tasting solutions or substances during painful procedures.[34]

For a child with behavior problems, nitrous oxide sedation allows the surgeon to perform local anesthesia and carry out the surgical procedure with the child almost completely immobile.

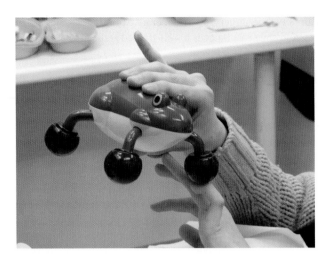

FIGURE 19.3   The vibrating frog used in our department. After 5 minutes, the end of the digit is numbed.

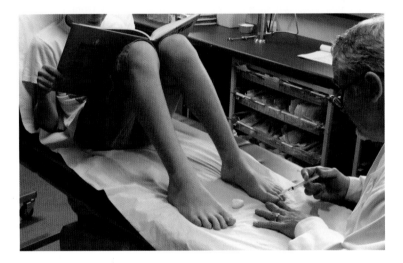

FIGURE 19.4   Distraction and confidence are a must.

Dealing with Postoperative Pain

Once the procedure is done, the first two questions of the parents will be "When will the anesthetic effect stop?" and "What should we do if the child has pain?"

Optimal management of postoperative pain requires an understanding of the pathophysiology of pain, methods available to reduce pain, invasiveness of the procedure, and patient factors associated with increased pain, such as anxiety, depression, catastrophizing, and neuroticism.[35]

Long-lasting anesthetics should be used. After the end of the procedure, the surgeon should inject bupivacaine 0.5% exactly in the same manner as for the distal digital block. This will be painless because of the previous lidocaine block and this will also act as a volumetric tourniquet by pressing on the digital proper arteries, thus limiting the risk of postoperative bleeding. But the most important issue is that bupivacaine acts for up to 8 hours.[36] Another option is to inject ropivacaine 5 mg/mL, if available, in the meantime to regain full sensation over 10 hours. Ropivacaine is now considered as the reference drug for regional anesthesia in pediatric patients, mainly because it is less toxic than bupivacaine and provides excellent postoperative analgesia even when used at low concentrations.[37]

Painkillers should be adequately prescribed. The inflammation and the postoperative pain will last for roughly 48 hours. Pain should be completely covered for during this period. The first thing to explain to the parents is that the limb should be kept elevated for the next 2 days. This will avoid edema and throbbing.

The type and power of painkiller will depend upon the procedure performed, the age of the patient, and his/her tolerance to pain. Nail biopsies (nail bed punch, nail matrix punch, tangential excision of a LM) do not induce a lot of pain, except the lateral longitudinal biopsy. For the first ones, regular painkillers such as paracetamol work well. Diclofenac is an alternative and has been shown to be safe for children.[38] However, there is high evidence that ibuprofen 400 mg is superior to paracetamol 1000 mg.[39] Several reports mention that paracetamol with codeine offers equivalent analgesia to ibuprofen in children with extreme injuries.[40–42] Prescription of ibuprofen postoperatively does not increase the risk of bleeding.[43,44] Considering opioids, the overall evidence regarding tramadol for postoperative pain in children is currently low or very low.[45] Morphine was much less efficient in reducing pain after tonsillectomy than ibuprofen.[46] The best pain relief in children seems now to be a combination of ibuprofen with paracetamol.[47]

Removal of the Dressing

Young children fear pain from sticky dressings that are abruptly pulled out. This is why the immediate postoperative dressing should be adapted to nail surgery. Applying large amounts of ointment covered with nonadherent dressing, such as petrolatum-coated gauze (Tulle gras®, Bactigras®, Adaptic®, Jelonet®) will protect the wound from drying and will allow an easy and painless removal. Telfa® is another option. Mepitel® is a porous, semitransparent, low-adherent, flexible polyamide net coated with soft silicone. It is not absorbent, but contains apertures of approximately 1 mm in diameter that allow the passage of exudate into a secondary absorbent dressing. It is expensive, but if available, it works wonderfully.

If done so, the dressing will not stick to the wound even though there is almost always some bleeding into the dressing. The dressing should be removed on the second day postsurgery. Sometimes, early removal is necessary after 24 hours if bleeding is severe, because the impregnated gauze of the bulky dressing dries and becomes stiff, and may cause unpleasant or painful compression. If left in place for too long, such dry and hard dressings may induce superficial erosion on the skin of the proximal and/or lateral nail folds.[48] In case of adherence, never try to pull, but soak the dressing in lukewarm water until it detaches spontaneously. Hydrogen peroxide is also a very good option, but the child should be informed that some light heat might occur.

Surgical Procedures

There are no specific surgical procedures for children. Anesthesia procedures are identical to the ones performed in adults (distal digital block and wing block).

Surgical procedures are identical to the ones performed in adults. The various biopsy techniques that are performed for diagnosis in children are listed in the following sections.

Punch Biopsy of the Nail Bed

Punch biopsy of the nail bed is mainly indicated in onycholytic or distal hyperkeratotic psoriasis and LP. Nail bed biopsy can be performed with or without prior partial nail avulsion. The punch should be pushed until bone contact (Figure 19.5) takes place. Its size should not be greater than 3 mm in diameter, to avoid any secondary scarring and onycholysis. The fragile specimen should be harvested delicately with sharp, curved scissors and not pulled out with forceps. In psoriatic onycholysis, the nail bed biopsy has almost always a nonspecific image under the microscope, even if performed at the most proximal edge of the onycholysis.

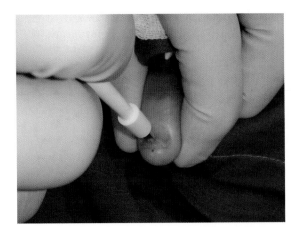

FIGURE 19.5 Nail bed punch biopsy, here for a distal subungual hyperkeratosis. The punch should be pushed until bone contact happens. Histology revealed psoriasis.

Lateral Longitudinal Biopsy

Lateral longitudinal biopsy is mostly indicated in nail diseases presenting with alterations of the surface of the nail plate, notably LP in children (Figure 19.6a). In order to collect relevant microscopic information, this biopsy should be performed on a nail exhibiting a lateral involvement with marked clinical signs (Figure 19.6b and c). Pathologists favor this technique as it allows the study of the whole nail apparatus: proximal nail fold, matrix, nail bed, nail plate and hyponychium. Its main drawback, though, is the permanent narrowing of the nail due to the partial amputation of the lateral horn of the matrix (Figure 19.7a and b), which should be discussed with the parents. Postoperative risks include lateral deviation if the specimen exceeds 3 mm[49] and nail spicule formation if some nail matrix tissue is left after incomplete detachment of the matrix from the bone at the proximal tip of the biopsy. This technique is also suitable for LM of the lateral third of the nail plate.

Punch Matrix Biopsy

Before embarking on any systemic treatments, especially steroids that may impair the child's growth, it is recommended to confirm the diagnosis of nail LP with a punch matrix biopsy, even if the clinical features are obvious. Two lateral incisions are performed in order to allow retraction of the proximal nail fold. The proximal nail plate is avulsed in a lateral way. A punch biopsy is performed within the median part of the matrix. The nail plate is put back in place and secured to the lateral fold. Some authors recommend biopsy of both nail bed and nail matrix.[3]

The same technique may be used to excise a narrow LM in children. Most of the time, nail pigmentation originates from the distal matrix (95% of cases) and in this case postoperative sequelae will be a thinned nail plate. If the pigment location is in the proximal matrix, a postoperative dystrophy with longitudinal fissure is expected[50] (Figure 19.8a and b).

If the pigmented macule on the matrix fits in a 3 mm punch, the specimen is harvested at the level of the periosteum with fine curved fine-tipped scissors and the defect is not sutured[51] (Figure 19.9a and b). If the shape of the pigment is longitudinally oriented, a narrow ellipse is performed and delicate lateral undermining allows suturing of the defect with 5/0 sutures (Figure 19.10a through c). In all instances, the pigmented area must be removed completely, as this should be an excisional biopsy, allowing the pathologist to fully examine the lesion.

Shave Biopsy for Wide LM

This technique is indicated in wide pigmented LM. It consists of a tangential excision of the matrix epidermis and a small layer of dermis (Figure 19.11a through c). Haneke[52] first described the shave

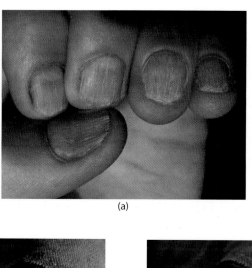

(a)

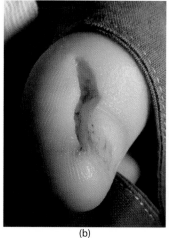

(b)

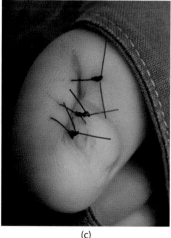

(c)

FIGURE 19.6 (a) Prominent onychorrhexia in a child, involving 20 nails. Note the inflammatory red lunula. (b) The great toe was chosen as biopsy site because it showed severe lateral involvement. Note the proximal curve of the incision to ensure removal of the lateral horn of the matrix. (c) Reapproximation with loose stitches.

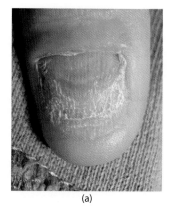

(a)

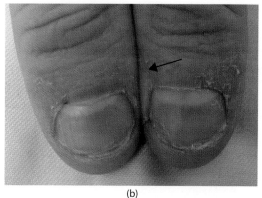

(b)

FIGURE 19.7 (a) Severe lichen planus of the left thumb. As the condition was monodactylic a biopsy was required before embarking with intramuscular systemic steroids. (b) Two years after treatment. One can see the scar from the lateral longitudinal biopsy on the medial side of the left thumb (arrow). Compare with the contralateral nail.

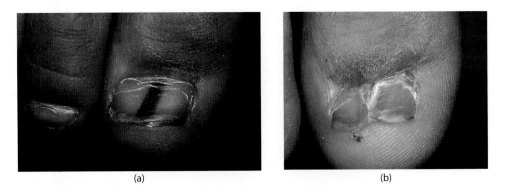

(a)   (b)

FIGURE 19.8   (a) Dark longitudinal melanonychia in a child. (b) The pigmented macule was unfortunately located proximally, leaving thus a split in the nail. Histology revealed a nevus. (Courtesy of André J.)

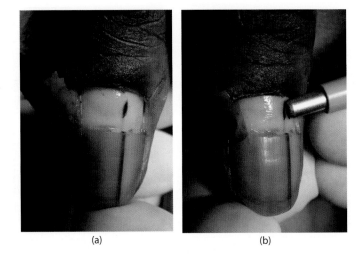

(a)   (b)

FIGURE 19.9   (a) Distally located pigmented macule. (b) The pigmented macule is removed in a 3 mm punch. Histology revealed a lentigo.

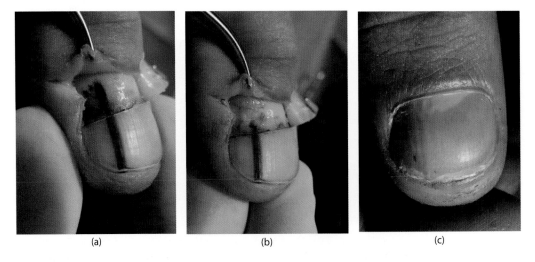

(a)   (b)   (c)

FIGURE 19.10   (a) The pigmented macule is elliptic and longitudinally oriented. (b) It is excised within a longitudinal ellipse and delicately sutured after undermining the lateral edges. (c) One year after operation.

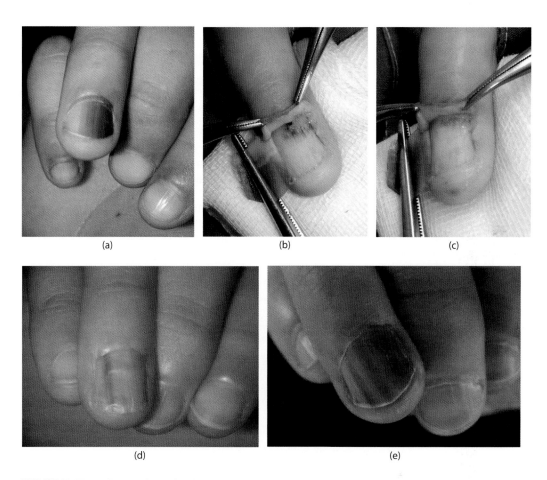

(a)   (b)   (c)

(d)   (e)

FIGURE 19.11   (a) Large (>6 mm) longitudinal melanonychia in a 7-year-old boy. (b) Avulsion reveals a wide pigmentation on the matrix. (c) The whole pigmented area is tangentially excised. Histology showed a nevus. (d) Six months after operation. (e) Two years after operation.

biopsy, and its main benefit is healing without scarring. Though the margins are difficult to assess, the pathologist is able to examine the entire lesion. Handling the thin specimen in the lab requires skilled technicians. In a large series of nail matrix tangential excisions, this technique has shown to provide adequate slides and allow an accurate diagnosis in all cases. Postoperative outcome was excellent, even after removal of a wide area of the distal and proximal matrix (Figure 19.11d). The major drawback of this technique is a high level of recurrent pigmentation, up to 75% after 2 years (Figure 19.11e). Its main advantage is that it prevents a mutilating surgery for large benign LM.[53]

REFERENCES

1. Tosti A, Piraccini BM, Cambiaghi S, Jorizzo M. Nail lichen planus in children: Clinical features, response to treatment, and long-term follow-up. *Arch Dermatol.* 2001; 137(8): 1027–1032.
2. Piraccini BM, Starace M. Nail disorders in infants and children. *Curr Opin Pediatr.* 2014; 26(4): 440–445.
3. Goettmann S, Zaraa I, Moulonguet I. Nail lichen planus: Epidemiological, clinical, pathological, therapeutic and prognosis study of 67 cases. *J Eur Acad Dermatol Venereol.* 2012; 26(10): 1304–1309.
4. Holzberg M, Ruben BS, Baran R. Psoriasis restricted to the nail in a 7-year-old child. Should biologics be an appropriate treatment modality when considering quality of life? *J Eur Acad Dermatol Venereol.* 2014; 28(5): 668–670.

5. Läuchli S, Eichmann A, Baran R. Swelling of the proximal nail fold caused by underlying warts. *Dermatology.* 2001; 202(4): 328–329.

6. Piraccini BM, Fanti PA, Iorizzo M, Tosti A. Juvenile xanthogranuloma of the proximal nail fold. *Pediatr Dermatol.* 2003; 20(4): 307–308.

7. Chang P, Baran R, Villanueva C et al. Juvenile xanthogranuloma beneath a fingernail. *Cutis.* 1996; 58(2): 173–174.

8. Frumkin A, Roytman M, Johnson SF. Juvenile xanthogranuloma underneath a toenail. *Cutis.* 1987; 40(3): 244–245.

9. Goettmann-Bonvallot S, André J, Belaich S. Longitudinal melanonychia in children: A clinical and histopathologic study of 40 cases. *J Am Acad Dermatol.* 1999; 41(1): 17–22.

10. Cooper C, Arva NC, Lee C et al. A clinical, histopathologic, and outcome study of melanonychia striata in childhood. *J Am Acad Dermatol.* 2015; 72(5): 773–779.

11. Tosti A, Piraccini BM, Cagalli A, Haneke E. In situ melanoma of the nail unit in children: Report of two cases in fair-skinned Caucasian children. *Pediatr Dermatol.* 2012; 29(1): 79–83.

12. Iorizzo M, Tosti A, Di Chiacchio N et al. Nail melanoma in children: Differential diagnosis and management. *Dermatol Surg.* 2008; 34(7): 974–978.

13. Antonovich DD, Grin C, Grant-Kels JM. Childhood subungual melanoma in situ in diffuse nail melanosis beginning as expanding longitudinal melanonychia. *Pediatr Dermatol.* 2005; 22(3): 210–212.

14. Tosti A, de Farias DC, Murrell DF. Nail involvement in epidermolysis bullosa. *Dermatol Clin.* 2010; 28(1): 153–157.

15. Tosti A, Piraccini BM, Scher RK. Isolated nail dystrophy suggestive of dominant dystrophic epidermolysis bullosa. *Pediatr Dermatol.* 2003; 20(5): 456–457.

16. Dharma B, Moss C, McGrath JA et al. Dominant dystrophic epidermolysis bullosa presenting as familial nail dystrophy. *Clin Exp Dermatol.* 2001; 26(1): 93–96.

17. Sheroan MM, Dilley DC, Lucas WJ, Vann WF. A prospective study of 2 sedation regimens in children: Chloral hydrate, meperidine, and hydroxyzine versus midazolam, meperidine, and hydroxyzine. *Anesth Prog.* 2006; 53(3): 83–90.

18. Day PF, Power AM, Hibbert SA, Paterson SA. Effectiveness of oral midazolam for paediatric dental care: A retrospective study in two specialist centres. *Eur Arch Paediatr Dent.* 2006; 7(4): 228–235.

19. Lourenço-Matharu L, Ashley PF, Furness S. Sedation of children undergoing dental treatment. *Cochrane Database Syst Rev.* 2012; (3): CD003877.

20. Shoroghi M, Arbabi S, Farahbakhsh F et al. Perioperative effects of oral midazolam premedication in children undergoing skin laser treatment. A double-blinded randomized placebo-controlled trial. *Acta Cir Bras.* 2011; 26(4): 303–309.

21. Arts SE, Abu-Saad HH, Champion GD et al. Age-related response to lidocaine-prilocaine (EMLA) emulsion and effect of music distraction on the pain of intravenous cannulation. *Pediatrics.* 1994; 93(5): 797–801.

22. Browne J, Fung M, Donnelly M, Cooney C. The use of EMLA reduces the pain associated with digital ring block for ingrowing toenail correction. *Eur J Anaesthesiol.* 2000; 17(3): 182–184.

23. Serour F, Ben-Yehuda Y, Boaz M. EMLA cream prior to digital nerve block for ingrown nail surgery does not reduce pain at injection of anesthetic solution. *Acta Anaesthesiol Scand.* 2002; 46(2): 203–206.

24. Burnweit C, Diana-Zerpa JA, Nahmad MH et al. Nitrous oxide analgesia for minor pediatric surgical procedures: An effective alternative to conscious sedation? *J Pediatr Surg.* 2004; 39(3): 495–499; discussion 495–499.

25. Lévêque C, Mikaeloff Y, Hamza J, Ponsot G. Efficacy and safety of inhalation premixed nitrous oxide and oxygen for the management of procedural diagnostic pain in neuropediatrics. *Arch Pediatr.* 2002; 9(9): 907–912.

26. Smith KC, Comite SL, Balasubramanian S et al. Vibration anesthesia: A noninvasive method of reducing discomfort prior to dermatologic procedures. *Dermatol Online J.* 2004; 10(2): 1.

27. Shilpapriya M, Jayanthi M, Reddy VN et al. Effectiveness of new vibration delivery system on pain associated with injection of local anesthesia in children. *J Indian Soc Pedod Prev Dent.* 2015; 33(3): 173–176.

28. Bahorski JS, Hauber RP, Hanks C et al. Mitigating procedural pain during venipuncture in a pediatric population: A randomized factorial study. *Int J Nurs Stud.* 2015; 52(10): 15534–15564. pii: S0020-7489(15)00191-1.

29. Cornelius P, Kendall J, Meek S, Rajan R. Alkalinisation of lignocaine to reduce the pain of digital nerve blockade. *J Accid Emerg Med.* 1996; 13(5): 339–340.

30. Cepeda MS, Tzortzopoulou A, Thackrey M et al. WITHDRAWN: Adjusting the pH of lidocaine for reducing pain on injection. *Cochrane Database Syst Rev.* 2015; (5): CD006581.

31. Colaric KB, Overton DT, Moore K. Pain reduction in lidocaine administration through buffering and warming. *Am J Emerg Med.* 1998; 16(4): 353–356.

32. Uman LS, Birnie KA, Noel M et al. Psychological interventions for needle-related procedural pain and distress in children and adolescents. *Cochrane Database Syst Rev.* 2013; (10): CD005179.

33. Sahiner NC, Bal MD. The effects of three different distraction methods on pain and anxiety in children. *J Child Health Care.* 2015. pii: 1367493515587062.

34. Harrison D, Yamada J, Adams-Webber T et al. Sweet tasting solutions for reduction of needle-related procedural pain in children aged one to 16 years. *Cochrane Database Syst Rev.* 2015; (5): CD008408.

35. Lovich-Sapola J, Smith CE, Brandt CP. Postoperative pain control. *Surg Clin North Am.* 2015; 95(2): 301–318.

36. Reichl M, Quinton D. Comparison of 1% lignocaine with 0.5% bupivacaine in digital ring blocks. *J Hand Surg Br.* 1987; 12(3): 375–376.

37. Mazoit JX, Dalens BJ. Ropivacaine in infants and children. *Curr Opin Anaesthesiol.* 2003; 16(3): 305–307.

38. Standing JF, Savage I, Pritchard D, Waddington M. Diclofenac for acute pain in children. *Cochrane Database Syst Rev.* 2015; (7): CD005538.

39. Bailey E, Worthington HV, van Wijk A et al. Ibuprofen and/or paracetamol (acetaminophen) for pain relief after surgical removal of lower wisdom teeth. *Cochrane Database Syst Rev.* 2013; (12): CD004624.

40. Stanhope B. Paracetamol/codeine probably had equivalent analgesia to ibuprofen in children with extremity injuries. *Arch Dis Child Educ Pract Ed.* 2010; 95(5): 167.

41. Braun CA. Ibuprofen provides similar pain relief but reduces adverse effects and improves function compared with acetaminophen plus codeine in children with uncomplicated fractures. *Evid Based Nurs.* 2010; 13(1): 10–11.

42. Friday JH, Kanegaye JT, McCaslin I et al. Ibuprofen provides analgesia equivalent to acetaminophen-codeine in the treatment of acute pain in children with extremity injuries: A randomized clinical trial. *Acad Emerg Med.* 2009; 16(8): 711–716.

43. Yaman H, Belada A, Yilmaz S. The effect of ibuprofen on postoperative hemorrhage following tonsillectomy in children. *Eur Arch Otorhinolaryngol.* 2011; 268(4): 615–617.

44. Mattos JL, Robison JG, Greenberg J, Yellon RF. Acetaminophen plus ibuprofen versus opioids for treatment of post-tonsillectomy pain in children. *Int J Pediatr Otorhinolaryngol.* 2014; 78(10): 1671–1676.

45. Schnabel A, Reichl SU, Meyer-Frießem C et al. Tramadol for postoperative pain treatment in children. *Cochrane Database Syst Rev.* 2015; (3): CD009574.

46. Kelly LE, Sommer DD, Ramakrishna J et al. Morphine or ibuprofen for post-tonsillectomy analgesia: A randomized trial. *Pediatrics.* 2015; 135(2): 307–3013.

47. Bailey E, Worthington HV, van Wijk A et al. Ibuprofen and/or paracetamol (acetaminophen) for pain relief after surgical removal of lower wisdom teeth. *Cochrane Database Syst Rev.* 2013; (12): CD004624.

48. Richert B, Dahdah M. Complications in nail surgery. In Nouri K (ed.), *Complications in Dermatologic Surgery.* Philadelphia, PA: Mosby Elsevier; 2008. pp. 137–158.

49. De Berker DA, Baran R. Acquired malalignment: A complication of lateral longitudinal nail biopsy. *Acta Derm Venereol.* 1998; 78: 468–470.

50. Baran R, Kechijian P. Longitudinal melanonychia (melanonychia striata): Diagnosis and management. *J Am Acad Dermatol.* 1989; 21: 1165–1175.

51. Jellinek N. Nail matrix biopsy of longitudinal melanonychia: Diagnostic algorithm including the matrix shave biopsy. *J Am Acad Dermatol.* 2007; 56: 803–810.

52. Haneke E, Baran R. Longitudinal melanonychia. *Dermatol Surg.* 2001; 27: 580–584.

53. Richert B, Theunis A, Norrenberg S, André J. Tangential excision of pigmented nail matrix lesions responsible for longitudinal melanonychia: Evaluation of the technique on a series of 30 patients. *J Am Acad Dermatol.* 2013; 69: 96–104.

20

Ultrasound of Pediatric Nails

Ximena Wortsman

Introduction

Ultrasound has been used for studying nails since the 1980s[1,2]; however, with the development of multichannel color Doppler ultrasound machines working with high and variable frequency, and linear and compact linear probes, the applications have increased. This is due to the improved definition for studying ungual and periungual structures.[3]

In comparison to other imaging modalities, ultrasound is a safe, nonradiating imaging technique that provides high definition imaging with a good balance between resolution and penetration, showing all the parts of the ungual unit from the plaque to the bony margin of the distal phalanx as well as the periungual structures, such as the distal insertion of the extensor tendon and the distal interphalangeal joint.[4]

The usage of ultrasound for studying nail pathologies includes a wide range of applications that include congenital and location alterations, tumors and pseudotumors, and inflammatory pathologies.[5]

Thus, this imaging modality provides a potent tool for supporting diagnosis and can avoid the potential cosmetic sequels derived from biopsies.[5,6]

Normal Anatomy

The nail is composed of the ungual plate, the nail bed, and the periungual tissue. The ungual plate has a dorsal and ventral plate and appears as a billaminar parallel hyperechoic structure with a hypoechoic space between the plates on ultrasound. The origin of the plates is far from the distal interphalangeal joint. The nail bed appears as a hypoechoic space between the nail plate and the hyperechoic linear bony margin of the distal phalanx. In the proximal part of the nail bed, there is a slightly hyperechoic area that corresponds to the matrix region. In children with a non-ossified skeleton, there is a hypoechoic structure attached to the bony margin of the distal phalanx that corresponds to cartilage. According to age, the ossification nucleus develops and finally the distal ossified epiphysis is fused with the rest of the distal phalanx.

The periungual region is composed of the proximal and lateral nail folds that shows skin with a non-glabrous appearance, which means that the epidermis presents itself as a monolaminar hyperechoic layer and the dermis as a hyperechoic band less bright than the epidermis. The proximal and lateral nail folds lack hypodermal fat. In the pulp of the finger, the skin turns to a glabrous type; therefore, the epidermis appears as a hyperechoic bilaminar layer, the dermis also shows a hyperechoic band, and the hypodermis presents a hypoechoic texture due to the fatty lobules. Some hyperechoic septa may be detected in between the fatty tissue.

The distal insertion of the extensor tendon shows a fibrillar hyperechoic pattern. The distal interphalangeal joint is an anechoic space in between the hyperechoic bony margins of the distal and middle phalanges.

On color Doppler, low velocity arterial and venous vessels can be detected in the nail bed closely attached to the bony margin of the distal phalanx. On the proximal nail fold, the distal part of the digital arteries can be detected (Figure 20.1).[5,6]

Technical Considerations

The ultrasound examination of the nail should be performed with the finger or toe fully extended. A copious amount of gel is applied to the surface to achieve good contact with the skin and transmission of the sound waves. A towel or pad underneath the digit may be useful when studying the thumbs.[5,6]

In children ≤4 years old, sedation is commonly used to avoid the movements that can generate artifacts on the screen. Chloral hydrate 50 mg/kg or melatonin, according to age, is given orally to the patient 30 minutes before the examination. This induces a short sleep in the child that provides a quiet environment for performing the examination. The parent or guardian signs an informed consent, and the child is monitored in the department using the modified Aldrete scale and discharged only when awake.[7]

Pathology

There are several applications for studying the nail by means of ultrasound; therefore, they have been divided according to their nature and origin.

Growth—Location Alterations, Congenital Conditions

Ingrowing Toenail

Also called onychocryptosis, this implies the embedding of a nail plate fragment into the lateral nail fold. In children ≤2 years old, the reported frequency is 2.4%; however, it can be more frequent in adolescents and young adults and can reach up to 20% of the consultations of family physicians for foot conditions. This may be due to anatomical alterations, regional trauma, or improper trimming of the nails.[8,9] On ultrasound, the nail plate fragment appears as a bilaminar hyperechoic structure in the lateral nail fold. Commonly, there is hypoechoic tissue surrounding the hyperechoic fragment due to inflammation and a granulomatous reaction (Figure 20.2).[5,6]

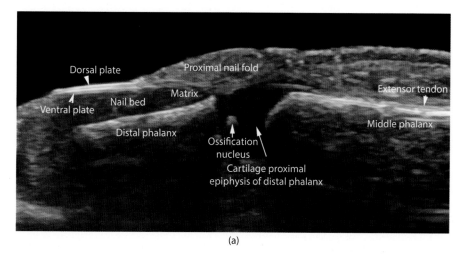

(a)

FIGURE 20.1 Normal ultrasound anatomy of the nail. (a) and (b) Gray-scale longitudinal views (with color filter). (a) Infant with non-ossified epiphysis of the distal phalanx.   (*Continued*)

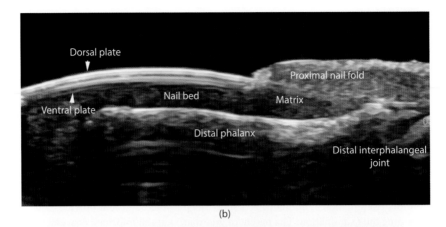

(b)

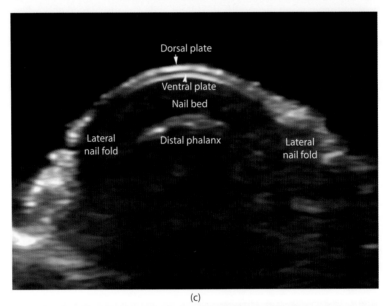

(c)

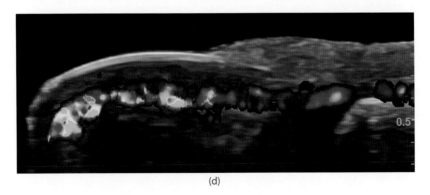

(d)

FIGURE 20.1 (*Continued*) Normal ultrasound anatomy of the nail. (b) Child with ossified epiphysis of the distal phalanx. (c) Gray-scale transverse view of the nail. (d) Color Doppler ultrasound (longitudinal view) demonstrates the normal
blood flow (colors) within the nail bed.

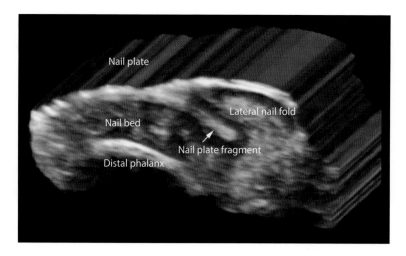

FIGURE 20.2 Onychocryptosis. Three-dimensional (3D) ultrasound (transverse view) shows hyperechoic linear structure that corresponds to nail plate fragment embedded in the lateral nail fold.

Onychomadesis

This is secondary to the arrest of nail formation in a period. On ultrasound, two or more nail plate fragments can be detected. Thickening and decreased echogenicity of the nail bed may also be seen (Figure 20.3).[5,6,10]

Retronychia

This location alteration has been reported in children, adolescents, and young adults.[11] It involves a posterior embedding of the hyperechoic nail plate into the proximal nail fold and can be detected on ultrasound.[10,12] Thickening and decreased echogenicity of the proximal nail fold is also a common finding. The distance between the origin of the nail plate and the base of the distal phalanx is decreased. Comparison with the contralateral finger during the examination may better disclose the anatomical changes (Figure 20.4).[5,6,10,12]

Congenital Malalignment

On ultrasound, thickening and decreased echogenicity of the nail bed is a common finding. Usually, the nail bed is hypovascular and the presence of onychocriptosis complicating the malalignment can be ruled out with sonography (Figure 20.5).[5,6]

Congenital Hypertrophic Lip of the Hallux

Ultrasound shows hypertrophy of the skin layers of the medial nail fold of the hallux, commonly accompanied by hypoechogenicity of the regional dermis; sometimes hyperechoic nail plate fragments may be found embedded in the medial nail folds.[5,6]

Ichtyosis

In this genetic cornification disorder pachyonychia congenita has been reported.[13,14] On ultrasound, thickening of the nail plate that lacks the hypoechoic interplate space may be detected. Additionally, thickening of the epidermis in the periungual region can be seen.[15]

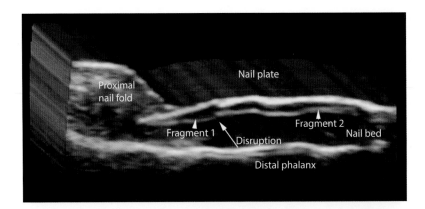

FIGURE 20.3 Onychomadesis. 3D ultrasound (longitudinal view) demonstrates two hyperechoic fragments of nail plates separated by a disruption area.

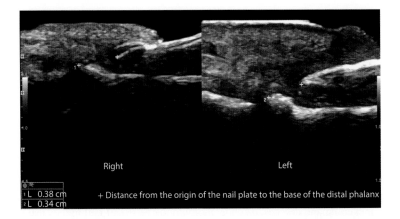

FIGURE 20.4 Retronychia. Gray-scale ultrasound (side by side comparison, right and left great toe; longitudinal views) shows decreased distance between the origin of the nail plate and the base of the distal phalanx on the left side. Notice the thickening and decreased echogenicity of the proximal nail fold and nail bed in the left great toe.

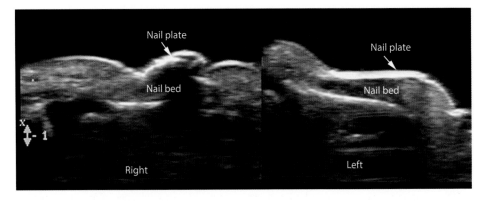

FIGURE 20.5 Congenital malalignment. Gray-scale ultrasound (longitudinal view, side by side, right to left, great toes) shows thickening and decreased echogenicity of the nail bed as well as thickening of the nail plate on the right side.

Cystic Fibrosis

This autosomal recessive condition results from mutations in the cystic fibrosis transmembrane conductance regulator gene (*CFTR*).[16] The clubbing present in cystic fibrosis has been under study and it has been postulated to be caused by fibrovascular hyperplasia of the underlying connective tissue of the nail bed.[17] Also, a high presence of electrolytes, such as sodium and chloride, has been reported in the nail bed .[18] Recently, the anatomical alterations seen on color Doppler ultrasound have been described. These are increased thickness and decreased echogenicity of the nail bed, upward displacement of the nail plate, and hypervascularity that is more prominent in the proximal part of the nail bed. No signs of increased blood flow have been detected in the lateral nail fold in these cases (Figure 20.6).[19]

Tumors and Pseudotumors

Many tumoral and pseudotumoral (i.e., mimicker) entities can affect the nail unit. The use of ultrasound can provide relevant anatomical data, such as the origin (ungual or periungual), the exact location, the affected parts of the nail unit, the size in all axes, the nature (solid or cystic), and the vascularity (hypovascular or hypervascular). We have selected the most common pediatric conditions that are referred for an ultrasound examination of the nail and for academic purposes these have been divided into the following categories:

Ungual Tumors

These are composed of primary conditions that originate from the nail.

Solid

Glomus Tumor   These benign entities are derived from the neuromyoarterial apparatus and their main symptom is the exquisite pain that is present in the majority of the cases. Glomus tumors are not frequent in infants; however, they have been reported in children ≥11 years old associated with neurofibromatosis type 1.[20] On ultrasound, a well-defined hypoechoic nodule that produces scalloping of the underlying bony margin of the distal phalanx is detected. Hypervascularity within the nodule is a common finding using color Doppler. Proximal locations in the nail bed are more frequent than distal ones (Figure 20.7).[5–7,21–24]

Fibrous Tumors   These are composed of a large heterogeneous group of tumors that may be congenital or acquired. They have been reported in children and have been described as being associated with tuberous sclerosis.[25,26] On ultrasound they present ill-defined hypoechoic structures, commonly eccentric in the nail bed. They tend to involve the periungual tissues and show hypovascularity. Nevertheless, angiofibromas can present inner low-velocity vessels. Also, fibrous tumors may produce scalloping of the bony margin of the distal phalanx (Figure 20.8).[5–7]

Onychomatricoma   These tumors are derived from the nail matrix and few cases have been described in children.[27] On ultrasound, they show ill-defined mixed echogenicity structures that involve the proximal nail bed, including the matrix region and also extending to the interplate space. They appear as hypoechoic structures with hyperechoic spots or lines that conform a band-like pattern. Frequently, they have an eccentric location in the nail bed and affect one of the matrix wings. On color Doppler, they tend to show hypovascularity. No signs of hypervascularity or scalloping of the bony margin have been detected (Figure 20.9).[5–7,28]

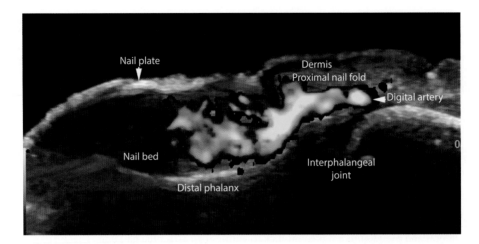

FIGURE 20.6 Cystic fibrosis. Power Doppler ultrasound (longitudinal view, left thumb) demonstrates increased thickness and decreased echogenicity of the nail bed, upward displacement of the nail plate, and hypervascularity in the proximal part of the nail bed. Also notice the decreased echogenicity of the dermis in the proximal nail fold.

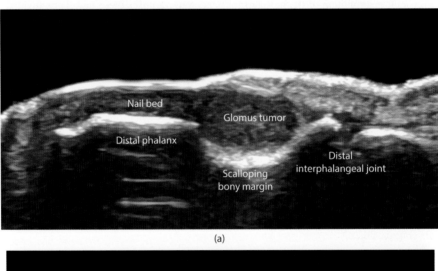

(a)

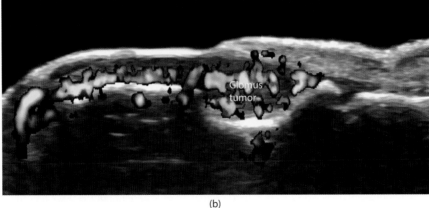

(b)

FIGURE 20.7 Glomus tumor. (a) Gray-scale and (b) Power Doppler demonstrates well-defined hypoechoic nodule in the proximal nail bed. Scalloping of the bony margin of the distal phalanx is also shown. Hypervascularity is observed within the tumor.

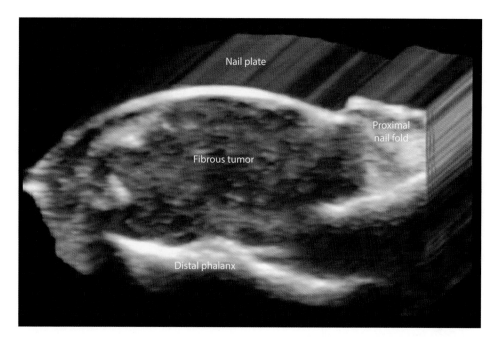

FIGURE 20.8 Fibrous tumor. 3D ultrasound (longitudinal view) shows lobulated and ill-defined hypoechoic mass in the nail bed that displaces the nail plate upward.

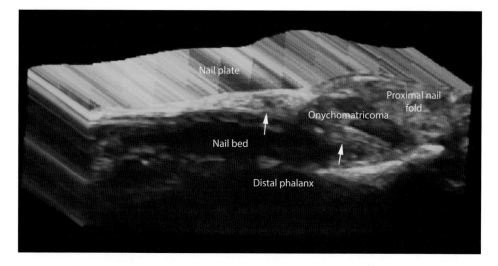

FIGURE 20.9 Onychomatricoma. 3D gray-scale ultrasound (longitudinal view) demonstrates ill-defined mixed echogenicity structure that involves the proximal nail bed, including the matrix region, and also extents to the interplate space with hyperechoic lines (arrows).

Cystic

Mucous Cyst These cystic structures contain mucoid material and degenerated collagen. On ultrasound, they present as well-defined oval- or round-shaped anechoic structures with posterior acoustic enhancement, an artifact typically seen in fluid-filled lesions. If the cyst involves the matrix region, secondary thickening and irregularities in the nail plate may be detected. Mucous cysts are avascular on color Doppler (Figure 20.10).[5,6]

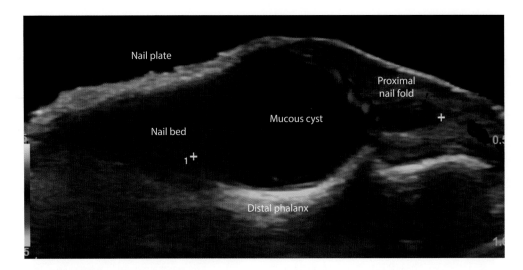

FIGURE 20.10   Mucous cyst. Color Doppler ultrasound (longitudinal view) shows well-defined round-shaped and slightly lobulated anechoic structure within the nail bed that involves the matrix region. No vascularity is detected within the cyst.

Ungual Pseudotumors

These are conditions that can mimic nail tumors. The following are those conditions that are most commonly derived for ultrasound examination in the pediatric population in our department:

Granuloma

These entities are composed of scarring and chronic inflammatory changes that produce a mass-like structure. On ultrasound, they appear as ill-defined hypoechoic hypovascular structures; however, the telangiectatic (vascular) variant may present hypervascularity with slow-flow vessels. Due to involvement of the matrix region, thickening, upward displacement, and irregularities of the nail plate may be seen. Usually no signs of abnormalities in the bony margin are detected (Figure 20.11).[5,6]

Warts

The cause of warts is infection by the human papilloma virus that generates a fibroepithelial and inflammatory reaction in the nail bed and periungual tissues. Commonly, the hyponychium and/or the lateral nail fold are affected. On ultrasound, they appear as hypoechoic fusiform structures with an eccentric location and secondary thickening and irregularities of the nail plate. Commonly, they are hypovascular in the nail bed; however, they may present hypervascularity in the periungual tissues. Rarely, subungual warts may show a nodular shape in the proximal nail bed (Figure 20.12).[5,6]

Periungual Tumors and Pseudotumors

These entities are derived from the periungual tissues and generate a secondary involvement of the nail bed.

Solid

Subungual Exostosis   Subungual exostoses in children have been described in up to 16% of the population in some series.[29] These tumors are an outgrowth of bone and/or cartilaginous tissue and the most common location is the big toe.[30] They are commonly sent for ultrasound examination because these lesions can mimic other pathologies, such as ungual tumors or onychomicosis. On ultrasound, there is a band-like hyperechoic structure that emerges from the surface of the bony margin of the distal phalanx and protrudes into the nail bed. Commonly, exostoses present an eccentric

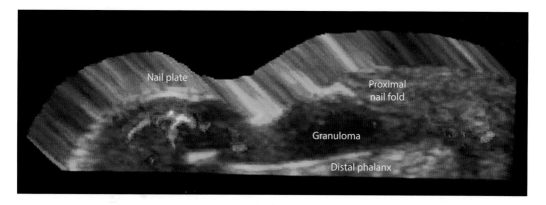

FIGURE 20.11 Granuloma. 3D power Doppler ultrasound (longitudinal view) demonstrates ill-defined hypoechoic hypovascular structure in the proximal nail bed.

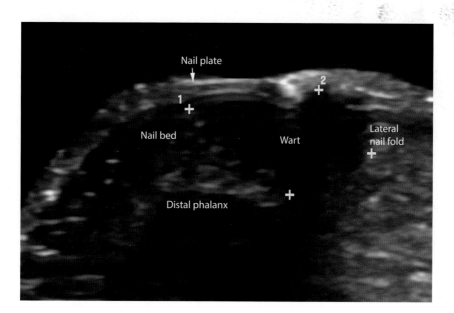

FIGURE 20.12 Wart. Gray-scale ultrasound (transverse view) demonstrates hypoechoic fusiform structure (between marks) with eccentric location involving the nail bed and lateral nail fold. Thickening of the nail plate in the same aspect is also detected.

location in the nail bed. An hypoechoic cap surrounding the hyperechoic band is detected in cases with a cartilaginous component. The nail bed is usually thickened and hypoechoic due to the secondary inflammatory and scarring process. The nail plate is commonly thickened and irregular in cases where the nail matrix is involved. On color Doppler, the nail bed usually appears as hypovascular; nevertheless, in cases with a significant inflammatory reaction hypervascularity may be detected (Figure 20.13).[5,6,21]

Periungual Fibrokeratomas These are fibrous polypoid structures that are located over the proximal part of the nail plate. On ultrasound, they appear as eccentric polypoid or oval hypoechoic lesions that commonly extend into the proximal nail bed and involve part of the matrix region. Fibrokeratomas may also involve the proximal and lateral nail folds. On color Doppler, they are usually hypovascular; however, they may present some low-velocity vessels (Figure 20.14).[5,6]

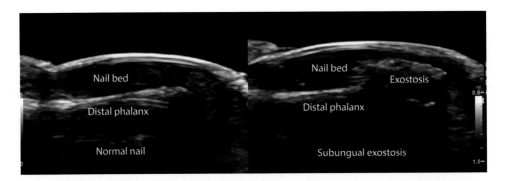

FIGURE 20.13 Subungual exostosis. Gray-scale ultrasound (side by side, left to right hallux comparison) shows band-like hyperechoic structure that emerges from the surface of the bony margin of the distal phalanx of the right big toe and protrudes into the nail bed.

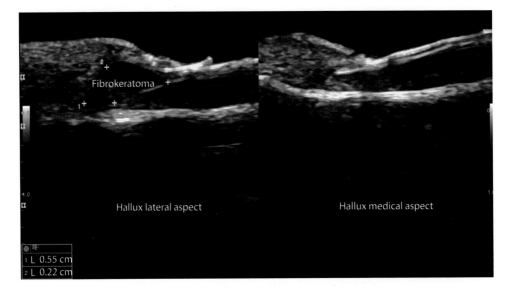

FIGURE 20.14 Fibrokeratoma. Gray-scale ultrasound (longitudinal view, side by side comparison, lateral to medial aspect of the right hallux) shows 5.5 x 2.2 mm hypoechoic structure (between markers) in the proximal nail fold on the lateral aspect.

Inflammatory Conditions

Fluid Collections, Phlegmon, Abscesses, and Fistulous Tracts

These may be produced by trauma and infection, particularly in immunosuppressed patients. On ultrasound fluid collections appear as anechoic avascular deposits in the nail bed that may contain hyperechoic bubbles of air that can show posterior reverberance and sometimes posterior acoustic shadowing artifacts. The free air can move according to variations in the position of the finger or toe. Phlegmons show as hypoechoic and heterogeneous areas within the nail bed or periungual tissues that can present regional hypervascularity (Figure 20.15). Abscesses usually show as anechoic fluid collections containing echoes due to debris and peripheral hypervascularity. A fistulous tract can be detected as an anechoic or hypoechoic tortuous structure that may connect the periungual tissues with the nail bed.[5,6]

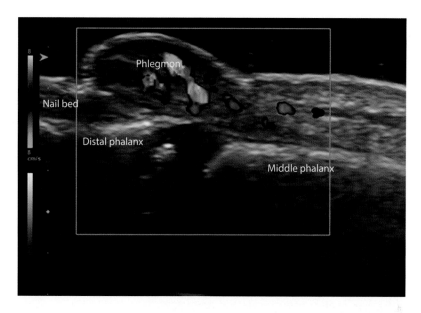

FIGURE 20.15   Phlegmon. Color Doppler ultrasound (longitudinal view, right middle finger) shows thickening and decreased echogenicity as well as increased blood flow in the proximal nail fold in a 2-year-old female patient. (Courtesy of Sanchez R.)

Foreign Bodies

These exogenous components can be secondary to trauma or surgery. Their echogenicity will vary according to the nature of the foreign body. Thus, organic materials such as splinters of wood or thorns appear as hyperechoic bilaminar structures. However, pieces of glass or metal can present itself as mono-laminar hyperechoic structures with a posterior reverberance artifact. Prosthetic or corrective devices usually show as hyperechoic bands.[5,6]

Psoriasis

In children, nail psoriasis has been described to be present in 12% to 39% of the pediatric population in some series.[31,32] It has been reported that ultrasound can show almost pathognomonic changes in nail psoriasis that may precede the appearance of cutaneous lesions. From early to late phases, the ultrasound changes are thickening and decreased echogenicity of the nail bed, loss of definition of the ventral plate, focal hyperechoic deposits in the ventral plate, thickening and loss of definition of the dorsal and ventral plates, thickened and wavy-shaped nail plates with thickening, and posterior acoustic shadowing in the nail bed (Figure 20.16). During the active stages, hypervascularity can be detected in the nail using color Doppler. Additionally, inflammatory changes in the distal interphalangeal joint, such as synovitis can show as an anechoic bulging of the joint. Decreased echogenicity of the extensor tendon (tendinopathy or enthesopathy) and erosion of the hyperechoic bony margins of the distal phalanx can also be detected.[5,6,33–37]

Conclusions

Ultrasound is a reliable noninvasive window to image the nail and its conditions. Its high definition, the wide range of anatomical data provided, and its safe nature make it a potent tool and appropriate imaging technique for studying the nails in the pediatric field.

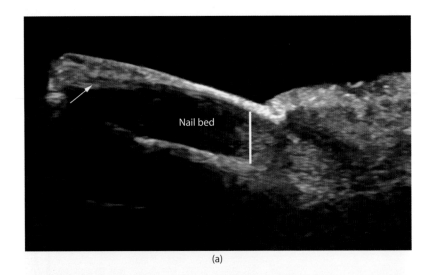

(a)

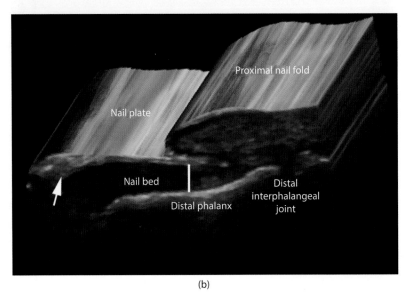

(b)

FIGURE 20.16 Psoriasis. (a) Gray-scale and (b) 3D reconstruction (longitudinal view) demonstrates focal hyperechoic deposit in the distal part of the ventral plate and thickening of the nail bed (vertical line).

REFERENCES

1. Finlay AY, Moseley H, Duggan TC. Ultrasound transmission time: An in vivo guide to nail thickness. *Br J Dermatol*. 1987; 117: 765–770.
2. Jemec GB, Serup J. Ultrasound structure of the human nail plate. *Arch Dermatol*. 1989; 125: 643–646.
3. Wortsman X, Jemec GB. Ultrasound imaging of nails. *Dermatol Clin*. 2006; 24: 323–328.
4. Wortsman X. Ultrasound in dermatology: Why, how, and when? *Semin Ultrasound CT MR*. 2013; 34: 177–195.
5. Thomas L, Vaudaine M, Wortsman X et al. Imaging the nail unit. In Baran R, de Berker D, Holzberg M, Thomas L (eds.), *Baran and Dawber's Diseases of the Nails and Their Management*, Fourth Edition. Chichester, United Kingdom: Wiley-Blackwell; 2012. pp. 132–153.
6. Wortsman X. Sonography of the nail. In Wortsman X, Jemec GBE (eds.), *Dermatologic Ultrasound with Clinical and Histologic Correlations*, First Edition. New York, NY: Springer; 2013. pp. 419–476.
7. Wortsman X. Common applications of dermatologic sonography. *J Ultrasound Med*. 2012; 31: 97–111.

8. Sarifakioglu E, Yilmaz AE, Gorpelioglu C. Nail alterations in 250 infant patients: A clinical study. *J Eur Acad Dermatol Venereol.* 2008; 22: 741–744.

9. Wagner G, Sachse MM. Congenital malalignment of the big toe nail. *J Dtsch Dermatol Ges.* 2012; 10: 326–330.

10. Wortsman X, Wortsman J, Guerrero R et al. Anatomical changes in retronychia and onychomadesis detected using ultrasound. *Dermatol Surg.* 2010; 36: 1615–1620.

11. Piraccini BM, Richert B, de Berker DA et al. Retronychia in children, adolescents, and young adults: A case series. *J Am Acad Dermatol.* 2014; 70: 388–390.

12. Wortsman X, Calderon P, Baran R. Finger retronychias detected early by 3D ultrasound examination. *J Eur Acad Dermatol Venereol.* 2012; 26: 254–256.

13. Reed WB, Stone VM, Boder E, Ziprkowski L. Hereditary syndromes with auditory and dermatological manifestations. *Arch Dermatol.* 1967; 95: 456–461.

14. Gruber R, Wilson NJ, Smith FJ et al. Increased pachyonychia congenita severity in patients with concurrent keratin and filaggrin mutations. *Br J Dermatol.* 2009; 161: 1391–1395.

15. Wortsman X, Aranibar L, Morales C. Postnatal 2- and 3-dimensional sonography of the skin and nail in congenital autosomal recessive ichthyosis correlated with cutaneous histologic findings. *J Ultrasound Med.* 2011; 30(10): 1437–1439.

16. Wenk KS, Higgins KB, Greer KE. Cystic fibrosis presenting with dermatitis. *Arch Dermatol.* 2010; 146: 171–174.

17. Holzberg M. The nail in systemic diseases. In Baran R, de Berker D, Holzberg M, Thomas L (eds.), *Baran and Dawber's Diseases of the Nail and Their Management,* Third Edition. Chichester, United Kingdom: Wiley-Blackwell; 2012. pp. 316–388.

18. Roomans GM, Afzelius BA, Kollberg H, Forslind B. Electrolytes in nails analysed by X-ray microanalysis in electron microscopy. Considerations on a new method for the diagnosis of cystic fibrosis. *Acta Paediatr Scand.* 1978; 67: 89–94.

19. Wortsman X, Alvarez S. Colour Doppler ultrasound findings in the nail in cystic fibrosis. *J Eur Acad Dermatol Venereol.* 2014; 30: 149–151.

20. Stewart DR, Sloan JL, Yao L et al. Diagnosis, management, and complications of glomus tumours of the digits in neurofibromatosis type 1. *J Med Genet.* 2010; 47: 525–532.

21. Wortsman X, Wortsman J, Soto R et al. Benign tumors and pseudotumors of the nail: A novel application of sonography. *J Ultrasound Med.* 2010; 29: 803–816.

22. Chiang YP, Hsu CY, Lien WC, Chang YJ. Ultrasonographic appearance of subungual glomus tumors. *J Clin Ultrasound.* 2014; 42: 336–340.

23. Wortsman X, Jemec GB. Role of high-variable frequency ultrasound in preoperative diagnosis of glomus tumors: A pilot study. *Am J Clin Dermatol.* 2009; 10: 23–27.

24. Matsunaga A, Ochiai T, Abe I et al. Subungual glomus tumour: Evaluation of ultrasound imaging in preoperative assessment. *Eur J Dermatol.* 2007; 17: 67–69.

25. Hollmann TJ, Bovée JV, Fletcher CD. Digital fibromyxoma (superficial acral fibromyxoma): A detailed characterization of 124 cases. *Am J Surg Pathol.* 2012; 36: 789–798.

26. Arora V, Nijjar IS, Singh J, Sandhu PS. Tuberous sclerosis—A multisystem disease. *Indian J Pediatr.* 2008; 75: 77–79.

27. Piraccini BM, Antonucci A, Rech G et al. Onychomatricoma: First description in a child. *Pediatr Dermatol.* 2007; 24: 46–48.

28. Soto R, Wortsman X, Corredoira Y. Onychomatricoma: Clinical and sonographic findings. *Arch Dermatol.* 2009; 145: 1461–1462.

29. Davis DA, Cohen PR. Subungual exostosis: Case report and review of the literature. *Pediatr Dermatol.* 1996; 13: 212–218.

30. Letts M, Davidson D, Nizalik E. Subungual exostosis: Diagnosis and treatment in children. *J Trauma.* 1998; 44: 346–349.

31. Moustou AE, Kakourou T, Masouri S et al. Childhood and adolescent psoriasis in Greece: A retrospective analysis of 842 patients. *Int J Dermatol.* 2014; 53: 1447–1453.

32. Mercy K, Kwasny M, Cordoro KM et al. Clinical manifestations of pediatric psoriasis: Results of a multicenter study in the United States. *Pediatr Dermatol.* 2013; 30: 424–428.

33. Wortsman X, Holm EA, Jemec GBE et al. 15 MHz high resolution ultrasound examination of psoriatic nails. *Revista Chilena de Radiologia.* 2004; 10: 6–9.

34. Gutierrez M, Wortsman X, Filippucci E et al. High-frequency sonography in the evaluation of psoriasis: Nail and skin involvement. *J Ultrasound Med.* 2009; 28: 1569–1574.

35. Sandobal C, Carbó E, Iribas J et al. Ultrasound nail imaging on patients with psoriasis and psoriatic arthritis compared with rheumatoid arthritis and control subjects. *J Clin Rheumatol.* 2014; 20: 21–24.

36. Aydin SZ, Castillo-Gallego C, Ash ZR et al. Ultrasonographic assessment of nail in psoriatic disease shows a link between onychopathy and distal interphalangeal joint extensor tendon enthesopathy. *Dermatology.* 2012; 225: 231–235.

37. Gisondi P, Idolazzi L, Girolomoni G. Ultrasonography reveals nail thickening in patients with chronic plaque psoriasis. *Arch Dermatol Res.* 2012; 304: 727–732.

21

Magnetic Resonance Imaging of Pediatric Nails

Jean-Luc Drapé, Marc Al Ahmar, and Valérie Merzoug

Introduction

Magnetic resonance imaging (MRI) has proven its relevance in the imaging of adult ungual diseases but remains limited in children.[1] Imaging is rarely performed and consists mainly of conventional radiographs and occasionally, ultrasonography. In our institution, we conducted MRI for 50 children, with ages ranging from 6 to 15 years, from 1996 to 2015. Examination consisted of 25 fingers among 9 thumbs and 25 toes; 18 were great toes. Two etiologies dominated the indications: traumatic lesions and exostosis. The remaining indications consisted of tumor, infectious, and congenital abnormalities. We will first discuss the specific technical aspect of MRI in children, the normal nail apparatus anatomy, and our two primary indications. The other indications will be briefly reviewed at the end of this chapter.

MRI Technique

Just like ultrasonography, MRI is a non-irradiant examination that makes itself particularly adapted for the pediatric population. Compared to ultrasonography, it offers a higher spontaneous contrast of components of the nail unit, and allows analysis of the surrounding environment, such as the distal phalanx and the distal interphalangeal joint, the latter being partially accessible in ultrasound. One major disadvantage of the MRI is the requirement of a total immobilization of the hand or feet for 15–20 minutes; thus, it requires highly cooperative children. Only children who are 6 years old and above are explored in our series; for children below this age range sedation is considered (rectal phenobarbital, Nembutal®, rectal or per os chloral hydrate). Sedation is obtained for almost 1 hour. In some cases, parents are asked to enter the MRI room, to stay by their child's side during the examination process; this technique is commonly efficient.

The use of a circular surface microcoil of 4 cm in diameter is mandatory to obtain a sufficient signal-to-noise ratio for the analysis of these small extremities. Contention is important and requires the use of pads and straps. For fingers, the child is in prone position with the arm elevated above the head ("superman" position) to get an optimum position of the fingertip in the center of the magnet. For the examination of toes, prone position is also the preferred position, allowing better forefeet stability. The coil is centered on the dorsal aspect of the nail. The use of Vaseline gel on the nail provides a contrast with the ungual surface, allowing the appreciation of its thickness and deformity; these two elements are not spontaneously seen through MRI due to the lack of signal of the nail plate (Figure 21.1).

The sequences used are not specific for children but the acquisition time can be shortened in the case of incontrollable movements of the child. The most informative planes are the axial and the sagittal planes. The axial plane allows a veritable compartmental approach of the ungual apparatus, whereas in the sagittal plane the matrix recess and the interphalangeal joint are better visualized. The use of gadolinium intravenous injection should be avoided at all ages; its use should be limited to certain indications, mainly tumor and infectious diseases.

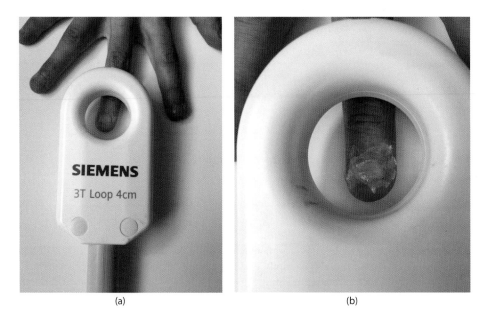

(a)   (b)

FIGURE 21.1 Surface microcoil. (a) The coil is centered above the fingertip and the other fingers are outspread. (b) A thin layer of Vaseline covers the surface of the fingertip to highlight the thickness of the nail plate.

MRI Anatomy of the Normal Nail Unit

Sagittal Plane

The nail plate is poorly hydrated and contains keratin, a scleroprotein with no MRI signal (Figure 21.2). The nail root presents a progressive distal thickening and is surrounded by the matrix. The signal of the matrix is identical to the cutaneous epithelium and to the nail bed epithelium. Its thickness can be measured (about 0.2 mm) and its curvature can be evaluated. The matrix recess is formed by the union of the dorsal and the ventral matrix; its exact limit is difficult to determine due to the absence of contrast with the surrounding sterile epithelium. The submatrix dermis layer extends deeply to the periosteum of the base of the distal phalanx. The dermis of the nail bed presents a thin layer of superficial derma with low signal and a thick layer of deep derma with a higher and heterogeneous signal due to the presence of vascular arcades and of numerous glomus bodies. The submatrix area often presents itself as an oval shape zone of high signal intensity, noted also in the adult nail, which can be misinterpreted as a tumor lesion. The distal part of the nail bed (hyponychium) is covered by the free edge of the nail plate and is limited in depth by the phalangeal tuft. The thickness of the nail bed can be measured by its entire length between the deep aspect of the nail plate and the dorsal cortex of the distal phalanx. The eponychium or posterior nail fold is best analyzed on sagittal slices; in its depth lays the interphalangeal joint and the insertion of the extensor tendon on the base of the distal phalanx. The articular cartilage and the growth cartilage of the base of the distal phalanx are better depicted on the sagittal plane. The fusion of the growth plate is variable and depends on the gender of the children; it is established between 12 and 15 years. The volar plate is interposed between the interphalangeal joint and the deep flexor tendon. The pulp area, although, distant to the nail unit, is a part of the systematic analysis of nail disorders. The signal of the fatty lobules of the hypoderm contrasts with the low signal of the septa and of the superficial derma. The pulp epidermis presents a higher signal, identical to all other epithelium. Vascular and nervous structures (Paccini nodules) may produce more or less heterogeneous signal of the pulp. The insertion of the deep flexor tendon is located on the palmar aspect of the distal phalanx.

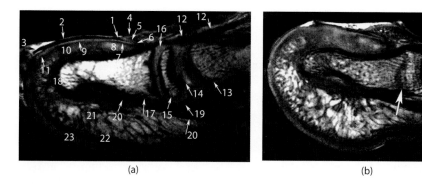

FIGURE 21.2 (a) Sagittal slice of a normal nail unit (11-year-old boy). Nail plate: 1: Nail root; 2: Mid part; 3: Free edge; 4: Eponychium; 5: Dorsal matrix; 6: Matrix cul-de-sac; 7: Ventral matrix; 8: Submatrical area; 9: Nail bed epithelium; 10: Nail bed dermis; 11: Hyponychium; 12: Terminal band extensor tendon; 13: Head middle phalanx; 14: Distal interphalangeal joint; 15: Epiphysis of the distal phalanx; 16: Physeal cartilage; 17: Distal phalanx; 18: Tuft; 19: Volar plate; 20: Flexor digitorum profondus tendon; 21: Pulp hyodermis fat; 22: Pulp dermis; 23: Pulp epidermis. (b) Sagittal slice of a normal nail unit (15-year-old boy). Note the quasi fusion the physeal cartilage (arrow).

Axial Plane

Axial slices are mandatory for determining the anatomical relationships of nail diseases with the matrix, the nail bed, the nail folds, and the pulp area (Figure 21.3). The transverse curvature of the matrix recess is well analyzed, and its lateral horns are linked to the distal phalanx by the matricophalangeal ligaments. The eponychium covers a major part of the matrix tissue. The distal slices show the individualization of the lateral folds, which coat the lateral borders of the nail plate. These borders are in continuity with the interosseous Flint's ligament, extending from the base of the distal phalanx to the tuft. They delineate the rima ungualum, a passage area between the nail bed and the pulp. Vascular arcades as well as certain nail disorders cross the rima ungualum. The two dermal layers of the nail bed are particularly visible on axial slices. The papillary crests of the nail bed epithelium are difficult to detect in the nails of normal children; they are seen only in cases of pathological hypertrophy.

Coronal plane is of little help in the nail apparatus analysis (slices are tangent to most anatomical structures with partial volume artifact). Coronal slices can be used as a complementary sequence for the analysis of an interphalangeal arthropathy or a distal phalanx bone lesion with a lateral extension. A magnetic resonance angiogram (MRA) after gadolinium injection in the coronal plane can be helpful to assess the architecture and the dynamic enhancement of vascular malformations and glomus tumors.

Trauma

Post-traumatic ungual dystrophy is a frequent cause of pediatric nail consultation and a primary MRI indication. Crush injury mechanism is by far the most frequent etiology. Children are often seen well after the initial trauma and after inappropriate treatment in early childhood. In such cases, the middle finger is mainly involved.[2] Conventional X-rays are performed to assess the traumatic bony sequela of the distal phalanx and to evaluate the interphalangeal joint. They can also reveal radiopaque foreign bodies. Ultrasonography has the advantage of detecting non-radiopaque foreign bodies but is insufficient in evaluating the matrix.[3]

MRI is capable of detecting foreign bodies, sometimes associated with a granulomatous reaction or epidermoid cyst. The cyst presents a specific signal with a regular peripheral wall, a thickness and a

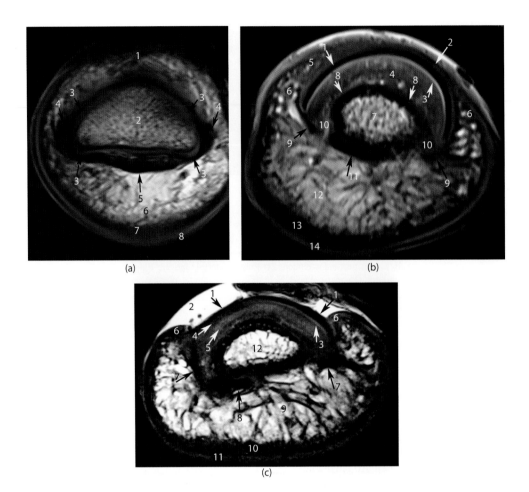

FIGURE 21.3 Axial slices of the nail unit (9-year-old girl). (a) Level of the eponychium: 1: Epoychium; 2: Epiphysis distal phalanx; 3: Physeal cartilage; 4: Matricophalangeal ligament; 5: Flexor Digitorum Profondus tendon; 6: Pulp hypodermis; 7: Pulp dermis; 8: Pulp epidermis. (b) Level of the nail matrix: 1: Nail plate; 2: Dorsal matrix; 3: Ventral matrix; 4: Submatrical dermis, 5: Eponychium; 6: Lateral nail fold; 7: Distal phalanx; 8: Periosteum; 9: Flint's ligament; 10: Rima ungualum; 11: Flexor digitorum profundus tendon; 12: Pulp hypodermis; 13: Pulp dermis; 14: Pulp epidermis. (c) Level of the mid part of the nail bed: 1: Nail plate; 2: Vaselin; 3: Nail bed epithelium; 4: Nail bed superficial dermis; 5: Nail bed deep dermis; 6: Lateral nail fold; 7: Flint's ligament; 8: Tuft; 9: Pulp hypodermis; 10: Pulp dermis; 11: Pulp epidermis; 12: Distal phalanx.

signal similar to that of a normal epithelium. Its center shows an area of heterogeneous mixed high signal intensities on T1- and T2-weighted images and more specific areas of low signal intensities on T1- and T2-weighted images suggestive of the diagnosis.[1,4,5] They consist of keratin lamellae in the center of the lesion. Gadolinium uptake is variable and heterogeneous (Figure 21.4). Inflammatory reaction may occur in the case of cyst rupture. MRI depicts the relationships between the cyst and the matrix tissue and an eventual intraosseous component.[6]

MRI is the only imaging technique that allows a complete and exhaustive examination of the matrix, the nail bed, the distal phalanx, and the pulp. Imaging of the matrix tissue is difficult and requires an adapted technique with the use of three-dimensional (3D) sequences providing thin millimetric continuous slices mandatory for the study of the 0.2-mm-thick matrix tissue. Spatial resolution must be sufficient enough to distinguish the root of the nail plate and the dorsal and ventral matrix. Thus, it is possible to differentiate fibrous traumatic sequelae that affect solely the matrix associated with distal nail plate dystrophy (Figures 21.5 and 21.6) from most distal lesions involving

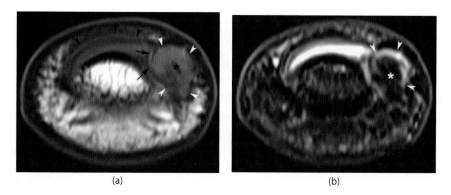

(a) (b)

FIGURE 21.4 Post-trauma epidermoid cyst of the fourth finger in a 13-year-old girl. (a) Axial T1-weighted slice: the cyst (white arrowheads) is seated in the lateral aspect of the posterior nail fold and displaces the underlying nail matrix (arrows). The center of the cyst (*) presents a low signal. Normal nail matrix (black arrowheads). (b) Axial T2-weighted slice: the keratin filled center with a low signal is better depicted (*). The surrounding epithelium presents a high signal (arrowheads).

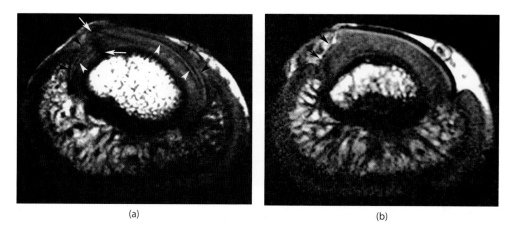

(a) (b)

FIGURE 21.5 Matrix trauma of the big toe in an 11-year-old boy. (a) Axial three-dimensional (3D) T2*-weighted slice at the level of the matrix cul-de-sac: focal scar tissue with low signal (arrows) involving both the dorsal matrix (black arrowheads) and the ventral matrix (white arrowheads). (b) Distal axial 3D T2*-weighted slice: nail dystrophy distal to the matrix injury (arrows).

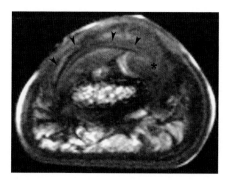

FIGURE 21.6 Nail matrix trauma of the fourth finger in a 9-year-old girl. Axial 3D T2*-weighted slice: More extensive injury of the nail matrix (arrowheads) replaced by scar tissue of 5-mm length (*).

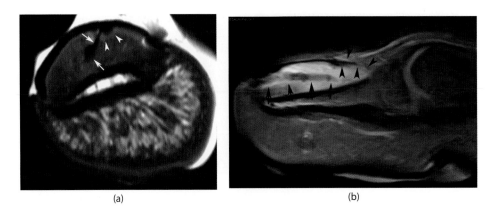

FIGURE 21.7 Nail bed trauma of the right thumb in a 15-year-old boy. (a) Axial 3D T2*-weighted slice: sagittal fissure of the nail bed (arrows) involving the epithelium and the dorsal mid part of the dermis. The epithelium is displaced by some hyperkeratosis of the nail plate (arrowheads). (b) Post-enhanced sagittal T1-weighted fat-saturated (FS) slice: the fissure of the nail bed (arrows) is distal to the nail matrix (arrowheads) and extends to the hyponychium.

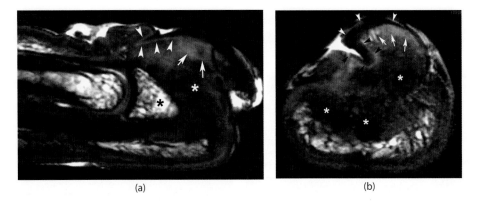

FIGURE 21.8 Nail bed trauma of the third finger in 14-year-old girl after skin graft. (a) Sagittal 3D T2*-weighted slice: Residual base of the distal phalanx (black star). Scar tissue of the nail bed with low signal (white star). The nail matrix is not injured (arrowheads). Thickening of the epithelium of the nail bed (arrows) and increased sagittal curve of the nail plate. (b) Axial 3D T2*-weighted slice: increased transverse curve of the nail plate (white arrowheads) with thickening of the underlying epithelium (arrows). Scar tissue of the nail bed (*). Deformity of the lateral aspect of the nail plate and the lateral nail fold (black arrowheads).

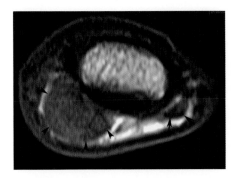

FIGURE 21.9 Post-trauma neuroma of the fifth finger in a 13-year-old girl. Axial T1-weighted slice: enlarged proper digital nerve (arrowheads) with hypertrophy of its nerve bundles in comparison to the contralateral nerve (arrows).

only the nail bed (Figure 21.7). MRI allows detection of ectopic matrix tissue. The quality of the reconstruction of the nail bed, after cutaneous graft in case of substance loss of the nail bed and the phalanx, can be followed up with MRI (Figure 21.8). Fibrotic zones with low signal intensity are accurately depicted. The pulp should also be checked with the possibility of a post-traumatic neuroma. The nerve and its fascicles are hypertrophied with a possible end-bulb shape (Figure 21.9). Gadolinium uptake is common.[7]

Exostosis

A recent meta-analysis demonstrated a high incidence of this disorder (up to 55%) in subjects less than 18 years old.[8] In case of suspicion of a subungual exostosis in front of a painful on palpation keratinized firm and telangiectatic subungual lesion, posteroanterior and lateral plain films are performed, eventually completed with oblique views.[9] The big toe was mainly affected, as it is not a true osteochondroma but rather a post-traumatic osteocartilaginous metaplasia related to the bizarre parosteal osteochondromatous proliferation (BPOP or Nora's lesion).[10,11] It consists of distal phalanx surface bone osteocartilaginous proliferation lying on the cortex. Unlike in real osteochondroma, classically there is no continuity between the cortical bone and the spongious bone on plain films (Figure 21.10). However, in certain conditions, rarely in the big toe, continuity can be found, making the diagnosis of a true osteochondroma discussed here (Figure 21.11a). Microtraumatic lesions of the big toe are less frequent in children as compared to adults.[10] X-rays may guide the diagnosis, showing a juxta-epiphyseal location in true osteochondroma and a more distal location on the dorsal aspect of the phalangeal tuft in exostosis; MRI is indicated when conventional radiographs are negative or not conclusive. In fact, the mineralization can be poor in the big toe, making it difficult to analyze (Figure 21.12a).[11] MRI identifies clearly the exact nature of the lesion and its maturation status. In osteochondroma, the ossification is mature with a fatty spongious bone and a hyalin cartilaginous regular cap (Figure 21.11b). In Nora's lesion, ossification is progressive and spongious tissue can be immature with a nonfatty low signal on T1-weighted images. T2-weighted images and post-gadolinium images reveal the reticular pattern of the spongious bone (Figure 21.12b and 12.13).[12] A cartilaginous cap is also present, but sometimes more irregular and heterogeneous due to its fibrocartilaginous component.[1] The thickness of the cap depends on the maturity stage of the lesion and is reduced in mature lesions.

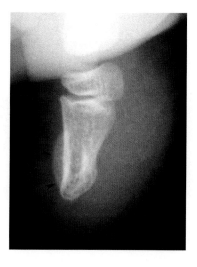

FIGURE 21.10 Subungual exostosis of the big toe in a 9-year-old boy. Lateral radiograph: parosteal ossification (arrowheads) without continuity with the underlying cortex and cancellous bone of the distal phalanx.

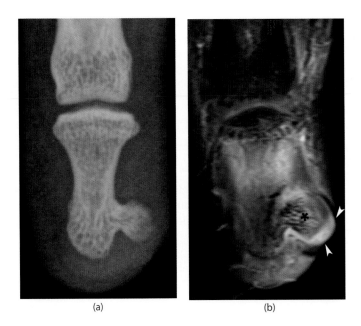

(a)   (b)

FIGURE 21.11 Subungual osteochondroma of the second finger in a 15-year-old girl. (a) Anterioposterior (AP) radiograph: lateral ossification with fingertip deformity and continuity of the cortex and the cancellous bone of the distal phalanx. (b) Coronal proton density FS slice: the osteochondroma is composed of mature cancellous bone (*), with the same signal than the distal phalanx, and a hyaline cartilage cap with a high signal (arrowheads).

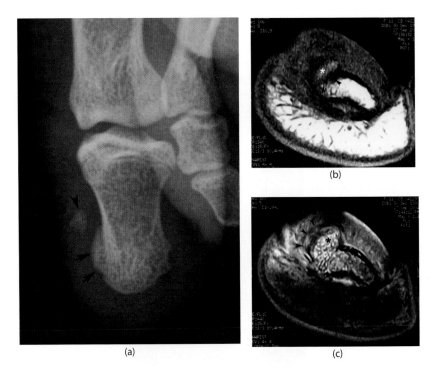

(a)   (c)

FIGURE 21.12 Subungual exostosis of the big toe in a 11-year-old girl. (a) Oblique view: slight hypertrophy of the tuft (arrows) and ossification of the soft tissue (arrowhead). (b) Axial T1-weighted slice: small mature fatty cancellous bone (*) lying on a continuous cortex (arrowheads). Thickening of the underlying nail bed. (c) Axial post-enhanced T1-weighted FS slice: the enhanced cancellous bone of the exostosis (*) is better depicted and larger than the fatty component. Note an irregular fibrocartilaginous cap with an intermediate signal (arrowheads).

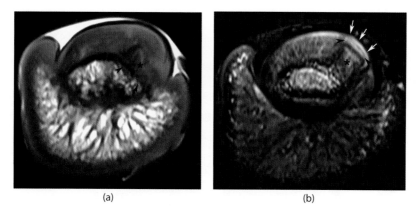

(a)   (b)

FIGURE 21.13 Subungual exostosis of the thumb with complete immature bone in a 15-year-old boy. (a) Axial T1-weighted slice: asymmetrical thickening of the nail bed (*) without visible bone formation. Note some irregularities of the cortex (arrowheads). (b) Axial T2-weighted slice: the cancellous bone is better depicted (*), whereas the cartilage cap (arrowheads) beneath the epithelium of the nail bed (arrows) is not.

Other Pathologies

Tumors

Fibrous Tumors

Periungual fibromas may be isolated or multiple in a child and may raise the diagnosis of tuberous sclerosis in multiple lesions, also called Koenen tumors. They are more frequent on the toes and may be similar to fibrokeratomas.[1,3] MRI is capable of detecting small fibrous tumors located in the matrix area beneath the posterior nail fold. The tumors demonstrate a peripheral rim of intermediate signal and a fibrous core of low signal (Figure 21.14). Axial slices accurately determine the location of the tumor, commonly above but also under or even within the nail plate.[12] More distal slices depict the nail plate groove in front of the tumor.

Glomus Tumors

Glomus tumors are hamartomas developing in middle-aged patients from the glomus bodies, particularly numerous in the nail bed. There is a high female predominance in this case. They are rare in infancy but some cases are reported in the available literature.[13–15] The diagnosis is delayed several years after clinical symptoms, which can be present as early as 2 years of age. The clinical diagnosis is based on the triad and may be incomplete in children: pain, cold, sensitivity, and positive pin test. Sometimes a reddish blue spot is visible under the nail plate and a nail dystrophy if the matrix is involved. Hildreth's test is difficult to conduct in children; it consists of a cuff/tourniquet placed at the base of the limb and it is considered positive if it reduces the symptoms. Fingertip tumors are more common than toe lesions.[14] Transillumination of the finger may reveal a bluish nodule. Radiographs may depict a bony erosion of the distal phalanx in 22%–36% of the cases.[16] Ultrasonography is more accurate than radiographs to detect a bony erosion and Dopper ultrasound highlight the vascular nature of the tumor. Lesions less than 2 mm are difficult to detect with ultrasound. MRI is the most accurate imaging modality in detecting glomus tumors, even in lesions less than 2 mm. In most cases the tumor presents a high signal on T2-weighted images and a peripheral pseudocapsule. The normal high signal of the submatrix dermis must not be confused with a glomus tumor. The presence of underlying bony erosion is helpful for the diagnosis. Intravenous injection of gadolinium is not always necessary but improves the accuracy, particularly in case of multiple lesions and in recurrence after surgery. Magnetic resonance angiography (MRA) should be added with an MIP (maximum intensity projection) reformatting of the fingertip (Figure 21.15). The

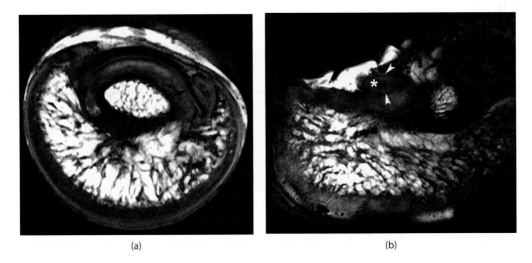

(a)   (b)

FIGURE 21.14 Fibrokeratoma of the big toe in a 14-year-old boy. (a) Axial 3D T2*-weighted slice: the oval-shaped tumor is seated at the origin of the lateral nail fold with a peripheral rim of intermediate signal and a fibrous core with a low signal. Note the displacement of the nail plate and the nail bed (arrows). (b) Sagittal 3D T2*-weighted slice: the tumor (*) is seated in the nail matrix cul-de-sac (arrowheads).

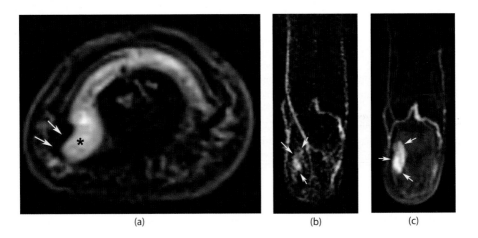

(a)   (b)   (c)

FIGURE 21.15 Glomus tumor of the third finger of a 10-year-old girl. (a) Axial T2-weighted slice: the glomus tumor is seated in the rima ungualum (*) and shifts the Flint's ligament (arrows). The extension toward the pulp is well depicted, whereas the limits in the nail bed are blurred. (b) Magnetic resonance (MR) angiography at an arterial phase: early enhancement of the tumor (arrows). (c) MR angiography at a delayed phase: the size of the tumor (arrows) is better assessed on this phase.

dynamic of the enhancement is assessed with an early enhancement at the arterial phase and a progressive filling in the delayed phases. Some rare glomus tumors may present a dominant mucoid component with a low and delayed enhancement.[16] Multiple glomus tumors may involve a single fingertip or several fingers; in these cases glomangiomatosis or the association with a neurofibromatosis type 1 should be discussed.[15,17]

Osteoid Osteoma

Osteoid osteoma of the distal phalanx is very rare in children and young adults. The index is mostly affected. It presents itself as a swelling of the distal phalanx and clubbing is seen as well. Nail thickening and enlargement can be associated with this. Inflammatory pain is usual but rare cases of painless lesions are reported in children.[18] Radiographs can identify a more or less calcified nidus surrounded by bony sclerosis and cortex hypertrophy. However, radiological findings may be atypical at the level of the distal phalanx with a bone sclerosis and periostitis of the tuft without a clear visible nidus, even on computed tomography (CT) scan. A premature fusion of the adjacent epiphysis is described.[1] MRI may be helpful in difficult cases and highlights the bone edema of the distal phalanx and the associated periostitis and inflammatory reaction of the nail bed. The nail bed may be extensively thickened with an increased curvature of the nail plate. Dynamic intravenous gadolinium injection is accurate to locate the nidus, which enhances early at the arterial phase (Figure 21.16).[19]

Infection

Radiographs are performed to detect foreign bodies, osteitis or osteoarthritis, and other arthropathy. MRI is rarely indicated in infectious conditions, it is performed mainly to detect an osteitis of the distal phalanx.[9,20] MRI may be useful in case of subacute or chronic paronychia with previous negative cultures, in order to guide a biopsy. A thickening of the eponychium and the matrix recess may be associated to the rupture of the cuticle (Figure 21.17). The intravenous injection of gadolinium confirms necrotic collections surrounded by an enhanced peripheral rim.

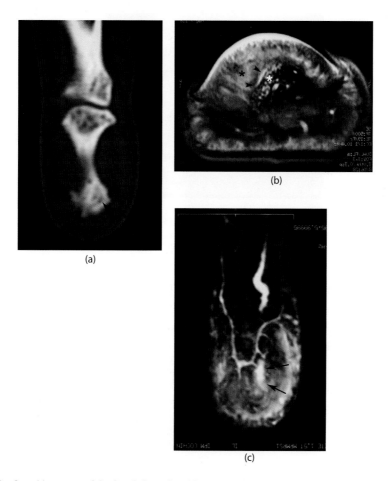

(a)

(b)

(c)

FIGURE 21.16 Osteoid osteoma of the fourth finger in a 15-year-old girl. (a) Coronal computed tomography (CT) slice: doubtful nidus of the tuft (arrow). (b) Axial post-enhanced T1-weighted slice: enhancement of the lateral aspect of the tuft (white star) and the periosteum (arrowheads) with asymmetrical inflammatory thickening of the nail bed (black star). (c) MR angiography, arterial phase: early enhancement of the nidus of the tuft (arrows).

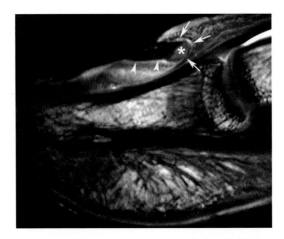

FIGURE 21.17   Subacute paronychia of the big toe in a 14-year-old girl. Sagittal 3D T2*-weighted slice: granuloma seated in the nail root (*) with bulging of the nail cul-de-sac (arrows) and subungual hyperkeratosis (arrowheads).

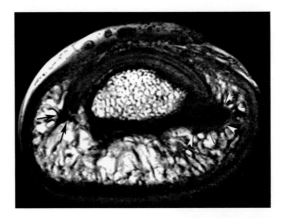

FIGURE 21.18   Congenital malalignment of the big toenail. Axial 3D T2*-weighted slice: Hypertrophy of the lateral ligament and its dorsal extension to the matrix (arrowheads) on the lateral aspect of the toe in comparison to the contralateral ligament (arrows).

Congenital Malalignment of the Big Toe

It was first described by P.D. Samman (1978) as a great toenail dystrophy.[21] MRI is not necessary for the diagnosis but was helpful to understand the mechanism of this disease. It presents as a lateral deviation of the nail plate with respect to the phalanx and may be complicated paronychia, onychogryphosis, and lateral nail ingrowing.[22] MRI demonstrated that this congenital abnormality is caused by a lateral rotation of the matrix due to an increased tension by the ligamentous elements and hypertrophy of the lateral matricophalangeal ligament (Figure 21.18).[22,23]

Conclusions

MRI of the nail apparatus in children is a technical challenge but is accessible with the most powerful and newest MRI scanners. The main indications are the post-traumatic nail dystrophies and the subungual tumors.

REFERENCES

1. Baran R, Haneke E, Drapé JL et al. Tumours of the nail apparatus and adjacent tissues. In Baran R, Dawber RPR (eds.), *Diseases of the Nails and Their Management*, Third Edition. Oxford, United Kingdom: Blackwell Scientific Publications; 2008. pp. 515–630.

2. Salazard B, Launay F, Descouches C et al. Les traumatismes des phalanges distales chez l'enfant. *Rev Chir Orthop Reparatrice Appar Mot*. 2004; 90: 621–627.

3. Richert B and André J. Nail disorders in children: Diagnosis and management. *Am J Clin Dermatol*. 2011; 12(2): 101–112.

4. Baek HJ, Lee SJ, Cho KH et al. Subungual tumors: Clinicopathologic correlation with US and MR imaging findings. *Radiographics*. 2010; 30(6): 1621–1636.

5. Horcajadas AB, Lafuente JL, de la Crue Burgos R et al. Ultrasound and MR findings in tumor and tumor-like lesions of the fingers. *Eur Radiol*. 2003; 13(4): 672–685.

6. Nakajo M, Ohkubo K, Nandate T et al. Intraosseous epidermal cyst of the distal phalanx of the thumb: Radiographic and magnetic resonance imaging findings. *Radiat Med*. 2005; 23(2): 128–132.

7. Ahlawat S, Belzberg AJ, Montgomery E, Fayad LM. MRI features of peripheral traumatic neuromas. *Eur Radiol*. 2016; 26(4): 1204–1212.

8. DaCambra MP, Gupta SK, Ferri-de-Barros F. Subungual exostosis of the toes: A systematic review. *Clin Orthop Relat Res*. 2014; 472: 1251–1259.

9. Goettmann S. Les messages clés en pathologie unguéale. *Presse Med*. 2014; 43: 1267–1278.

10. Lee SK, Jung MS, Lee YH et al. Two distinctive subungual pathologies: Subungual exostosis and sub-ungual osteochondroma. *Foot Ankle Int*. 2007; 28: 595–601.

11. Fikry T, Dkhissi M, Harfaoui A et al. Les exostoses sous-unguéales. Etude rétrospective d'une série de 28 cas. *Acta Orthop Belg*. 1998; 64(1): 35–40.

12. Goettmann S, Drape JL, Idy-Peretti I et al. Magnetic resonance imaging: A new tool in the diagnosis of tumours of the nail apparatus. *Br J Dermatol*. 1994; 130(6): 701–710.

13. Rabarin F, Saint Cast Y, Fouque PA et al. Tumeurs glomiques des extrémités de l'enfant, une cause rare de douleur chronique. A propos de deux cas cliniques. *Chir Main*. 2010; 29: 270–273.

14. Delecourt C, Léonard JC, Morin C et al. Une tumeur glomique de l'orteil: Une observation pédiatrique. *Rev Chir Orthop Reparatrice Appar Mot*. 2008; 94(8): 777–779.

15. Dahlin LB, Müller G, Anagnostaki L, Nordborg K. Glomus tumours in the long finger and in the thumb of a young patient with neurofibromatosis-1 (Nf-1). *J Plast Surg Hand Surg*. 2013; 47: 238–240.

16. Drapé JL, Idy-Peretti I, Goettmann S et al. Standard and high resolution magnetic resonance imaging of glomus tumors of toes and fingertips. *J Am Acad Dermatol*. 1996; 35(4): 550–555.

17. Tami I, Schibli S, Baldi Balmelli S et al. Glomangiomatosis on the hand. A case report. *Handchir Mikrochir Plast Chir*. 2009; 41(1): 52–55.

18. De Smet L, Spaepen D, Zachee B, Fabry G. Painless osteoid osteoma of the finger in a child. Case report. *Chir Main*. 1998; 17(2): 143–146.

19. Teixeira PA, Chanson A, Beaumont M et al. Dynamic MR imaging of osteoid osteomas: Correlation of semiquantitative and quantitative perfusion parameters with patient symptoms and treatment outcome. *Eur Radiol*. 2013; 23(9): 2602–2611.

20. Wulkan AJ, Tosti A. Pediatric nail conditions. *Clin Dermatol*. 2013; 31: 564–572.

21. Samman PD. Great toenail dystrophy. *Clin Exp Dermatol*. 1978; 3: 81–82.

22. Wagner G, Sachse M. Congenital malalignment of the big toenail. *J Dtsch Dermatol Ges*. 2012; 10(5): 326–330.

23. Baran R, Grognard C, Duhard E, Drapé JL. Congenital malalignment of the great toenail. An enigma resolved by a new surgical treatment. *Br J Dermatol*. 1998; 139(Suppl 51): 72.

Index